T0190281

EFFECTIVE TEACHING

Instructional Methods and Strategies for Occupational Therapy Education

EFFECTIVE TEACHING

Instructional Methods and Strategies for Occupational Therapy Education

EDITOR

Whitney Henderson, OTD, MOT, OTR/L
Associate Clinical Professor
Department of Occupational Therapy
University of Missouri
Columbia, Missouri

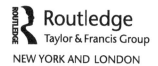

Routledge
Taylor & Francis Group

NEW YORK AND LONDON

First published 2021 by SLACK Incorporated

Published in 2024 by Routledge
605 Third Avenue, New York, NY 10158

and by Routledge
4 Park Square, Milton Park, Abingdon, Oxon, OX14 4RN

Routledge is an imprint of the Taylor & Francis Group, an informa business

Cover Artist: Justin Dalton

Library of Congress Cataloging-in-Publication Data

Names: Henderson, Whitney, editor.
Title: Effective teaching : instructional methods and strategies for
   occupational therapy education / editor, Whitney Henderson.
Other titles: Effective teaching (Henderson)
Description: Thorofare, NJ : SLACK Incorporated, [2021] | Includes
   bibliographical references and index.
Identifiers: LCCN 2021005765 (print) | ISBN 9781630916794 (paperback)
Subjects: MESH: Occupational Therapy--education | Teaching
Classification: LCC RM735.32 (print) | NLM WB 18
   | DDC 615.8/515076--dc23
LC record available at https://lccn.loc.gov/2021005765

ISBN: 9781630916794 (pbk)
ISBN: 9781003523956 (ebk)

DOI: 10.4324/9781003523956

DEDICATION

To my late grandmothers, Janis and Myrna—full of fiery strength and love.

CONTENTS

ACKNOWLEDGMENTS

First and foremost, I would like to thank God for giving me the patience, strength, endurance, courage, and opportunity to write this book. Without His grace, mercy, and blessing, I would not have achieved this task.

Importantly, I would like to thank my mom and dad for the characteristics they modeled to me throughout my life; characteristics that no doubt served me well during the process of writing this book. I would also like to thank my brother and my friends for their endless laughs, reassurance, and inspiration. I only hope I have impacted your life a fraction of your impact on mine. I love each of you so much.

I am forever grateful for my colleagues at the University of Missouri for their continuous encouragement and support of my professional and personal growth and their willingness to take extra responsibilities and provide feedback when needed. I would particularly like to acknowledge Dr. Winnie Dunn for her enduring mentorship throughout this entire project and Dr. Anna Boone for her consistent commitment to designated writing and coffee times. In addition, I am very appreciative of my colleagues that contributed to the chapters of this book. Their many talents are spread throughout these pages.

Another huge thank you to my students at the University of Missouri; many of which accepted my new attempts to incorporate many of the methods found in this book into their courses. Thank you for your participation, feedback, questions, challenges, support, enthusiasm, and patience. You make me a better educator and a better person. I would like to give a special acknowledgement to those students that assisted in this project—Bailey Baucum, Kelli Bayne, Bailey Bremser, Paige Headlee, Casey Hinkle, Haley Homan, Bethany Irlmeier, Natalie Pelletier, Breanna Perry, and Lyndi Plattner. This project does not get completed without each of your important contributions.

I would also like to recognize my Orangetheory Fitness family. Thank you to the coaches, staff, and members for supporting my crazy schedule and for being a motivating force and bright light in my day. Keep crushing your goals!

Lastly, thank you to SLACK Incorporated for trusting me with the opportunity to write this book, particularly Brien Cummings for his support throughout the process.

About the Editor

Whitney Henderson, OTD, MOT, OTR/L, is an associate clinical professor in the Department of Occupational Therapy at the University of Missouri. She teaches a variety of courses across the curriculum, including Human Development and Occupation, Principles of Assessment, Human Motion and Occupation, and Adult Practice. She also provides supervision to students during adult practicum experiences and engages in research in areas of occupational therapy education and adult neurological rehabilitation.

Henderson graduated from the University of Missouri with a bachelor's degree (2006) and master's degree (2008) in occupational therapy. In addition, she completed a postprofessional Doctorate of Occupational Therapy from Creighton University (2017). Henderson worked in an acute care setting with individuals with neurological conditions and burn injuries for 5 years prior to entering academia. She also has experience working in skilled nursing facilities.

In addition to teaching, Henderson coaches at Orangetheory Fitness. She enjoys spending time with her family, friends, and two West Highland terriers (CJ and Paulie), participating in church activities, attending sporting events and concerts, and traveling to various parts of the world.

For more information about the editor and resources for evidence-based teaching, please visit www.thinkwide.space.

Contributing Authors

Bailey Baucum, MOT, OTR/L (Chapter 4)
Department of Occupational Therapy
University of Missouri
Columbia, Missouri

Kelli Bayne, MOT, OTR/L (Chapter 6)
Department of Occupational Therapy
University of Missouri
Columbia, Missouri

Bailey Bremser, MOT, OTR/L (Chapter 7)
Department of Occupational Therapy
University of Missouri
Columbia, Missouri

Cynthia Clough, PhD, OT/L (Chapter 9)
Assistant Professor
Occupational Therapy Program
Mount Mary University
Milwaukee, Wisconsin

Megan Edwards Collins, PhD, OTR/L, CAPS, CFPS (Chapter 14)
Assistant Professor
Occupational Therapy Department
Winston-Salem State University
Winston-Salem, North Carolina

Meredith Gronski, OTD, OTR/L, CLA (Chapter 12)
Director and Assistant Professor
Doctor of Occupational Therapy Program
Methodist University
Fayetteville, North Carolina

Paige Headlee, MOT, OTR/L (Chapter 4)
Department of Occupational Therapy
University of Missouri
Columbia, Missouri

Haley Homan, MOT, OTR/L (Chapter 6)
Occupational Therapist
Department of Special Services
Morgan County R-1 School
Stover, Missouri

Leigh Neier, PhD (Chapters 2 and 3)
Associate Teaching Professor
College of Education
University of Missouri
Columbia, Missouri

Stacy Neier, PhD (Chapter 2)
Senior Ignatian Lecturer
Quinlan School of Business
Loyola University Chicago
Chicago, Illinois

Lyndi Plattner, MOT, OTR/L (Chapter 4)
Department of Occupational Therapy
University of Missouri
Columbia, Missouri

INTRODUCTION

My path to occupational therapy is not an exciting one, as I knew I wanted to be an occupational therapist when I was in high school. My mom was a recreational therapist (and an occupational therapist at heart) and later a health care administrator, so I was literally born and raised in a nursing home. In college, I switched my major to premedicine twice, but quickly turned my studies and efforts back to the profession that captured my attention at such an early age.

I also knew I wanted to teach at an early age. My mom often tells stories of my pretend play of arranging stuffed animals in their seats before standing in front of the chalkboard to deliver the lesson of the day in my room. Several years later, my brother was born. He sometimes played the student role in my pretend classroom and certainly taught me how to capture and maintain an individual's attention and how to manage classroom behaviors (joking...partially). Throughout high school, I had the opportunity to assist in a third grade classroom, and in college, serve as a teaching assistant for a couple of courses. In practice, as many of you do, I often played the educator role with clients, families, and multidisciplinary teams and with the students I supervised on fieldwork and in volunteer and observation experiences. I further gained an appreciation and understanding of education through my postprofessional Doctorate of Occupational Therapy and through a dream team of mentors and colleagues at the University of Missouri and educators at Creighton University. Each of these experiences and opportunities, paired with my innate desire to teach, undoubtedly fueled my passion for both occupational therapy and education.

More importantly, I **love** instructional methods—really **love** instructional methods. I think this is where my creativity as an occupational therapy practitioner manifests itself as an occupational therapy educator. In one semester, I worked with a group of students to select and successfully (and sometimes unsuccessfully) implement over 15 instructional methods in a course. I **love** instructional methods because these methods are **fun** and **engaging**, foster *application-based learning*, and promote *collaboration, problem-solving, and self-directed learning*. In addition, I **love** that I no longer feel pressure to play the expert role or to endlessly prepare talking points and presentations like I once felt as a novice educator. Most of all, I **love** observing students from diverse backgrounds and experiences; all learning styles actually experience *deep learning* of and *connection* to concepts when I use engaging instructional methods. All that passion that has been growing and evolving manifests itself in every topic you will encounter. Turn the pages and have fun with your students.

Book Outline

Before moving through the pages of this book, I want to outline the layout of the chapters that follow this Introduction. In the first three chapters, we inspire educators to pursue teaching excellence and to reflect on their teaching practices through the provision of materials for evidence-based teaching, design thinking, and inclusive design. In Chapter 4, we further highlight how educators can achieve teaching excellence through the inclusion of students in curricular design.

The remainder of the chapters outline various instructional methods you can implement with a variety of students and the many different concepts found in your courses. We begin this portion of the book with a chapter on flipped classroom (Chapter 5). Once educators understand and implement this approach, they can use any of the instructional methods discussed in the remaining chapters of the book within their flipped classroom model.

Each of the chapters on instructional methods follows a similar outline. We hope this structure allows you to easily absorb the content and quickly access needed information as you are creating or revising your courses.

- **Basic Tenets:** Discusses an overview of the instructional method(s).
- **Background:** Provides a brief historical description of the instructional method(s).
- **Theory:** Highlights an educational theory or framework for implementation of the instructional method(s); many of these theories are applicable to various instructional methods; therefore, have these guiding resources in mind as you try instructional methods within or outside of this book.
- **Implementation:** Offers a step-by-step approach to create and implement the instructional method(s).
- **Additional Implementation Notes:** Provides any additional information an educator should consider when designing or implementing the method(s).
- **Tips and Tricks:** Offers short bullet points to maximize the benefit and success of the instructional method(s).
- **Opportunities for Feedback and Reflection:** Provides numerous ways educators can facilitate these critical skills during or after execution of the instructional method.
- **Application to Occupational Therapy Practice:** Gives two ways occupational therapy practitioners can use the instructional method in professional practice; as occupational therapy practitioners, we serve an educator role and desire to collaborate with clients, families, and communities. Similar to evidence-based teaching, we aim to achieve high-quality outcomes and provide client-centered care by fostering *active* participation, *cocreation* of interventions and recommendations, *autonomy* in decision-making, and *feedback and reflection* during the occupational therapy process. Therefore, we felt a brief section on Application to Occupational Therapy Practice in each chapter was beneficial to aid educators and students to operate as a facilitator (versus a transmitter of knowledge or expertise) to maximize client participation and independence in their **own** lives.
- **Advantages and Challenges:** Lists many benefits and challenges to using the instructional method(s).
- **Three Things You Can Do Tomorrow:** Lists three simple tasks you can use to implement various evidence-based instructional methods or strategies into your teaching practices.
- **Evidence Table:** Lastly, each of the chapters devoted to specific instructional methods provides an evidence table for you to reference. The table provides evidence about the instructional method(s) across different disciplines in health professional education. Following traditional professional guidelines, we only included quantitative articles published after 2010 in these tables. Because of the volume of the evidence supporting some of the methods, we limited some tables to systematic reviews or meta-analysis. If authors included a study in a systematic review, meta-analysis, or integrative review, we did not include the individual article in the evidence table. We provide a few notes at the end of some tables to provide transparency about our decision-making process. In addition, we would like to note that we did a broad review of the literature, but due to resources and scope of this book, we recognize we may have missed articles that would typically be found and included in a comprehensive analysis. It is our hope these tables still provide a large overview of the evidence available for each instructional method.

Goals

One of my primary goals for this book was to craft a text that was easy for educators to read, as well as one that was rich with resources and opportunities for engagement. As you read this book, I encourage you to complete the reflection activities strategically positioned throughout each chapter, pause and consider the important callouts, access the resources, and apply a few of the simple strategies to your teaching practices that we suggest at the end of each chapter.

If you are a new educator, welcome to a satisfying career in academia—you have made a great (but sometimes scary) choice. I hope the content of this book greatly facilitates your transition to teaching. If you are a seasoned educator, my desire is this book re-energizes your teaching practices and stirs many ideas for innovation.

Whether you are a novice or seasoned educator—thank you! Thank you for impacting the future of our great profession. Thank you for **loving** what you do, for being **bold** to try new ideas, for your **pursuit of excellence**, and for your **steadfast commitment** to your students and the scholarship of teaching and learning.

EVIDENCE-BASED TEACHING AND OCCUPATIONAL THERAPY EDUCATION

Whitney Henderson, OTD, MOT, OTR/L

In the current higher education landscape, the need for *evidence-based teaching* has never been more important. Key stakeholders, such as students, parents, society, administrators, policymakers, and accrediting and governing bodies, are demanding high-quality education that yields qualified graduates prepared to enter the workforce. Because of this increased accountability, educators find themselves in an environment where evidence-based teaching is required to produce adequate student learning outcomes. Buskist and Groccia (2011) synthesized definitions from a variety of health care–related fields and applied these definitions to higher education. The authors defined evidence-based teaching as "…the conscientious, explicit, and judicious integration of best available research on teaching technique and expertise within the context of student, teacher, department, college, university, and community characteristics" (Buskist & Groccia, 2011, p. 8). In other words, educators must use educational research to enhance educational practices.

Just as with other professional fields, such as medicine and agriculture, educators must embrace evidence as the foundation for their teaching practices. Despite having access to a growing body of knowledge and resources to support their teaching decisions, some educators are unaware that evidence-based approaches to teaching even exist. When educators truly engage in evidence-based teaching they critically read educational literature on teaching and learning and adopt instructional methods that are supported by evidence. They use resources, develop classroom activities based on research, and reflect on their teaching practices. Currently a majority of educators select instructional methods based on experimental, common sense, or anecdotal evidence. They also tend to teach the way they were taught. In an era of high accountability to produce students capable of engaging in lifelong learning, education is too important to be based on unfounded opinion or tradition. Similarly, you would not want your occupational therapist or physician to implement an intervention based on tradition, opinion, or anecdote. Therefore, we embrace the challenge to incorporate evidence-based teaching methods by plunging into educational literature to incorporate sound instructional methods to enhance our work, students, department, institution, and society.

Henderson, W. (Ed.). *Effective Teaching: Instructional Methods and Strategies for Occupational Therapy Education* (pp. 1-18).

Educational literature suggests there are two levels of evidence-based teaching. Davies (1999) reported the first level is to utilize existing evidence from the teaching and learning literature and research. Educators use the available evidence in a variety of ways:

- To inform teaching
- To focus students' attention on their areas of strengths and challenges
- To guide or improve program planning and outcomes
- To demonstrate achievement of student learning outcomes

Educators need to develop and use a set of skills that allows them to ask critical questions about what they are witnessing during the learning experience, locate evidence, critically appraise the evidence, and determine the relevance and applicability of the evidence to a situation. The second level of evidence-based teaching is to establish and disseminate sound evidence. Although implementing evidence-based teaching is important for educational practices, there remains a critical need for educators to further investigate the pragmatics and effectiveness of these teaching and learning methods across various contexts.

The term the *scholarship of teaching and learning (SoTL)* describes this notion—the systematic inquiry of how students learn, which educators use to inform the ways they teach. Similar to completing research in practice, educators identify a problem, review literature, implement a change, document and analyze the effects of this change, write and submit a manuscript, and prepare and present findings to further expand the educational literature. Educational researchers create evidence through various forms of assessment. They use observations, tests, and peer and course evaluations among other things to measure learning outcomes of students, groups, and cohorts or to measure the effectiveness of educational programs. There remains a need for educators and students to become both analysts of their own educational practice and critical informers of the scholastic community.

BENEFITS FOR EDUCATORS

Educators and students equally benefit when educators implement practices grounded by evidence and theory. By using or contributing to current evidence to select best teaching practices, educators can be confident their students will learn because research suggests particular methods are effective. Evidence-based teaching facilitates student engagement with and learning of course content, improves student performance, and supports long-term retention of skills and knowledge. They can use this body of knowledge to successfully implement strategies to demonstrate student achievement of high-quality learning outcomes. Additionally, educators use the collected data to determine teaching effectiveness for promotion and tenure. When educators employ methods supported by literature and theory in courses, they generate more student participation and engage in authentic communication with their students to develop trust and rapport (Figure 1-1). Educators experience great personal and professional gratification when they watch their students develop critical and creative thinking skills reflective of deep and high-level learning and progression of independent lifelong learning abilities.

Educators also profit when they engage in the SoTL. It is estimated that more than half of higher education institutions value engagement in the SoTL when determining if educators are qualified for promotion and tenure. In addition, as they increase involvement in the SoTL, they build a reputation and professional standing that could lead to professional opportunities (providing a keynote address at a conference) or leadership and administrative opportunities (leading a campus committee on student outcomes or serving as an assistant dean of assessment). Departments, schools, and institutions also benefit from evidence-based teaching because they demonstrate student achievement to meet regional and professional accrediting agency requirements. Evidence-based teaching often results in higher rates of student retention and better-prepared graduates to enter the workforce—critically important metrics in higher education.

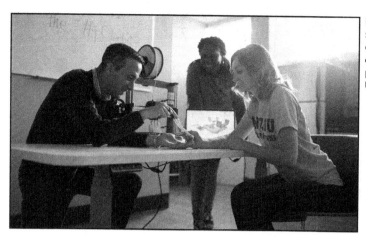

Figure 1-1. An educator and students engage in authentic communication during a learning experience. (Reproduced with permission from Keith Borgmeyer/ University of Missouri.)

BENEFITS FOR STUDENTS

Students also experience many important benefits when educators employ evidence-based teaching in course and curricular design. First and foremost, **students learn and retain more content!** Educational literature suggests they learn because educators implement a variety of methods sensitive to different learning needs and preferences, encourage the active co-construction of knowledge, and integrate learning with life experiences. When students believe they are learning, they experience more success, satisfaction, confidence, and happiness. In turn, they are motivated and excited to learn and take more responsibility for their own learning. They recognize they can learn inside and outside of the classroom and understand and discuss what types of learning strategies best meet their individual learning needs. Particularly in health professional education, students improve their ability to assess and reflect on situations in order to transfer knowledge to new encounters and to provide more effective and safe care when they are taught from an evidence-based perspective. Most importantly, students are better prepared to enter society as productive citizens capable of lifelong learning, critical thinking, collaborating, solving problems, and making challenging decisions.

LEARNER-CENTERED EDUCATION

One feature of evidence-based teaching is learner-centered education. We discuss learner-centered education because many characteristics of this educational practice align with the key features of evidence-based teaching. Over the past 3 decades, higher education is shifting from the traditional (and oftentimes, still dominant) view that an institution exists to deliver instruction to a view in which the institution produces student learning by whatever means works the best. While there is growing awareness of the importance and evidence in support of learner-centered education, some instructor-centered practices continue to dominate the higher education landscape. In *learner-centered education*, educators focus on the students and learning versus the instruction or subject and learning. They embrace an eclectic array of instructional methods, demonstrate an understanding of the students in their courses, and adapt to meet the collective and individual needs. In addition, educators provide resources and processes, which empower students to be autonomous learners in pursuit of educational and professional development and goals. Learner-centered education emphasizes a number of different features based on sound evidence for effective teaching and learning practices.

Figure 1-2. Students engage in active learning. (Reproduced with permission from Keith Borgmeyer/ University of Missouri.)

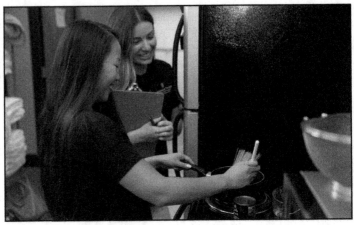

Active Learning

Many researchers and educators have expended much effort to move away from instructional methods that require the transmission of knowledge. They challenge the previous notion that educators efficiently transfer information to students who are open and passive containers ready to learn the content (e.g., sage on the stage). This method of instruction is recognized as *lecture-based learning*. Educators that use evidence-based teaching and learner-centered education to guide their practices spend proportionally less time lecturing and more time using active methods of instruction. In active learning, the students are dynamically involved in the educational process to engage in effective learning—deep, meaningful, and long lasting (Figure 1-2). If the students are spending a majority of their time listening in the classroom, they are not engaged in active learning. In comparison, if educators are spending a majority of their time preparing what they will be doing during class versus what their students will be doing, their top priority is not active learning. In active learning, the educator compels students to play a dynamic role that shifts from reliance on lectures to learning on their own or with peers. Educators select instructional methods insightful of the needs and characteristics of their students and require them to reflect on ideas and how they are integrating those ideas with prior and current knowledge.

Construction of Knowledge

According to evidence-based teaching and learner-centered education, students must also be active discoverers and constructors of their own knowledge and skills (rather than directed by an educator). Students arrive to courses with prior knowledge, beliefs, and attitudes from their previous learning or life experiences. They store this prior information in an abundance of interacting frameworks. In occupational therapy education, students enter their professional education with at least 12 to 15 years of experiences in classrooms. In addition, they often possess valuable volunteer, observation, and leadership experiences. An educator must effectively harness the ability to intentionally create contexts and situations that require students to connect what they are learning to what they already know from their experiences and educational pursuits. By building on foundational frameworks, the students construct new cognitive structures to process and apply new knowledge to various contexts. Educators also prompt students to confront their prior and current assumptions to aid in further professional and personal development to benefit their future careers. We want to caution educators that students entering graduate programs might possess firm convictions about how educators should teach. Their beliefs about how graduate education or what a classroom should "look like" are often not aligned with evidence-based teaching or learner-centered paradigms.

Collaboration and Responsibility

In traditional classrooms, educators are responsible for learning by making and implementing course decisions, controlling instructional methods, and creating educational contexts. They heavily hold power, as they are in charge of everything with no to little input from students. However, in learner-centered education, the educator and students collaboratively co-construct knowledge and co-produce learning. They learn and work together and mutually share power. The educator accomplishes a balance of power by offering choices, encouraging participation in decision-making opportunities, and establishing empowering environments. Because of these actions, the institution no longer owns the responsibility of learning (e.g., providing quality instruction via lecture and discussion), but instead shifts this important responsibility to students.

It is important to recognize not all students will embrace this role due to their prior experience as passive participants of their education. In addition, some students might initially lack the ability to make learning decisions but are capable of increasing involvement in this process with more experience. Despite these challenges, higher education typically views this collaborative partnership as a win-win because two parties own responsibility for the same outcome of learning. Even though neither partner is entirely in control, evidence suggests there is great potential to produce powerful outcomes.

Student Autonomy

Educators foster autonomy and motivation when they invite students to accept more responsibility for their own learning. In learner-centered education, students are often more motivated to learn knowledge and develop skills because they possess greater control of their education. Their beliefs, values, interests, and goals influence their motivation. When educators offer students options within certain parameters, they tap into the areas which drive motivation. In return, the students demonstrate increased engagement with the content and become more self-directed and independent learners.

Facilitation

In evidence-based teaching and learner-centered education, educators do less telling and lecturing and do more facilitating. In other words, they serve as a *guide on the side*. Educators design an optimal learning environment or experience, which requires students to engage in higher order thinking by applying information to make discoveries and solve problems. They encourage active participation and create learning communities where students interact with and learn from each other. In addition, they model expected behaviors and skills, adapt to meet their students' needs and preferences, and scaffold content and experiences to progress students to autonomous learning. Lastly, educators provide opportunities for reflection and offer feedback about achievement of learning goals.

Reflection

In these paradigms, educators encourage students to reflect on content and experiences during the teaching and learning process. The ability to reflect is particularly important for occupational therapy as educators strive to develop students capable of being reflective practitioners in their future careers. When educators provide opportunities for reflection, they assist students to develop the metacognitive skills to recognize and confront their prior and current knowledge and to determine good or difficult aspects of a situation to further adapt and learn. The students become aware of the ways they learn and begin to appreciate the ways their peers learn when they share their experiences. Educators equally benefit from student reflection, as they can identify gaps in knowledge, understand how to scaffold content, confront misconceptions, and appreciate interests and strengths.

The Teaching Practices Inventory serves as a good starting source for reflection!

Educators must also integrate reflection on their teaching into their contemporary educational practices. In higher education, literature considers reflection an essential skill for educators' professional competence. Educators use this critical skill to self-examine and self-evaluate what they do to further enhance their teaching and learning. They act more deliberately and intentionally when making curricular or course design decisions and challenge assumptions and beliefs to better meet the needs of their students. They also consider multiple resources and options during the learning process and seek opportunities and supports for professional growth. Similar to students, educators can engage in reflection in multiple ways, such as seeking student feedback, writing in a journal, and setting professional goals based on strengths and areas for improvement.

Evaluation and Feedback

In the current higher education landscape, it is becoming more critical that institutions and educators identify what specifically they have learned. Educational literature and academic experience suggests evaluation is the most challenging component for educators to design and implement effectively and consistently. In traditional teacher-centered courses, educators typically use summative evaluation to assess what their students achieved to date. An example of summative feedback is a course grade, and this mechanism often interferes with student learning. Once this type of evaluation has been completed, there are minimal opportunities for students to demonstrate further learning. In learner-centered education, educators implement formative and summative evaluative methods. In formative evaluation, they assess their students' current knowledge, performance, and skills to provide numerous opportunities for feedback—a key element to formative evaluation. In addition, educators use this method to facilitate improvements in learning by extending beyond recognition of correct and incorrect responses to discussion and feedback on the students' lines of thinking that led to those responses. Students begin to learn about and become more aware of their own thinking in relation to professional standards.

As previously mentioned, feedback is a critical component for evidence-based teaching and learner-centered education. Interestingly and contrary to what educators might believe, researchers in the Harvard Assessment Project found a majority of students reported learning significantly more with several highly structured quizzes and short assignments (Figure 1-3). They preferred this method of formative evaluation because they received quick feedback to further improve their learning throughout the remainder of the course. Hence, educators need to provide more feedback throughout the educational process. In addition, they should give specific and developmentally appropriate feedback because students do not benefit from general statements of "great work" or "expand here." It is also important for educators to understand that they do not need to grade every learning task. Students equally benefit from self-assessment, peer feedback, and practice tests. When educators implement a strong version of learner-centered education, they actually consult and collaborate with their students when selecting feedback and evaluation mechanisms. Students take more ownership of their education when they have a voice in how they demonstrate what they have learned.

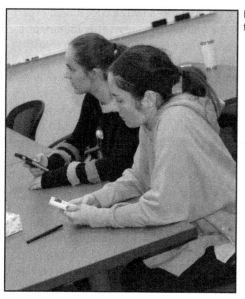

Figure 1-3. Students complete a short quiz with formative feedback using technology.

ASSESSMENT OF LEARNING

As previously mentioned, accrediting agencies increasingly pressure institutions and programs to systematically assess student learning outcomes. These entities are not concerned with teacher productivity but learning productivity. Many faculty evaluation systems assess performance in terms of teaching. These methods rarely assess if students are actually learning and often do not demand evidence of learning. In addition, good scores on teaching evaluations or educators increasing time spent on improving their teaching do not automatically translate to student learning. In our current climate, educators are expected to demonstrate student mastery of standards set by accrediting bodies (e.g., Accreditation Council for Occupational Therapy Education [ACOTE]). With a large number of standards and an ever-changing profession and health care system, it is impossible for educators to teach students everything they need to know in class. Therefore, educators should use their valuable class time to teach concepts the students deem important and engage them in high levels of application-based learning. From a learner-centered perspective, educators view effective learning more in terms of personal relevance to students versus achieving standards set by outside agencies.

Given what is at stake, it remains imperative that researchers and educators continue to explore ways to develop and assess students' competencies and talents. In order to achieve this mission, educators begin with the important step of creating explicit and high-level learning objectives. This is known as *backward design*. While this is not the focus of this book, this is often where the design process begins, and we encourage you to further access resources related to backward design and construction of learning objectives. However, in Chapter 2, we offer an innovative framework that extends backward design to facilitate student engagement in deep learning.

> Use Bloom's taxonomy resources to write high-level learning objectives!

Books
Gronlund's Writing Instructional Objectives by Gronlund & Brookhart
Understanding by Design by Wiggins & McTighe

The accreditation standards and curricular expectations serve as a guide for identifying teaching and learning priorities. Educators use learning objectives to inform other decisions, such as the careful selection of concepts, assignments, learning activities, and assessments. They leave an impression on the course by identifying what they expect their students to learn, how their students will be changed by the educational experience, and what their students should be able to do by the end of the course. It is important for educators to write high-level objectives for deep learning to occur (e.g., formulate, judge, justify). Students learn best when they clearly understand the learning objectives and view these goals as personally and professionally relevant. These components are the fuel for students to meaningful apply knowledge and skills for long-lasting learning.

Avoid the use of assessment to demonstrate that content is rigorous and complex! Students become demotivated because they view the grade reflective of ability and not effort.

In the next step, educators use the established objectives to guide their assessment of student learning. They think about what and how they are going to assess what the students learn before developing the learning activities or instructional methods or before introducing the content. Some scholars suggest the selection and implementation of selection methods has the greatest impact on students because it indicates what the educator believes is most important to learn and provides the target for successful learning. From a learner-centered perspective, Saulnier and colleagues (2008) provide several guidelines for creating methods of assessment that promote learning. They propose for educators to:

- Focus students on the learning process by describing the learning objective or outcome and explaining the design of effective learning activities and teaching methods
- Build confidence and decrease stress and anxiety of the educational experience by providing examples, creating low-stakes situations for assessment, and allowing opportunities to revisit learning activities
- Provide situations that prepare students to engage in high levels of learning in order to perform well on assessments (e.g., practice)
- Use formative feedback regularly (see Evaluation and Feedback section) and direct feedback toward performance by using language that describes more than it assesses
- Compare assessments to exemplary examples found in literature

After educators have selected ways to assess student learning, they begin to select learning and instructional methods that facilitate active and engaged learning. The more students uncover topics themselves (rather than listening to the educator cover), the more likely they are to achieve higher-level learning outcomes. The aim of this book is to provide you with a variety of instructional methods supported by evidence- and learner-centered principles that foster student learning.

PREDICTORS OF STUDENT PERFORMANCE

Higher education research and literature offers educators several principles predictive of student performance. It is important to recognize none of the principles are contingent upon a certain personality type or teaching style. Therefore, any educator possesses the potential to enhance student performance when they develop and assimilate certain teaching and learning habits into the design of their classrooms and courses. They create effective learning when they encourage contact between the educator and student, facilitate cooperation among students, engage students in active learning, provide prompt feedback, highlight time on task, communicate high expectations, and respect the variety of talents and ways students learn (Table 1-1). Educators can implement each principle independently, but the effectiveness of learning greatly improves when they build experiences that incorporate each of the seven principles. In addition, these principles fit many different types of students, learning styles, and concepts. The authors encourage educators to seek various sources of support and resources inside and outside of their institution to successfully implement these valuable principles.

TABLE 1-1

Examples of Seven Principles for Effective Learning

PRINCIPLE	EXAMPLES
1. Encourage contact between educators and students	Use discussion seminars Implement focus groups for course feedback
2. Facilitate cooperation among students	Establish learning groups Implement methods that require collaborative work (e.g., team-based learning, jigsaw)
3. Engage students in active learning	Use debate Develop experiential learning opportunities
4. Provide prompt feedback	Use a game that provides formative feedback during play Integrate practice questions at end of class
5. Highlight time on task	Establish learning contract to determine appropriate amount of time on assignment Use accountability assignments to ensure time spent with content
6. Communicate high expectations	Collaborate with students to establish expectations for course Communicate ways to be successful in course in syllabus
7. Respect the variety of talents and learning styles	Implement variety of instructional methods to meet different needs Provide opportunities for students to discuss experiences

OCCUPATIONAL THERAPY EDUCATION

The philosophy of occupational therapy education includes distinct beliefs about teaching and learning while embracing the core values of the profession. According to the American Occupational Therapy Association (AOTA; 2015), educators aim to prepare "…occupational therapy practitioners to address the occupational needs of individuals, groups, communities, and populations" (p. 1) through the combination of didactic coursework and fieldwork experiences. In the current health care climate, occupational therapists are serving individuals with complex concerns in a variety of dynamic and challenging practice settings. To best address these needs, students learn to integrate the profession's values, theories, evidence, and ethics with the development of various skills (i.e., clinical reasoning, critical thinking, metacognition) to deliver occupation-based and client-centered services. Our profession encourages occupational therapy educators to use the best evidence and outcome data to provide a teaching-learning experience that adequately prepares students to be successful in practice. Therefore, we are charged to implement sophisticated teaching methods that match the multifaceted demands of occupational therapy practice.

Similar to the concept of the interaction between the person, environment, and occupation in practice, students (person) engage in dynamic transactions with various learning contexts (environment) during a variety of educational experiences (occupation). Comparable to characteristics of evidence-based teaching and learner-centered education, the AOTA (2015) suggests the educational experiences include:

TABLE 1-2

Signature Pedagogies in Occupational Therapy Education

SIGNATURE PEDAGOGY	DEFINITION	EXAMPLE
Relational Learning	Students learn through the human connection.	Educator-student or peer relationships in the classroom. Client-student relationship in a experiential learning or fieldwork experience.
Affective Learning	Students develop a personal and professional identity.	A learning experience in which a student experiences a shift in attitudes, beliefs, or values.
Highly Contextualized, Active Engagement	Students learn by doing.	Practicing transfers in a lab. Interviewing a community member when learning to develop an occupational profile.

Adapted from Schaber, P. (2014). Conference proceedings—keynote address: Searching for and identifying signature pedagogies in occupational therapy education. *American Journal of Occupational Therapy, 68,* S40-S44; Schwartz, B. M., & Gurung, A. R. (2012). *Evidence-based teaching for higher education.* American Psychological Association.

- "Active and diverse learning within and beyond the classroom environment
- A collaborative process that builds on prior knowledge and experience
- Continuous professional judgment, evaluation, and self-reflection
- Lifelong learning" (p. 1)

Although these values are readily seen across disciplines, occupational therapy education demonstrates certain ways of implementing these values, which make our profession's educational experiences unique from others. This is called *signature pedagogy*; the ways of teaching future practitioners their profession. Educators use signature pedagogies to determine how and what pieces of knowledge or skills are most important to convey and what values and beliefs are representative of the profession. For example, in occupational therapy education, we value the use of natural environments to foster student learning (e.g., developing a health and wellness program at a senior center or designing an inclusive playground at a preschool). Following a comprehensive review of the literature, Schaber (2014) identified three signature pedagogies in occupational therapy education (Table 1-2).

In occupational therapy educational literature, scholars present several interesting findings that align with notions discussed throughout this chapter. Schaber (2014) reported occupational therapy educators typically implement these signature pedagogies by starting a class with an introduction or short lecture and then guiding an active learning activity. Similarly, Hooper and colleagues (2013) reported experiential or active learning was the most prominent educational approach in occupational therapy education, and other literature suggests educators use a hodgepodge of teaching methods ranging from role play to games to simulation. In a survey, Henderson and colleagues (2017) also found that occupational therapy educators use a variety of active teaching methods. However, educators continued to report the frequent use of lecture despite rating the value of this teaching strategy for developing professional reasoning low. Although Krishnagiri and colleagues (2019) found occupational therapy educators use several active learning methods to convey occupation, lecture remained in the top five instructional methods for teaching our profession's core value. Higher education literature has indicated the use of lecture (instructor-based education) no longer adequately prepares students for entry to the workforce. Although our signature pedagogies reflect characteristics of evidence-based teaching, there remains a need for occupational therapy educators to move beyond lecture-based learning to further use of evidence to inform what **and** how they teach.

STATE OF OCCUPATIONAL THERAPY EDUCATION RESEARCH

Although research in occupational therapy education remains relatively new, we have witnessed great growth since the turn of the 21st century. In collaboration with the AOTA, educators, clinicians, and leaders in occupational therapy programs have provided a foundation of research to advance curricula and fieldwork. With this information, educators can improve their understanding of how to best prepare occupational therapists and occupational therapy assistants to effectively meet the needs of society. Occupational therapy education will continue to see significant advancements in teaching and learning practices as educators continue to bring new energy and innovation.

In recent years, occupational therapy educators have had more opportunities and resources to be producers and consumers of educational research. In 2018, the AOTA (2018) revised the *Occupational Therapy Education Research Agenda* to provide educators with a conceptual framework to guide their questions and integrate their inquiry in areas where more research was needed. This revised document included the addition of a priority to the six original research priorities established in the 2014 agenda. The seven research priorities for occupational therapy education include:

1. "Theory building
2. Signature pedagogies
3. Instructional methods
4. Learner characteristics and competencies
5. Socialization to the profession
6. Faculty development and resources
7. Promotion of diversity, inclusion, and equity throughout the education pipeline and curricula" (AOTA, 2018, p. 1)

In addition to the research agenda, the AOTA established an annual Education Summit in 2013, a conference specifically designed for occupational therapy educators. Educators also have access to an encouraging body of written work that affords opportunities to engage in evidence-based teaching. In 2014, *The American Journal of Occupational Therapy* produced the inaugural publication of an education supplement. Three years later, Eastern Kentucky established the *Journal of Occupational Therapy Education*; a peer-reviewed journal devoted to occupational therapy education research and information. Similarly, in each issue, *The Open Journal of Occupational Therapy* highlights various Topics in Education; however, Hooper (2016) reported nearly half of the journal's publications are related to education. These illustrations demonstrate the maturation of the body of science supporting occupational therapy education.

When reviewing the last 2 decades of literature, we can clearly view the progression of occupational therapy education research. Hooper and colleagues (2013) conducted a systematic mapping review of literature from 2000 to 2009 to understand and summarize the occupational therapy education research landscape. During this time frame, occupational therapy education researchers were primarily focused on educational approaches and teaching methods and examined these topics in local learning environments. In addition, these studies were primarily conceptual and descriptive papers that were more qualitative in nature and rarely used a conceptual framework. Researchers also favored the use of assessment methods that measured changes in students' attitudes and perceptions. Since this time, experts have noted several features that highlight the growth of evidence in occupational therapy education literature. These features include research that is theoretically driven and includes perspectives from multiple stakeholders, the emergence of refined assessment methods and longitudinal studies, and the expansion of topics that address more novel areas of occupational therapy education.

Although context-specific and descriptive studies provide value, several occupational therapy education researchers propose developing more rigorous studies and moving studies beyond the local learning environment. As educators take these steps forward, we need to clearly describe the learning context and carefully state and align the research questions with the research agenda and educational issues that impact a variety of occupational therapy programs. In addition, there remains a need for occupational therapy education research to be aligned with educational theories from higher education and SoTL literature. As occupational therapy educators, there is much to learn from these resources rather than creating our own educational theories. However, they must carefully translate these theories into our educational practices that are reflective of the professional philosophies and ways of knowing. This action is similar to what practitioners do in occupational therapy practice. For example, they use a cognitive-behavioral frame of reference from psychology literature, but determine how to use it with the individuals they serve in occupational therapy practice. As educators continue to translate these theories into the occupational therapy education, it is important they select outcome measures that align with learning and practice performance. Together these actions will continue to strengthen and diversify the research that guides educators' decisions in evidence-based teaching.

ACCREDITATION COUNCIL FOR OCCUPATIONAL THERAPY EDUCATION

The educational requirements have significantly changed since the conception of the occupational therapy profession, expanding from certificates to various levels of graduate degrees. As previously mentioned, accreditation entities have a significant impact on occupational therapy educators inside and outside the context of the classroom. Occupational therapy programs and higher institutions pursue accreditation to demonstrate they offer a quality education by achieving certain **minimal** standards. Accreditation entities assist programs to identify areas of improvement as well as provide assurance to the public and to students that a program has established objectives, has a plan to achieve those objectives, and accomplishes those objectives now and in the future. As you are likely aware, ACOTE accredits occupational therapy assistant and occupational therapy programs.

ACOTE (2007) describes four specific purposes for the accreditation process; three of which directly relate to roles and responsibilities related to teaching and learning:

1. Encourage continuous self-analysis and improvement with goal of **assuring students receive a quality education**
2. Determine if the occupational therapy program **achieves educational standards**
3. Encourage faculty to stay **abreast on new practice trends and developments for incorporation into occupational therapy education**

The profession's accrediting body requires educators to describe the learning process for each educational standard in Section B: Content Requirements and provide evidence that students have adequately achieved each standard. Currently, there are 55 B standards for associate and baccalaureate degree–level occupational therapy assistant programs, and 61 B standards for master's and doctoral degree–level occupational therapy programs. The *2018 ACOTE Standards and Interpretive Guide* presents the first educational standards for baccalaureate degree–level occupational therapy assistant programs and a marked decrease in the number of educational standards (B standards) for doctoral (110), master's (103), and associate (88) degree–level programs from the *2011 ACOTE Standards and Interpretive Guide.*

TABLE 1-3	
Accreditation Council for Occupational Therapy Education Standards Related to Evidence-Based Teaching	
STANDARD	**BRIEF DESCRIPTION**
A.2.3	The program director and faculty must possess academic and experiential qualification and backgrounds that meet program objectives, must document their expertise in areas of teaching and knowledge of content delivery method, and must hold expertise for appropriate curriculum design, content delivery, and program evaluation.
A.5.5	The instructional design must reflect the curriculum to ensure appropriate content delivery.
A.5.7	Each course must have a written syllabus with course objectives and learning activities that reflect the course content required by standards. In addition, the educator must identify the instructional method and assessment strategy used to achieve each course objective.
A.6.2	The program director and faculty that teach two or more courses must have a written professional growth and development plan.

In addition to the educational standards, our accrediting entity maintains a standard that each program must meet a certain benchmark for students passing the National Board for Certification in Occupational Therapy exam (A.6.4) and must also conduct regular evaluation consistent with their curriculum design, objectives, and competencies (A.3.5; A.5.5). In this era of accountability, occupational therapy educators experience pressure to meet these important standards under challenging circumstances in which there are more standards to meet, maxed out degree credit hours, and increased faculty workloads, among other things. However, by using evidence-based teaching methods and by engaging in the SoTL, educators can incorporate **current educational trends** to ensure they are working more effectively and to confirm that **students are learning and receiving a high-quality education**.

In addition to the educational standards, ACOTE (2018) outlines general requirements (also known as the A Standards: General Requirements) that require engagement in evidence-based teaching or the SoTL. Table 1-3 highlights four of these important standards. Educators are invited to further review the A standards to understand the specific requirements for the type of occupational therapy program in which they teach (see Table 1-3). It is important for both experienced and novice occupational therapy educators to stay abreast on current evidence and requirements and to continuously seek resources and support for teaching and learning processes.

OCCUPATIONAL THERAPY EDUCATORS

The need for qualified educators continues to grow for two reasons. First, there is demand for occupational therapy practitioners in the current health care climate. Second, there are more occupational therapy programs in the United States. Many occupational therapy educators transition from clinical practice to academia. On average, occupational therapy educators enter academia 10 to 12 years after graduation. Although occupational therapy practitioners often play the educator role in practice, they are often not adequately prepared for the shift to higher education and frequently experience insecurities about moving from a master clinician to a novice educator. Numerous educators in higher education have advanced degrees in their specific area of content. However, few of these educators possess formal training in teaching and learning and even less have adequate time to locate research to guide their selection of teaching methods (i.e., evidence-based teaching), as they often struggle balancing various roles and responsibilities. For example, in the *2018 to 2019 AOTA Faculty Workforce Survey*, 58% of educators reported their highest degree in occupational therapy or occupational science with only 16% of the highest degree in the realm of education. Because of these challenges, educators in occupational therapy resort to selecting teaching methods based either how they were taught or on what did or did not work the last time they taught something themselves. Since these actions are not necessarily supported by evidence, occupational therapy educators are challenged to **accelerate their development of teaching and scholarship roles** to adequately meet the demands of academia and society.

Occupational therapy educators serve numerous roles in the academic setting. In the 2010 survey, occupational therapy educators reported spending 52% of their time in teaching, 14% in scholarship, 11% in service, and 23% in other activities, such as advisement and administration (AOTA, 2010). Furthermore, in 2018 to 2019, 59% of occupational therapy educators and 52% of occupational therapy assistant educators reported spending 5 to 14 hours in the classroom per week. This statistic does not appear to include time spent developing teaching methods, selecting readings, and grading assignments. Despite spending a majority of their time in teaching, Gupta and Bilics (2014) stated only 16% of occupational therapy educators reported frequently engaging in education research or the SoTL that would support or advance their teaching practices. However, 90% of the occupational therapy educators in this survey reported examining available literature and applying this information to their teaching (evidence-based teaching). This statistic shows promise, as it suggests occupational therapy educators are improving engagement in evidence-based teaching. In addition, approximately half of occupational therapy programs are housed in institutions that value teaching over high-intensity research, and these programs traditionally recognize the importance of scholarly activities related to education. Although teaching is an essential function of occupational therapy educators and is valued by occupational therapy programs, there remains a need to invest time in scholarship to inform educational practices.

Similar to the transition to teaching, a majority of health professions faculty are relatively new to scholarship activities. The AOTA (2016) suggests that every occupational therapy practitioner has the responsibility to contribute "...to building the evidence base for occupational therapy practice and occupational therapy education" (p. 1). Despite this important position, occupational therapy educators often enter academia with a desire to teach (not to perform research), experience lower confidence in their research skills, and are often employed at institutions that do not have optimal infrastructure to support research. Although engaging in evidence-based teaching is an important first step, the next action for faculty would be to truly invest in the SoTL by applying literature, collecting and analyzing data, and disseminating findings about how to prepare students to be professionals capable of advancing the profession. In this same study, 52% of occupational therapy educators reported that they did not complete education research. When further analyzed, 69% of early career educators (0 to 9 years) "never" or "seldom" engaged in education research. If there is a desire to enrich occupational therapy education, stakeholders and educators must recognize the need to mature from an educator to a scholar, particularly a scholar in the field of teaching and learning.

Several of our professional documents embrace the role of the occupational therapy educator as a scholar of teaching and learning (Table 1-4). We can trace key elements of evidence-based teaching in a document developed by the Commission on Education (Dickerson, 2004) titled, *Role Competencies for a Professional-Level Occupational Therapist Faculty Member in an Academic Setting*. For example, "demonstrate the ability to effectively judge new materials, literature, and educational materials that enhance the lifelong learning of future occupational therapy practitioners" (p. 649) and "demonstrate the expertise to develop course objectives, course materials, and educational experiences that promote optimal learning for students" (p. 650). In the following years, the AOTA

TABLE 1-4

Documents Related to Teaching and Learning in Occupational Therapy Education

- *2018 (ACOTE) Standards and Interpretive Guide*
- *A Descriptive Review of Occupational Therapy Education*
- *Occupational Therapy Education Research Agenda—Revised*
- *Philosophy of Occupational Therapy Education*
- *Role Competencies for a Professional-Level Occupational Therapist Faculty Member in an Academic Setting*
- *Specialized Knowledge and Skills of Occupational Therapy Educators of the Future*

(2009) created an additional document titled, *Specialized Knowledge and Skills of Occupational Therapy Educators of the Future*, to describe the role of occupational therapy professionals as educators and to highlight the characteristics they should possess to fulfill the profession's vision.

In addition to these documents, the AOTA's Ad Hoc Committee–Future of Occupational Therapy Education provided recommendations to address challenges with the transition to the entry-level doctorate for occupational therapy and entry-level baccalaureate for occupational therapy assistant education. Several of the committee's recommendations specify strategies to support occupational therapy educators as scholars of teaching and learning. For example, the committee recommended developing a Center for Educational Excellence that offers resources and research support and provides opportunities for educators to develop skills and knowledge to conduct education research. We also recognize the AOTA's efforts to support educators, which include preconference workshops (e.g., practitioners considering a transition from professional practice to academia and the SoTL program) and the Academic Education Special Interest Section's development of a mentorship program for new educators and academic fieldwork coordinators. All of the recommendations and support move occupational therapy education toward a more scholarly approach to teaching and learning, which in turn creates evidence to support better student outcomes and data for accreditation and society.

SUMMARY

Occupational therapy educators craft learning experiences, assessment methods, courses, and curriculum. Similar to occupational therapy practice, educators create experiences for students (clients) with the goal of collecting outcomes to demonstrate effectiveness. It is essential educators develop skills and obtain support for implementing evidence-based teaching methods, performing assessments to understand the learning needs of their students, and demonstrating achievement of learning outcomes to many stakeholders. Educators use accreditation standards to guide teaching and learning priorities and evaluations. They spend a great deal of time contemplating learning objectives and assessment methods. Once the educator has thoughtfully considered these areas, they determine how to teach important concepts. This textbook provides educators with a variety of evidence-based instructional methods to achieve their desired learning outcomes and to produce students prepared to meaningfully contribute to society. We will all be inspired by the energy evidence-based teaching creates during the educational experience.

THREE THINGS YOU CAN DO TOMORROW TO IMPLEMENT EVIDENCE-BASED TEACHING WITH YOUR STUDENTS

1. Set aside 1 hour each week to read teaching and learning literature and research.
2. Complete the Teaching Practices Inventory and reflect on results.
3. Discuss evidence-based teaching with colleagues or seek out resources if your institution has a teaching and learning center.

REFERENCES

Accreditation Council for Occupational Therapy Education. (2007). Accreditation council for occupational therapy education accreditation manual [PDF document]. Retrieved from https://www.aota.org/~/media/Corporate/Files/EducationCareers/Accredit/Policies/47631/I%20Introduction.pdf

Accreditation Council for Occupational Therapy Education. (2018). 2018 accreditation council for occupational therapy education (ACOTE) standards and interpretive guide [PDF document]. Retrieved from https://www.aota.org/~/media/Corporate/Files/EducationCareers/Accredit/StandardsReview/2018-ACOTE-Standards-Interpretive-Guide.pdf

American Occupational Therapy Association. (2009). Specialized knowledge and skills of occupational therapy educators of the future. *American Journal of Occupational Therapy, 63*(6), 804-818.

American Occupational Therapy Association. (2010). Faculty workforce survey [PDF document]. Retrieved from https://www.aota.org/~/media/Corporate/Files/EducationCareers/Educators/OTEdData/2010%20Faculty%20Survey%20Report.pdf

American Occupational Therapy Association. (2015). Philosophy of occupational therapy education. *American Journal of Occupational Therapy, 69*(Suppl. 3), 6913410052. http://dx.doi.org/10.5014/ajot.2015.696S17

American Occupational Therapy Association. (2016). Scholarship in occupational therapy. *American Journal of Occupational Therapy, 70*(Suppl 2), 7012410080p1-7012410080p1.

American Occupational Therapy Association. (2018). Occupational therapy education research agenda—revised. *American Journal of Occupational Therapy, 72*(Suppl 2), 7212420070p1-7212420070p5.

Buskist, W., & Groccia, J. E. (2011). *Evidence-based teaching: New directions for teaching and learning, number 128.* John Wiley & Sons.

Dickerson, A. E. (2004). Role competencies for a professional-level occupational therapist faculty member in an academic setting. *American Journal of Occupational Therapy, 58*(6), 649-650.

Davies, P. (1999). What is evidence-based education? *British Journal of Educational Studies, 47*(2), 108-121. http://dx.doi.org/10.1111/1467-8527.00106

Gupta, J., & Bilics, A. (2014). Brief report—Scholarship and research in occupational therapy education. *American Journal of Occupational Therapy, 68,* S87-S92. http://dx.doi.org/10.5014/ajot.2014.012880

Henderson, W., Coppard, B., & Qi, Y. (2017). Identifying instructional methods for development of clinical reasoning in entry-level occupational therapy education: A mixed methods design. *Journal of Occupational Therapy Education, 1*(2). https://doi.org/10/26681/jote.2017.010201

Hooper, B. (2016). Broadening the scope and impact of occupational therapy education research by merging two research agendas: A new research agenda matrix. *Open Journal of Occupational Therapy, 4*(3), Article 1. http://dx.doi.org.10.15453/2168-6408.1305

Hooper, B., King, R., Wood, W., Bilics, A., & Gupta, J. (2013). An international systematic mapping review of educational approaches and teaching methods in occupational therapy. *British Journal of Occupational Therapy, 76*(1), 9-22. http://dx.doi.org.10.4276/030802213X13576469254612

Krishnagiri, S., Hooper, B., Price, P., Taff, S. D., Bilics, A. (2019). A national survey of learning activities and instructional strategies used to teach occupation: implication for signature pedagogies. *American Journal of Occupational Therapy, 73,* 7305205080. https://doi.org/10.5014.ajot.2019.032789

Saulnier, B. M., Laundry, J. P., Longenecker, H. E., & Wagner, T. A. (2008). From teaching to learning: learner-centered teaching and assessment in information systems education. *Journal of Information Systems Education, 19*(2), 169-174.

Schaber, P. (2014). Conference Proceedings—Keynote address: Searching for and identifying signature pedagogies in occupational therapy education. *American Journal of Occupational Therapy, 68,* S40-S44. http://dx.doi.org/10.5014/ajot.2014.685S08

Schwartz, B. M., & Gurung, A. R. (2012). *Evidence-based teaching for higher education.* American Psychological Association.

BIBLIOGRAPHY

Accreditation Council for Occupational Therapy Education. (2011). 2011 accreditation council for occupational therapy education (ACOTE) standards and interpretive guide [PDF document]. Retrieved from https://www.aota.org/~/media/Corporate/Files/EducationCareers/Accredit/Standards/2011-Standards-and-Interpretive-Guide.pdf

Accreditation Council for Occupational Therapy Education. (2017). ACOTE 2027 mandate [PDF document]. Retrieved from https://www.aota.org/~/media/Corporate/Files/EducationCareers/Accredit/ACOTE-2027-Mandate-Background-Materials.pdf

Ambrose, S. A., Bridges, M. W., DiPietro, M., Lovett, M. C., & Norman, M. K. (2010). *How learning works: Seven research-based principles for smart teaching*. Jossey-Bass Inc.

American Occupational Therapy Association. (2016). A descriptive review of occupational therapy education. *American Journal of Occupational Therapy, 70*(Suppl 1), 7012410040p1-7012410040p10.

Benson, P. (2012). Learner-centered teaching. In A. Burns & J. C. Richards (Eds.), *The Cambridge guide to pedagogy and practice in second language teaching* (pp. 30-37). Cambridge University Press.

Bondoc, S. (2005). Occupational therapy and evidence-based education. *Education Special Interest Section Quarterly, 15*(4), 1-4.

Brackenbury, T. (2012). A qualitative examination of connections between learner-centered teaching and past significant learning experiences. *Journal of the Scholarship of Teaching and Learning, 12*(4), 12-28.

Bruniges, M. (2005). An evidence-based approach to teaching and learning. Retrieved from http://research.acer.edu.au/research_conference_2005/15

Burke, J. P., & Harvison, N. (2015). Guest editorial—Evolution of a revolution in occupational therapy education. *American Journal of Occupational Therapy, 69*(Suppl. 2), 6912170010. http://dx.doi.org/10.5014/ajot.2015.695S01

Cabatan, M. C. C., Grajo, L. C., & Sana, E. A. (2019). A scoping review of challenges and the adaptation process in the academia: Implications for occupational therapy educators. *Open Journal of Occupational Therapy, 7*(1), Article 8. https://doi.org/10.15453/2168-6408.1523

Cheang, K. I. (2009). Effect of learner-centered teaching on motivation and learning strategies in a third-year pharmacotherapy course. *American Journal of Pharmaceutical Education, 73*(3), Article 42. http://doi.org/10.5688/aj730342

Cheng, A., Morse, K. J., Arab, A. A., Runnacles, J., & Eppich, W. (2016). Learner-centered debriefing for health care simulation education: Lessons for faculty development. *Simulation in Healthcare, 11*(1), 32-40.

Chickering, A. W., & Gamson, A. F. (1987). Seven principles for good practice in undergraduate education. *AAHE Bulletin, 39*, 3-7.

Coker, P. (2010). Effects of an experiential learning program on the clinical reasoning and critical thinking skills of occupational therapy students. *Journal of Allied Health, 39*(4), 280-286.

Commission of Education. (2019). Report of the COE faculty workforce task group [PDF document]. Retrieved from https://www.aota.org/~/media/Corporate/Files/Secure/Governance/RA/2019-fall-meeting/COE-Task-Group-on-Faculty-Workforce-September-2019.pdf

Doabler, C. T., Nelson, N. J., Kennedy, P. C., Stoolmiller, M., Fien, H., Clarke, B., Gearin, B., Smolkowski, K., & Baker, S. K. (2018). Investigating the longitudinal effects of a core mathematics program on evidence-based teaching practices in mathematics. *Learning Disability Quarterly, 41*(3), 144-158. http://dx.doi.org/10.1177/0731948718756040

Donohoe, A. (2019). The blended reflective inquiry educators framework; origins, development, and utilization. *Nurse Education in Practice, 38*, 96-104. https://doi.org/10.1016/j.nepr.2019.06.008

Falzarano, M., & Zipp, G. P. (2012). Perceptions of mentoring of full-time occupational therapy faculty in the United States. *Occupational Therapy International, 19*, 117-126.

Fleming-Castaldy, R. P., & Gillen, G. (2013). The issue is—Ensuring that education, certification, and practice are evidence-based. *American Journal of Occupational Therapy, 67*, 364-369. http://dx.doi.org/10.5014/ajot.2013.006973

Gronlund, N. D., & Brookhart, S. M. (2008). *Gronlund's writing instructional objectives* (8th ed.). Pearson.

Holland, T., Sherman, S. B., & Harris, S. (2018). Paired teaching: A professional development model for adopting evidence-based practices. *College Teaching, 66*(3), 148-157. http://dx.doi.org/10.1080/87567555.2018.1463506

Hooper, B., Mitcham, M. D., Taff, S. D., Price, P., Krishnagiri, S., & Bilics, A. (2015). This issue is—Energizing occupation as the center of teaching and learning. *American Journal of Occupational Therapy 69*(Suppl. 2), 6912360010. http://dx.doi.org/10.5014/ajot.2015.018242

Hooper, B., & Rodger, S. (2016). She said, she said: A conversation about growing education research in occupational therapy. *Open Journal of Occupational Therapy, 4*(3), Article 12. http://dx.doi.org.10.15453/2168-6408.1307

Hunter, W. J. (2017). Evidence-based teaching in the 21st century: The missing link. *Canadian Journal of Education, 40*(2), 1-6.

Journal of Occupational Therapy Education. (n.d.). About this journal. Retrieved https://encompass.eku.edu/jote/about.html

Kramer, P., Ideishi, R. I., Kearney, P., Cohen, M. E., Ames, J. O., Shea, G. B., Schemm, R., & Blumberg, P. (2007). Achieving curricular themes through learner-centered teaching. *Occupational Therapy in Health Care, 21*(1-2), 185-198. https://doi.org/10.1080/J003v21n01_14

Krishnagiri, S., Hooper, B., Price, P., Taff, S. D., Bilics, A. (2017). Explicit or hidden? Exploring how occupation is taught in occupational therapy curricula in the United States. *American Journal of Occupational Therapy, 71*, 7102230020. https://doi.org/10.5014/ajot.2017.024174

Light, R. J. (2001). *Making the most of college: Students speak their minds.* Harvard University Press.

Lockhart-Keene, L., & Potivn, M. C. (2018). Occupational therapy adjunct faculty self-perceptions of readiness to teach. *Open Journal of Occupational Therapy, 6*(2), Article 14. https://doi.org/10.15453/2168-6408.1415

Malott, K. M., Hall, K. H., Sheely-Moore, A., Krell, M. M., & Cardaciotto, L. (2014). Evidence-based teaching in higher education: Application to counselor education. *Counselor Education & Supervision, 53*, 294-305. http://dx.doi.org/10.1002/j.1556-6978.2014.00064.x

Neistadt, M. E. (1999). Educational interpretation of "cooperative learning as an approach to pedagogy". *American Journal of Occupational Therapy, 53*(1), 41-43. http://dx.doi.org/10.5014/ajot.53.1.41

Ordinetz, S. A. (2009). Perceptions and attitudes of occupational therapy faculty towards the scholarship of teaching (Doctoral dissertation). Retrieved from Capella University. (3379000).

Otty, R., & Wrightsman, W. (2013). Marking the move: Transitioning from practitioner to academic. *OT Practice, 18*(4), 13-17. http://dx.doi.org/10.7138/otp.2013.184f2

Paris, C., & Combs, B. (2006). Lived meanings: what teachers mean when they say they are learner-centered. *Teachers and Teaching: Theory and Practice, 12*(5), 571-592. http://dx.doi.org/10.1080/13540600600832296

Pierce, J. W., & Kalman, D. L. (2003). Applying learner-centered principles in teacher education. *Theory into Practice, 42*(4), 127-132.

Sabel, J. L., Dauer, J. T., Forbes, C. T. (2017). Introductory biology students' use of enhanced answer keys and reflection questions to engage in metacognition and enhance understanding. *Life Sciences Education, 16*(40), 1-12. http://dx.doi.org/10.1187/cbe.16-10-0298

Schulman, L. S. (2005). Signature pedagogies in the professions. *Daedalus, 134,* 52-29. http://dx.doi.org/10.1162/0011526054622015

Shandomo, H. M. (2010). The role of critical reflection in teacher education. *School-University Partnerships, 4*(1), 101-113.

Simon, R. L., Krug, G., & Grajo, L. C. (2019). Developing a mentorship program for new educators and academic fieldwork coordinators using a community approach. *SIS Quarterly Practice Connections, 4*(2), 11-13.

Stevens, K. R., & Cassidy, V. R. (1999). *Evidence-based teaching: Current research in nursing education.* National League for Nursing Press.

Stoykov, M. E., Skarupski, K. A., Foucher, K., & Chubinskaya, S. (2017). Junior investigators thinking about quitting research: A survey. *American Journal of Occupational Therapy, 71*, 7102280010. https://doi.org.10.5014/ajot.2017.019448

Thomas, A., Bossers, A., Lee, M., & Lysaght, R. (2016). Occupational therapy education research: Results of a national survey. *American Journal of Occupational Therapy, 70*, 7005230010. http://dx.doi.org/10.5014/ajot.2016.018259

Toppino, T. C., & Cohen, M. S. (2010). Metacognitive control and spaced practice: Clarifying what people do and why. *Journal of Experimental Psychology: Learning, Memory, and Cognition, 36*(6), 1480-1491. https://doi.org.10.1037/a0020949

Whetten, D. A. (2007). Principles of effective course design: what I wish I had known about learning-centered teaching 30 years ago. *Journal of Management Education, 31*(3), 339-357. http://dx.doi.org/10.1177/1052562906298445

Wieman, C., & Gilbert, S. (2014). The teaching practice inventory: a new tool for characterizing college and university teaching in mathematics and science. *CBE-Life Sciences Education, 13*, 552-569.

Wiggins, G. P., & McTighe, J. (2005). *Understanding by design* (2nd ed.). Association for Supervision and Curriculum Development.

DESIGN THINKING FOR TEACHING EXCELLENCE

Leigh Neier, PhD
Stacy Neier, PhD

"IF IT'S NOT BROKE, WHY FIX IT?"

The phrase, "If it's not broke, why fix it," is a common adage. Essentially, the mantra supports the thinking if there is no perceived problem with a certain object or situation, the act of problem-solving is not worth the time. Instead of embracing the ambiguity that comes with change, the traditional, safe path is good enough. However, is good enough **good enough** in the pursuit of teaching excellence?

In recent years, institutions, administrators, and faculty have given increased attention to teaching effectiveness, or teaching for learning. Indeed, public inquiry regarding faculty teaching responsibilities has reinvigorated a desire from institutions to examine teaching practices and to consider new means for evaluating effective teaching. Examining teaching excellence is especially critical for occupational therapy education programs, given the increased need to recruit, retain, and graduate qualified professionals into the growing health care field.

At the same time, college students continue to encounter stereotypical college classrooms: A classroom experience where the educator conveys content and the student receives information. This traditional formula perpetuates the longstanding notion that the educator's expertise and knowledge are all that matters; the educator is the star of the show and the students are the audience.

It is not uncommon for educators to arrive to class with prepared talking points or PowerPoint slides, confident they will meet what they perceive their students' learning and engagement needs to be. It is also not uncommon for many educators to arrive to class with only a mental script. After teaching their content repeatedly, educators occasionally boast they do not need to prepare for class. After all, they have taught their content numerous times.

Henderson, W. (Ed.). *Effective Teaching: Instructional Methods
and Strategies for Occupational Therapy Education* (pp. 19-30).
© 2021 Taylor & Francis Group.

Perhaps their talking points and slides are materials they have previously used and received favorable course evaluations. Perhaps they have never received constructive or negative feedback from students or peer evaluators. Or, perhaps the educator cannot imagine teaching their content in any other format; there are only so many ways to examine occupational therapy, right? In other words, if it's not broke, why fix it?

The act of college teaching has historically centered on conveying knowledge from educator to student, a formula that does not consider the reciprocity (e.g., knowledge from student to teacher), which research demonstrates is needed for long-term recall of course materials. Such reciprocity is also needed to create relevance between the course content and the students' environments outside of and within the classroom and beyond their educational experience. With little to no incentive to revise—let alone revolutionize—their teaching practices, many educators default to the rationale that there is little to no need to rethink their teaching because this is simply the way it has always been done.

Yet, in the most sophisticated, connected era of our time, educators have the enormous potential to rethink default settings. By rethinking default settings, educators must reconsider if they are meeting, or even acknowledging, their students' actual needs, or do their teaching practices center on what they **perceive** those needs to be? Design-inspired educators recognize experimentation itself as a best practice, as they do not fear change and see value in taking risks. Educators must shift their mindsets by reprogramming their teaching practice to focus more on process and less on product or outcome. To achieve a risk-taking, process-over-product mindset, educators need a framework to rewire the art of teaching and the science of course design. Design Thinking provides a blueprint for needed change in the college classroom.

Originally pioneered by Stanford University's Tim Brown and Barry Katz, Design Thinking is, at its core, about innovating, need finding, and problem solving. Built on the concept of human-centered design, Design Thinking begins by taking the perspective of the people for whom you are designing. The ultimate goal is to test and retest tailor-made ideas to meet actual individual needs, not merely the perceived needs of a large population. In other words, Design Thinking is the opposite of "if it's not broke, why fix it?"

This chapter will examine the potential for Design Thinking as a go-to tool for educators to reconsider their default settings inside and outside of the occupational therapy classroom. Through an examination of Design Thinking steps and design-inspired mindsets, we will provide examples and ideas to overhaul default settings to achieve deeper student learning and engagement. We will re-emphasize empathy's role in human-centered design, and argue that practicing and modeling empathy as an educator is perhaps the single most important part of applying the ideology of Design Thinking to your teaching practice. As an occupational therapy educator, adopting empathy into your teaching philosophy presents a perfect opportunity to model perspective taking with your students, who will need to reflect on the role empathy will play in their own client-centered practices. Through intentional course design, occupational therapy educators can leverage empathy to enhance student connectedness while also providing an excellent example for what empathy looks like and feels like in the field of occupational therapy.

Borrowed From Business:
Design Thinking and Higher Education

Design Thinking Outside of Higher Education

Historically, Design Thinking stems from industries and disciplines ranging from product development and advertising to health care systems. Stanford University's pioneering schoolwork in Design Thinking launched consultancies (such as the Innovation Design Engineering Organization, a design company dedicated to building positive influences worldwide) into the spotlight as innovation partners for the world's leading companies and brands. As both for-profit and nonprofit organizations began to experience sizable shifts in how customers, clients, and stakeholders at large experienced society's "wicked problems" (Brown, 2019, p. 262), decision makers from C-suite executives to front-line managers gradually realized **business as usual would not suffice**. The status quo was no longer an option to remain competitive. As the expectation economy increasingly challenges companies to quickly respond to lifestyle changes, product developers, engineers, advertisers, and health care specialists realize basic human needs are ignored. Losing sight of such needs simultaneously occurs as society conditions today's consumers—and students—to believe that bigger, better, and faster is the way to solve the world's most pressing problems. Yet, businesses and organizations needed an ideology that provided permission to overturn the status quo.

Accordingly, as an ideology, design thinkers celebrated Design Thinking for its ability to address—if not completely solve—the world's most pressing, complex problems. Design thinkers recognize that incremental adjustments to long-term strategies are no longer sustainable for purpose or profit. Consumers now require/demand innovation that "leads to a quest for more meaningful pursuits than 'getting and spending'" (Brown, 2019, p. 193). As such, a social contract between organizations and society has gripped strategic planning: A "we're all in this together" mindset means companies listen to society's needs, recognizing that citizen-consumers are primed to participate in a company's strategic decisions in countless, values-based ways. An almost identical social contract characterizes the mindset of the empowered clients. Client-centered occupational therapists recognize their clients as experts of their **own** well-being and care; therefore, occupational therapists invite—and expect—their clients, families, and communities to actively participate in their individualized care and rehabilitation plans. Like human-centered design thinkers, client-centered health care professionals prioritize the value of client voice in pursuit of optimal care.

Design Thinking in Higher Education: What It Is Not, Backward Design

As today's students— tomorrow's professionals— enter client-centered environments, institutions and educators must recognize these students transfer their expectation-economy experiences into how they navigate their needs on campus and in the classroom. Outside of the classroom, students require more satisfying, individualized experiences, expecting educators to also deliver on that expectation. With full buy-in to the mindset "we're all in this together" (Brown, 2019, p. 193), students expect—if not implore—educators to deliver more than a lecture-based curriculum. Occupational therapy students expect multifaceted coursework that supersedes content delivery. They expect to translate new knowledge into practical applications with real-world consequences. They expect connections with educators, professional mentors, and peers. They expect innovation and experiences that add value to their professional resumes.

Given heightened student expectations of educators, the role of Design Thinking in higher education may also be understood in comparison to backward course design, another popular pedagogical framework. Backward design is generally thought of as "what we want our students to learn" (York, n.d.). Backward design, notably championed by Grant Wiggins and Jay McTighe in *Understanding by Design*, conceives that "enduring understanding" requires a strategic edit of curriculum content. In terms of "if it's not broke, why fix it?", educators' knee-jerk reactions are often expressed in the classroom as "trying to cover as much content as possible and assessing students when the teaching ends" (Lang, 2019; Nestor & Nestor, 2013). Therefore, backward design invites the educator to ask, "what is worth being familiar with and what is important to know and do?" Backward design, while a step forward to produce more teaching for learning, requires continuous fidelity to a linear sequence of steps. For example, if an educator outlines learning outcomes at the start of their curriculum planning, they isolate potential learning outcomes to this predetermined list. Then, their assessments are based on the learning outcomes. Yet, these up-front decisions oppose students' self-reported needs within the backward design approach.

Design Thinking, as described in the pages that follow, instead enables an iterative process that can **extend** backward design or independently operate as a pedagogical framework. More specifically, design thinkers balance the art and science between convergent and divergent thinking. Where backward design maintains a linear, deductive logic, Design Thinking promises educators autonomy in **creating** choices and **making** choices **while** the classroom activities unfold. Design Thinking gives permission to address content that may have evaded the pages of the syllabus or instructional methods. While this approach may feel jarring, the freedom it brings is not without constraints. Although backward design establishes resources and technology before coursework begins, Design Thinking allows for space to *explore and discover* through midcourse adjustments. Therefore, students' actual needs are grounded in the constant pursuit of desirability, viability, and feasibility instead of a linear path—not simply the default settings of semesters past.

WHY WE NEED EPISTEMOLOGY NOW MORE THAN EVER

The Innovation Design Engineering Organization, a global design and innovation company, established the importance of a social contract. In Design Thinking, the organization champions "all of us are smarter than any of us" (Brown, 2019, p. 37). As Bass (2012) theorizes, our postcourse era challenges us to more effectively embrace the "participatory culture" already present in our classroom. As institutions (and occupational therapy programs) more frequently include high-impact courses—including service-learning, research-based courses, and experiential capstones— in course catalogs, Design Thinking brings the messy, unstructured context of "real-world" decisions into the classroom. Within the Design Thinking ideology, students both design and decide. Students' exposure to controversies brought on by society's headlines and ethical dilemmas requires students to learn to exercise reflective judgment and reasoning skills. At a time when undergraduate and graduate students practice reasoning with a mostly structured problem, educators risk underpreparing students for how breakthrough innovation happens. Practicing Design Thinking in college teaching, therefore, means students may experience the joy of *intelligent confusion* and stray away from *ignorant certainty*. Design Thinking holds potential to transform aspiring occupational therapy students into citizen designers who take action and do not fear risk taking.

DESIGN THINKING FOR DEEPER LEARNING

Design Thinking's primary goal in college teaching is to reposition the student at the center of course design (see Chapter 4). Philosophically, though, Design Thinking, seeks to increase student learning by creating deeper connections to the course content and classroom community. To achieve deeper learning, educators must commit to more than sharing information with students and asking students to test their understanding of that knowledge. Instead, deeper learning asks educators to prioritize their student engagement, intrinsic motivation, and real-world applications of course material. Table 2-1 outlines six categories to consider to achieve deeper learning in the classroom and the skills/outcomes associated with each.

As you reflect on the meaning of deeper learning in occupational therapy, consider pairing your description(s) of deeper learning alongside your teaching philosophy in your course syllabus. Visibly committing to deeper learning by sharing your teaching philosophy in your syllabus is a powerful way to assure students you hold yourself accountable to the complexities of teaching and learning.

TABLE 2-1

Deeper Learning Categories and Student-Centered Outcomes

DEEPER LEARNING CATEGORY	STUDENT-CENTERED OUTCOMES
Master Academic Content	Students make connections between ideas and areas of study.
Think Critically and Solve Complex Problems	Students analyze problems, determine solutions, and strategize how to address the issue.
Work Collaboratively	Students focus on forming teams, identifying leaders, having open-minded conversations, taking on individual responsibilities, and reflecting on the process of solving the problem.
Effective Communication	Students practice clear, concise, and persuasive styles of written and verbal communication.
Learning How to Learn	Students become self-directed and take ownership of the learning process.
Develop Academic Mindsets	Students recognize the value of lifelong learning and commit to thinking curiously about the world around them.

START HERE: DESIGN-INSPIRED TEACHING AND COURSE DESIGN IN FIVE STAGES

In the practice of teaching and learning, human-centered design focuses on building deep empathy for our students, generating new student-centered ideas to rethink business as usual, and test-driving those new ideas to add value to the student experience and motivate deeper learning (Figure 2-1).

Because the Design Thinking steps are critical to understand the process of risk-taking and change, let's examine each step individually as it pertains to the college teaching. Although each stage is itself a landmark for a design-inspired educator, Brown (2019) states, ". . . the continuum of innovation is best thought of as a system of overlapping spaces rather than a sequence of orderly steps" (p. 22). Therefore, each stage of Design Thinking should not feel prescriptive but instead represent a part of the process where inspiration, ideation, and implementation overlap often.

Stage 1: Empathize From the Perspective of Your Students

Empathy, the practice of perspective taking to inform action, is the heart and soul of the Design Thinking process and occupational therapy practice. The act of empathetically thinking from the perspective of our students requires educators to ask curious questions about their students, their lives, and their academic aspirations. In effect, empathizing to more closely understand student needs then require educators to listen for, or at the very least recognize, their students' needs, desires,

Figure 2-1. Design Thinking in five stages. Stages do not necessarily occur in linear order. (Reproduced with permission from Stanford University's d.school. Note: Since the time of chapter submission, Stanford University's d.school announced its transition to a revised model of Design Thinking. You can read more about the new model here: https://www.ideou.com/blogs/inspiration/david-kelley-on-the-8-design-abilities-of-creative-problem-solvers.)

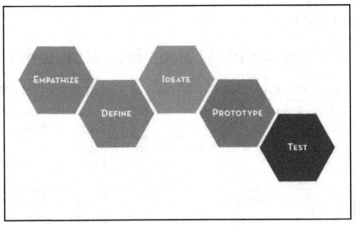

fears, and demands on their time **outside** of our classrooms. Speaking with students informally, before or after class or during office hours, is one of the best ways for educators to practice perspective taking. A desire to empathize with our students means taking time to listen and learn about our students' education or career goals, their uncertainties about the future, their campus leadership positions or employment status, and their psychosocial well-being.

Similar to working with clients in occupational therapy practice, each story a student shares is a data point to drive course design. The opportunity to learn more about our students' *lived experiences* gives educators the power to put empathy into action by using student perspectives to redesign our course structure, policies, and practices.

For example, a before-class conversation with a student provides information about the student's concern that they will miss their bus after class, which means they will be late for work. The student simply wants to make you aware of the reason they may pack up early on Thursdays. As an empathetic educator, this student's story offers an opportunity to reflect on how many other students might also have this actual need. The educator considers what it might be like to "walk a day in the life of their students," trying to find balance between academic, professional, and family obligations. Through empathy-driven reflections, educators intentionally consider contextual variables that may impact the learning environment. By acknowledging these variables, the educator places their course within the context of the students' lives and leans on empathy to examine the student experience.

We will subsequently re-examine empathy's distinct role in human-centered design to conclude the chapter.

Stage 2: Define Your Students' Needs

The hand-off from empathy to defining students' needs requires we use knowledge about our learners to build a different, arguably better, course. Defining students' needs and subsequently using these data points to recalibrate your course content and assignments, for example, does not mean that you relinquish control over course content. Likewise, recognizing students' needs does not mean tweaking **every** aspect in pursuit of a tailor-made product. Instead, though, defining students' needs and using that information to make decisions to shift classroom culture empowers students as valued members of the teaching and learning process.

Drawing upon the example above, after empathetically listening to the student's concerns about campus transportation, the educator decides to move the end-of-class announcements—a default setting the educator has used for years—to the beginning of the class. In deciding to restructure this part of the course design, the educator sees the potential to command the class' full attention instead losing attention toward the end of class. Although restructuring the timing of these announcements requires breaking the default setting of closing class time with announcements, in committing to this small course redesign, the educator demonstrates a commitment to empathy and meeting actual student needs. By defining our students' needs and acting on the information we gain through walking a day in the life of our students, educators can make data-driven decisions reflective of actual students' needs.

Stage 3: Challenge Assumptions and Create Ideas

When educators operate on default settings, opportunities to take risks and implement small changes to our teaching are easy to overlook. Likewise, new ideas require time and energy and may not provide a return on either investment.

Design Thinking is an opportunity to think differently about the challenges educators perceive as barriers, and instead consider new ideas to reinvent course design and re-engage with students. Gallagher and Thordarson (2018) provide design-inspired educators a useful tool to challenge assumptions and encourage ideation. As you contemplate a new idea but fear you have tried a similar approach that failed, ask yourself why that idea failed. However, do not just ask why the idea failed one time. Instead, ask yourself why the idea failed **five times**. In doing so, you shift from problem solving to recognizing and seeking opportunities. The end result will be a more purposeful learning experience for your students.

For example, perhaps you previously experimented with small group work, but at midsemester, you do not believe the groups are functioning as you had envisioned. Table 2-2 outlines an example of Gallagher and Thordarson's tool to challenge assumptions and create ideas.

By asking "why" five times to diagnose the small groups' dynamics, the educator challenges the assumptions behind their observations of the inoperable small groups. By challenging these assumptions, the educator determines the dysfunction may not be attributed to the small groups or group members; rather, the less-than-optimal dynamics in each small group are likely the result of the educator's insistence on maintaining a predetermined course pace to match the calendar, not to optimize student learning. The educator realizes their biggest challenge is a default setting rooted in the architecture of the course: It is too hard to change the syllabus after the students have the "final" copy in hand.

By confronting the challenge of maintaining complete dedication to the syllabus, the educator commits to giving the students more time to connect with one another and to establish expectations, roles, and responsibilities. The educator invested time and energy into challenging the assumptions about the small groups and reworking the original vision for group interactions, but the return on the investment promises to be stronger connections among group members and collective output from each group.

Some challenges to course or teaching redesign are more limiting than others. Brown (2019) identifies three important constraints to process and apply during the ideate phase of Design Thinking: "Feasibility, what is functionally possible within the foreseeable future; viability, what is likely to become part of a sustainable business model; and desirability, what makes sense to and for people" (Brown, 2019, p. 24). Design-inspired educators recognize the value in assessing for feasibility, viability, and desirability when challenging assumptions and creating new ideas. By recognizing these constraints, design-inspired educators build a stronger foundation to prototype and test drive their new ideas.

TABLE 2-2

Ask "Why" Five Times to
Challenge Assumptions and Create Ideas

WHY?	EDUCATOR'S OBSERVATION
1. Why do the small groups not function as I envisioned?	The small groups do not function the way I envisioned because I did not give the group members enough time to get to know one another and establish group norms.
2. Why did I not give the group members enough time to get to know one another and establish group norms?	I did not give the group members adequate time to get to know one another and establish group norms because I was too focused on the first group activity.
3. Why was I too focused on the first group activity?	I was too focused on the first group activity because I wanted the students to use their class time to work, not to get to know one another.
4. Why did I want the students to use their class time to work instead of getting to know one another?	I wanted the students to use their class time to work instead of getting to know one another because I didn't want to get off track of our class schedule.
5. Why did I not want to get off track of our class schedule?	I did not want to get off track of our class schedule because that might mean I have to adjust the rest of the syllabus.

Stage 4: Prototype and Test Drive Your Ideas

The prototyping process places the design-inspired educator in the driver's seat to officially test drive their new ideas. Restructured syllabi, revised assignments, flexible course policies, or even reformatted office hours are examples of where innovation and teaching meet actual student need. While launching new prototypes, educators should practice *transparency* with students. Clear, consistent communication with students is important to effectively integrate new innovations into the course design. Sharing the new vision for change and rationale for executing prototyped ideas in pursuit of deeper learning invites students to be a part of the prototyping process. By inviting students to provide formative feedback, educators can evaluate their prototypes and, eventually, determine the extent to which their test drive was successful.

For example, drawing on the small group example, a design-inspired educator decides to test drive an idea to enhance dialogue around the course readings. Default settings for course readings traditionally require all readings to be the responsibility of individual students; all readings are "fair game" for exams. However, the educator decides to test drive the jigsaw method (Chapter 8) to promote deeper learning, particularly mastering academic content and working collaboratively (see Table 2-1). The jigsaw method prompts each small group to concentrate on a specific part of the reading. As a class, the small groups will then "jigsaw" their summaries, questions, and conclusions about the respective portions of the article to complete the "puzzle." After two jigsaw sessions during the third and fourth weeks of the semester, the educator asks students to complete a two-question survey to gauge the students' perceptions of the jigsaw method and to determine the extent to which the students believe the jigsaw method contributed to their learning.

Students expect they will be given an opportunity to provide end-of-semester course feedback. Although summative evaluations are important in their own right, student feedback specific to the prototype invites educators to course correct when necessary or continue along their new, innovative path.

Stage 5: Test and Try Out Your Solutions

As the test drive continues, educators should keep notes in a teaching journal and annotate their current syllabus. Tracking detailed observations about what worked, what did not work, and why or why not is critical for later recall. Alongside formative and summative student feedback, anecdotal evidence from conversations with students or student emails adds another dimension to deciding which prototypes best aligned with goals for deeper learning and increased student engagement.

Risk and uncertainty are inherent to Design Thinking in college teaching. In fact, the process may feel chaotic at times; though you are test driving new ideas, you may not feel like you are in the driver seat at all. Yet, when we combine the powers of curiosity, creativity, and innovation to overcome the status quo, the benefits of course redesign far outweigh the risks.

"FAIL EARLY TO SUCCEED SOONER"

Brown (2019) practices the concept, "Fail early to succeed sooner" (p. 23). This basic approach to continuous feedback gives you the power to course correct at any time based on student feedback. Traditional evaluations provide limited snapshots of the students' collective course experience and may not speak to specific teaching and learning strategies. Asking students to provide feedback, either via in-class discussion or anonymous surveys, provides the data points needed to make informed decisions about your idea and its implementation. Whether the student feedback is negative, neutral, or overwhelmingly positive, the act of obtaining student feedback at important mile-markers reiterates your commitment to teaching and learning and the experience you are working to provide based on student need.

After administering the two-question survey about the jigsaw method, the educator interpreted the results as mixed—at best. It was clear some students appreciated the chance to focus specifically on a single part of the article, while others felt uncertainty in fully relying on another group's interpretation of the article. From the student feedback, the educator realizes a "one size fits all" model for analysis and synthesis of course materials may not exist for this group of students. Committed to meeting actual student need, the educator decides to provide students a choice in how they process their course readings: On days where course readings will be a part of the in-class discussion, students can choose to jigsaw the article in response to the prompt or work independently to complete the in-class assignment. The educator's solution is the result of innovative, empathetic thinking based on the stages of defining student need, ideation, and prototyping. When the test drive proved partially successful, the educator adapted the idea to individualized, actual student need. The educator's solution to provide students a choice adheres to the tenets of self-determination theory to meet the students' needs for autonomy, competence, and connectedness (see Chapter 12). By thinking innovatively about the process of teaching and learning, the design-inspired teacher has increased intrinsic motivation, empowering students to take control of their learning.

Design Thinking in Practice:
Never Fall in Love With Your Syllabus

Design Thinking requires intention and action to engineer the type of course design and student experience innovative educators seek to provide. In other words, Design Thinking requires practice, patience, and more practice—all the more reason to never fall in love with your syllabus. Innovative educators empathize, define, ideate, prototype, test, and retest often, without fear of change or failure. A well-organized syllabus can provide an important road map for students to reference throughout their time in your course. However, if educators confine themselves to the parameters of a syllabus they created before assessing their needs, they miss the opportunity to place the students at the heart of their teaching practice. Reorientating your syllabus for deeper learning means communicating intentions clearly and consistently. Let students know you will never change course policies, due dates, or expectations without discussing the changes as a class. Rather, as partners in the process of teaching and learning, the syllabus will be a living document—each change or adaptation a reflection of what the educator and students decide is important to their future as occupational therapy professionals.

The Heart and Soul of Design Thinking:
There Is No Innovation Without Empathy

In 2016, third grade teacher Kyle Schwartz asked her students a very simple question. Within the first few weeks of class, Schwartz asked her students to complete this phrase: "I wish my teacher knew. . ."

The students completed the exercise on notecards, providing personal details of their lives, ranging from missing deployed loved ones, feelings of loneliness at lunch, to not owning supplies needed to complete homework. Some students shared their adoration for pets and sports.

Schwartz's activity to fully know her students and their needs represents the best of Design Thinking for teaching excellence. Schwartz's empathy for her students as real people, not simply students, gave her an unmistakable power to connect with their actual, individualized needs to move from problem solving to opportunity seeking. She viewed each notecard as an opportunity to support her students' personal and academic success. She arranged for school counseling sessions for students with deployed parents, forged new lunchtime friendships, pooled extra school supplies, and of course, created intentional conversations with students to learn more about their pets and sports.

Is it possible that teaching excellence in Schwartz's third grade classroom mirrors teaching excellence in occupational therapy? As students come to our classrooms with more diverse lived experiences, financial needs, desires for belongingness, trauma, and career goals, a traditional, "one size fits all" approach may no longer be relevant. Likewise, the role of empathy in college teaching cannot be understated. Brown (2018) reminds educators of empathy's significance:

> As I often tell teachers—some of our most important leaders—we can't always ask our students to take off the armor at home, or even on their way to school, because their emotional and physical safety may require self-protections. But what we can do, and what we are ethically called to do, is create a safe space in our schools and classrooms where all students can walk in and, for that day or hour, take off the crushing weight of their armor, hang it on a rack, and open their heart to truly be seen. (p. 13)

Design Thinking provides an evidence-based approach to pursue excellence in college teaching with one destination in mind: Student-centered need discovered through empathy and met through innovation. Design Thinking for teaching excellence represents a shift from what is. . .to what could be. Perhaps the truest mark of teaching excellence, then, is the degree to which students are inspired to approach the world and its grand challenges as opportunity seekers. By modeling design-inspired principles, without fear of setback or failure, educators empower their students to think from a place of human-centered design, and it all starts with empathy.

THREE THINGS YOU CAN DO TOMORROW TO IMPLEMENT DESIGN THINKING WITH YOUR STUDENTS

These examples are small, but powerful changes to move your course from good to better to great, while maintaining the integrity of student-centered course design. We have prototyped these student-centered ideas in our teaching practices, but the sky is the limit for your innovative ideas to meet your students' actual needs in the field of occupational therapy.

1. Make your syllabus a destination document. A student-centered syllabus is more than a place for students to find due dates and course policies (see Chapter 3). Although that information is important, how might you repurpose your syllabus to include key images, models, quotes, charts, or even emojis? The addition of important visuals to your syllabus adds depth and creates a destination document for course **content**, not simply course **information**. Encourage students to rely on the course syllabus during in-class discussions and as a tool to complete assignments. Provide extra space throughout the syllabus for students to track important findings or reflect on their learning or the overall course culture.

2. A picture is worth a thousand words. Default settings often mean PowerPoint slides are cluttered with bulleted lists and lengthy sentences, an express invitation for students to take notes through **our** eyes, not their own. What if less is more when it comes to the information included on PowerPoint slides? Or, how might we rethink PowerPoint-centered presentations altogether and instead seek out novel, accessible image-based resources, such as Canva? Instead of summarizing, analyzing, and interpreting content for students with titled slides, bulleted lists, and complex tables and charts, insert photos or images to represent the ideas you want to convey. By using photos to tell the story of your content, students adapt to taking their own notes, interpreting concepts and conclusions in their own words. By reacting to the image alongside your narrative, students will have a visual to draw on when they are asked to recall central concepts.

3. Start with the "why" on the first day. Students many times attend the first day of class with preconceived expectations: A word-for-word review of the syllabus and an overview of the course content (i.e., course outcomes, assignments, assigned readings). What if not one of those words comes up on the first day of class? What if there is no mention of the words syllabus, course overview, policies, or projects? Instead, start with the "why" on the first day. Provide context for where your course fits in the world, drawing the students' attention to headlines, policy debates, economic impact, or other seemingly far-off concepts that speak to the heart of why your course content matters now more than ever before.

REFERENCES

Bass, R. (2012, March 21). Disrupting ourselves: The problem of learning in higher education. *Educause Review, 47*(2), 23-33. https://er.educause.edu/articles/2012/3/disrupting-ourselves-the-problem-of-learning-in-higher-education

Brown, B. (2018). *Dare to lead: Brave work, tough conversations, whole hearts.* Random House.

Brown, T. (2019). *Change by design, revised and updated: How design thinking transforms organizations and inspires innovation.* HarperCollins Publishers.

Gallagher, A., & Thordarson, K. (2018). *Design thinking for school leaders: Five roles and mindsets that ignite positive change.* Association for Supervision and Curriculum Development.

Lang, J. M. (2019, January 4). How to teach a good first day of class. *The Chronicle of Higher Education.* https://www.chronicle.com/interactives/advice-firstday

Nestor, M., & Nestor, C. E. (2013, November 24). Alignment and backward design [Video]. YouTube. https://www.youtube.com/watch?v=ZTv2HR2ckto

York, J. (n.d.). Designing with the end in mind: Introduction to backward design [Webinar]. University of Illinois at Urbana-Champaign. https://citl.illinois.edu/citl-101/online-strategy-development/develop-or-revise-an-online-course/online-course-in-a-box/designing-your-course/bigpicture/designing-with-the-end-in-mind

BIBLIOGRAPHY

Bain, K. (2004). *What the best college teachers do.* Harvard University Press.

Cavanagh, S. R. (2016). *The spark of learning: Energizing the college classroom with the science of emotion.* West Virginia University Press.

Gardner, E. B., Calderwood, P. E., & Torosyan, R. (2007). Dangerous pedagogy. *Journal of the Assembly for Expanded Perspectives on Learning, 13*(1), 5.

King, P. M., & Kitchener, K. S. (1994). *Developing reflective judgment: Understanding and promoting intellectual growth and critical thinking in adolescents and adults.* Jossey-Bass Inc.

Lang, J. M. (2016). *Small teaching: Everyday lessons from the science of learning.* Jossey-Bass Inc.

Mason, H., Mattin, D., Luthy, M., & Dumitrescu, D. (2015). *Trend-driven innovation.* Wiley.

ORS Impact. (2013). Deeper learning advocacy cluster evaluation key findings. https://hewlett.org/wp-content/uploads/2016/08/Hewlett%20Deeper%20Learning%20Key%20Learning%20Memo.PDF

Rudnitsky, A., Ellis, G. W., DiBartolo, P. M., & Shea, K. M. (2014). Developing a faculty learning community grounded in the science of how people learn. In J. Groccia & L. Cruz (Eds.), *To improve the academy: Resources for faculty, instructional, and organizational development* (pp. 127-143). Jossey-Bass Inc.

Shaw, P. A., Cole, B., & Russell, J. L. (2014). Determining our own tempos: Exploring slow pedagogy, curriculum, assessment, and professional development. In J. Groccia & L. Cruz (Eds.), *To improve the academy: Resources for faculty, instructional, and organizational development* (pp. 319-334). Jossey-Bass Inc.

Stachowiak, B. (Host). (2019, October 10). Design thinking in teaching and research (No. 278) [Audio podcast episode]. In teaching in higher ed. https://teachinginhighered.com/podcast/design-thinking-in-teaching-and-research/

Wiggins, G., & McTighe, J. (2005). *Understanding by design.* Association for Supervision & Curriculum Development.

EXCELLENCE IN INCLUSIVE TEACHING

Leigh Neier, PhD

Faculty conversations about diversity, equity, and inclusion in college teaching are commonplace across campuses nationwide. As institutions seek to recruit, enroll, and retain diverse student populations, educators are called to prioritize diversity, equity, and inclusion in their course design and interactions with students. Educators must (re)commit to inclusive teaching practices to foster a sense of community among all students and work toward increasing student success outcomes.

Although initiatives to advance diversity, equity, and inclusion pervade higher education, professional development focused on culturally responsive teaching practices is less universal. A critical starting point to manage diversity and inclusion in the classroom is to build capacity for inclusive teaching. In doing so, educators will create classroom cultures where students of all identities feel valued and capable.

DIVERSITY, EQUITY, AND INCLUSION IN OCCUPATIONAL THERAPY

As the landscapes of society and health care continue to change, occupational therapy education programs must respond by better preparing students for the skills and experiences needed to thrive in diverse health care and community contexts. Focused recruitment efforts suggest occupational therapy educator programs recognize the need to diversify their student populations. However, stronger, targeted recruitment efforts will be meaningless if programs cannot retain underrepresented minority students and/or students of color. Therefore, occupational therapy programs and educators must consistently prioritize inclusion efforts. Although inclusion efforts should be pervasive throughout the program's culture, such efforts are particularly meaningful in the classroom, where most student interactions take place.

Henderson, W. (Ed.). *Effective Teaching: Instructional Methods and Strategies for Occupational Therapy Education* (pp. 31-41).
© 2021 Taylor & Francis Group.

Recruitment and retention efforts have the potential to diversify student populations who will one day serve diverse communities. Currently, the demographics of our profession do not represent the individuals and communities we serve. The clients, families, communities, and interdisciplinary teams with which occupational therapists collaborate are increasingly more diverse. The *2015 American Occupational Therapy Association (AOTA) Salary and Workforce Survey* demonstrated there remains a dramatic difference between the diversity of our profession and the diversity of the country. For example, approximately 60% of the United States population is White compared to 85% of the occupational therapy profession. Similarly, approximately 18% are Hispanic or Latino and 13% are Black, but within the occupational therapy profession, we see only 6% total Latino or Black practitioners.

One of the five pillars of our profession's current vision reports, "…we are intentionally inclusive and equitable and embrace diversity in all its forms" (AOTA, 2019, para. 2). As occupational therapy educators, our goal is to produce students prepared to achieve the vision of our profession. Therefore, educators must demonstrate and embrace diversity, equity, and inclusion in our classrooms and programs. Although a number of occupational therapy programs are attempting to increase diversity within their programs, there remains a vital need to make our profession more reflective of society.

By diversifying the occupational therapy profession, aspiring professionals, practitioners, and communities benefit from increased access to varied ideas, skills, experiences, and knowledge. Our students will also benefit from learning and collaborating in diverse academic environments. Establishing a teaching practice that values diversity, equity, and inclusion begins by recognizing the differences between each term. For the purposes of this chapter, diversity, equity, and inclusion are defined as the following:

- **Diversity:** The various mix or combinations of human differences (e.g., personality, learning styles, life experiences) and group/social differences (e.g., race/ethnicity, class, gender/gender identity, sexual orientation, country of origin, and ability as well as cultural, political, religious, or other affiliations) that can be engaged in the service of learning and working together (University of Missouri, 2018).

- **Equity:** The creation of opportunities for historically underrepresented populations to have equal access and equitable opportunity to participate in educational programs designed to reduce the academic/opportunity gap in student success and completion. To advance equity is to allocate resources, programs, and opportunities to staff, faculty, and students to address historical imbalances (University of Missouri, 2018).

- **Inclusion:** The active, intentional, and ongoing engagement with diversity—in people, in the curriculum, in the cocurriculum, and in communities (intellectual, social, cultural, geographical) with which individuals might connect—in ways that increase one's awareness, content knowledge, cognitive sophistication, and emphatic understanding of the complex ways individuals interact with and within systems and institutions (University of Missouri, 2018).

Educators can benefit from professional development to enhance their awareness and understanding of diversity, equity, and inclusion and strategies to maintain inclusive classrooms. Such professional development provides educators the opportunity to reflect on their beliefs, attitudes, and behaviors when working with diverse student populations. Yet, even when campuses and leaders invest time and resources into professional development, why do educators continue to view diversity, equity, and inclusion as tenuous, if not divisive, topics in the classroom? They sometimes inadvertently (or advertently) avoid conversations about diversity. Likewise, scholarship pertaining to diversity in teaching finds intricate, multilayered reasons why educators avoid discussions of diversity with students. Educators rationalize avoiding the topic due to:

- Lack of familiarity with the scope of diversity's definition
- Limited opportunity to provide real-world connections when narrow heterogeneity exists in the student audience
- Limited knowledge of teaching methods to engage ever-growing diverse student audiences
- Lack of self-efficacy to oversee potential emotional responses that arise from difficult dialogues

Avoiding a conversation about inclusive teaching extends educator privilege, especially for those individuals who identify with the majority campus demographics. Brown (2018) asserts:

> People are opting out of vital conversations about diversity and inclusivity because they fear looking wrong, saying something wrong, or being wrong. Choosing our own comfort over hard conversations is the epitome of privilege, and it corrodes trust and moves us away from meaningful and lasting change. (p. 9)

This chapter will not analyze every relevant aspect of diversity, equity, and inclusion to college teaching. Rather, the purpose of this chapter is to contribute foundational, meaningful ideas and action items for educators to implement in their course design and classrooms. In redesigning courses and teaching practices to prioritize diversity, equity, and inclusion, educators send a message to their students: *Culturally responsive teaching matters.* By implementing pedagogies that recognize the significance of including students' cultural references in all aspects of learning, educators acknowledge, respond to, and celebrate students' cultural and social identities. Educators create more equitable access to their content and coursework for all students, not just students who identify with the majority population. In turn, increased student success—academic, personal, and social—follows as students gain agency over their experiences in and beyond the classroom.

This examination of culturally responsive teaching focuses on:

- The importance of student belongingness and mattering in academic settings
- The importance of knowing/using preferred student names and pronouns
- The importance of classroom climate for brave conversations

The Importance of Student Belongingness in Academic Settings

In addition to a student's academic and professional goals, the need for belongingness is among the most significant factors to shape the college experience. All people share a strong need to belong. Abraham Maslow's frequently referenced hierarchy of needs positions belongingness as a basic human motivation—placing love and belonging just above safety and physiological needs.

Belongingness is about connection: Humans are hardwired to feel connection with others. Strayhorn (2012) frames sense of belonging as:

> . . .a basic human need and motivation, sufficient to influence behavior. In terms of college, sense of belonging refers to students' perceived social support on campus, a feeling or sensation of connectedness, the experience of mattering or feeling cared about, accepted, respected, valued by, and important to the group (e.g., campus community) or others on campus (e.g., faculty, peers). It's a cognitive evaluation that typically leads to an affective response or behavior. (p. 3)

When a student feels their need to belong is satisfied, the student's experience is characterized by positive emotions, including an increased sense of joy and happiness. Likewise, increased academic performance and satisfaction with the college experience are possible when a student feels they belong.

Conversely, lack of belongingness is associated with marginalization and alienation, both of which undercut a college student's academic experience and classroom performance. Students who do not view themselves as belonging to the campus community or classroom are more likely to experience dissatisfaction, depression, and lower levels of self-esteem. Disconnected students experience decreased interest and engagement in educational settings when they do not feel connection to the learning environment. Diminishing motivations and impaired development leads to decreased performance on tests and assignments, which have implications on self-efficacy and self-esteem in the academic environment.

Belongingness among students with diverse social, gender, ethnic, and racial identities is the subject of ongoing research to determine what campus support systems and inputs are necessary to maximize the student experience. For underrepresented students and minority student groups, educators should recognize the need for belongingness is amplified in environments where individuals may feel disconnected as a function of their identities. In such environments, marginalized students strive to "fit in" but must confront unwelcoming or unsupportive contexts. Students of color; LGBTQ+ students; minorities and women in science, technology, engineering and math fields; first-generation college students; Latinx students; and other international students are especially impacted by the need for belongingness as they "perceive themselves as marginal to the mainstream of life [of college]" (Hurtado & Carter, 1997, p. 324).

The most important place an educator impacts their students is in the classroom. It is here where they must consider marginality and mattering. *Marginality* is correlated with self-consciousness and irritability. Notably, marginality maintains a steady presence in the college experience of students from minority and underrepresented groups. Conversely, students from majority groups may experience marginality as they transition to college or professional programs; however, these feelings are short-lived. Seminal research on marginality underscores the importance for educators to spend time early in the semester building community and setting the tone for the social and emotional climate in the classroom. Subsequent sections of this chapter will examine best practices and offer practical ideas to prioritize your classroom's social and emotional climate. This practice will benefit all students, but particularly those whose feelings of marginality will be longlasting.

Professors should also consider how mattering aligns with their teaching philosophies and practices. *Mattering* refers to a student's belief that they matter to someone else. The five aspects of mattering provide additional context from which to analyze students' belongingness needs:

1. **Attention:** A student feels noticed.
2. **Importance:** A student feels cared for.
3. **Ego Extension:** A student feels that a teacher will be proud of their accomplishments and support their failures.
4. **Dependence:** A student feels they are needed.
5. **Appreciation:** A student feels their efforts are appreciated by others.

The dimensions of mattering are also connected to students' feelings of validation. An examination of the college experience demonstrates the need for validation—a powerful tool during the first few weeks of class. *Validation*, or "an enabling, confirming, and supportive process initiated by in- and out-of-class agents that foster academic and interpersonal development" (Rendon, 1994, p. 44), leads to increased feelings of self-efficacy and self-worth. Additionally, students who feel validated are more likely to believe they have something to contribute to the academic community. Because minority and underrepresented students are less likely to feel adequate in the academic environment, validating students as contributing members of the learning community has the potential to motivate individual belongingness and collective inclusion.

Although more research is needed on the educator's specific role in meeting students' needs for belongingness, especially faculty-student interactions within specific minority and underrepresented student groups, prioritizing belongingness is essential for effective, inclusive teaching. Two strategies to foster stronger sense of belonging in all students are presented in the subsequent sections:

Namely, a commitment to knowing/using preferred student names and pronouns and establishing a classroom climate that supports brave conversations. Both inclusive teaching methods align with best practice in culturally responsive teaching, namely the tenets of:

- Learning within the context of culture
- Learner-centered instruction
- Culturally mediated instruction
- The educator as the facilitator

The Importance of Knowing/Using Preferred Student Names and Pronouns

To increase feelings of mattering in the classroom, educators should consider the importance of knowing their students' preferred names and pronouns. Cooper and colleagues (2017) identified nine reasons why knowing student names is an important part of culturally responsive teaching and building an inclusive classroom environment:

1. Students feel more valued.
2. Students feel more invested in the course.
3. Students feel more comfortable getting help.
4. Students feel more comfortable talking to the educator.
5. Students feel enhanced performance in the course of confidence in the material.
6. Students feel the educator cares.
7. Students feel it builds student-educator relationships.
8. Students feel it builds classroom community.
9. Students feel that educators are more likely to provide students with letters of recommendation or mentoring.

To establish a culture where preferred names and pronouns are important, educators should consider adding language to their syllabi to recognize the diverse identities in the classroom. The following is a sample of a *Commitment to Inclusion Syllabus Statement*:

> One of my top priorities as your instructor is to cultivate and maintain an inclusive learning community, where diversity is valued and equity is a priority. Professional courtesy is especially important with respect to individuals and topics regarding differences of race, culture, religion, politics, sexual orientation, gender, gender variance, and nationality. The course roster I receive only provides a student's legal name. I will gladly honor your request to address you by your preferred name and/or gender pronoun/s. Please reach out to me either via email or in person if you would like to speak further about your preferred name and/or pronouns. I value your lived experiences and look forward to learning more about you and your goals for our course.

Additionally, to underscore the importance of student names in the classroom, educators should consider asking students to create and use name tents every day in class. Name tents are an effective tool to create connections between educators and students, but the visual aid also provides peers the opportunity to learn their classmates' names.

In addition to creating a welcoming classroom climate, students who believe their educators know their names are more likely to come to class, participate during class, and attend office hours. Although additional research is needed to determine the influence of knowing student names on academic performance, commitment to learning preferred student names and pronouns is a basic example of culturally responsive teaching with potential for lasting, positive impacts on classroom climate.

TABLE 3-1

Discussions Versus Debates Versus Dialogues

DISCUSSIONS...	DEBATES...	DIALOGUES...
• Identify generally held or collective truths and frameworks • Present answers and solutions • Avoid the affective domain • Achieve preset outcomes or learning objectives	• Focus on right or wrong. • Identify areas of weakness • Discount the validity of feelings • Conclude that different points of view are invalid or inferior	• Include opportunities to challenge collective truths and may destabilize the realities participants hold true • Search for shared meaning • Promote nonjudgmental listening to understand diverse points of view • Challenge participants to reconsider preconceived conclusions

The Importance of Classroom Climate and Brave Conversations

Students perceive limited opportunities to build authentic relationships with their diverse peers. Research suggests students are often ill-prepared to engage in civil discussions with others whose lived experiences or identities are different from their own. For this reason, educators should invest time to build student capacity for difficult dialogues and brave conversations, particularly occupational therapy educators preparing students to enter the diverse workforce. The concept of difficult dialogues is often new to students and requires time to identify the distinctions between traditional discussions and the more nuanced debates and dialogues (Table 3-1). When educators design opportunities for more authentic engagement, modeling explicit expectations for discussions, debates, and dialogues, students benefit from a classroom climate where student voice and agency matter (see Chapter 9).

To foster stronger self-awareness among students, educators should support students to explore individual reasons for disconnect or discomfort during a class dialogue. The following questions are adapted from the University of Michigan (n.d.); these questions are powerful self-checks for students to process their feelings when participating in a group dialogue with diverse peers:

- Am I honoring my own experiences as valid **or** do I feel defensive about it?
- Can I trust others to respect differences **or** do I suspect others are trying to force me to change?
- Can I trust myself to be permeable and still maintain integrity **or** do I fear that hearing a different perspective will weaken my position?
- Am I willing to open myself to the pain of others (and my own pain) **or** am I resisting pain that I really do have to the strength to face?

In addition to building student capacity for difficult, collaborative dialogues, educators can enhance inclusion as a classroom practice by tailoring the concept of a brave space to their students' needs. Students may have varying degrees of familiarity with the idea of a classroom as a safe space. When a classroom is labeled as a safe space, the main goal is to make all students feel supported. Students may learn from exchanges with one another, but, by design, a safe space does not seek to promote new understandings by overcoming challenging, often preconceived notions, about others.

However, a brave space asks students to lean into the dialogue, even when uncomfortable, while also recognizing diverse individuals' lived experiences. Conducting class sessions in the spirit of a brave space means that everyone is accountable to sharing viewpoints to arrive at a new level of understanding, even if viewpoints are not closely aligned or misalign altogether. In a brave conversation, all members of the class should:

- Speak their truth
- Stay engaged
- Lean into discomfort
- Expect and accept nonclosure

Although physical and psychosocial safety should always remain top priorities, emphasizing a universally safe space, instead of a brave space, can provide the illusion that students do not need to engage in challenging conversation. As participants in a brave conversation, the educator and students recognize there will be some conflict between our self-identified comfort zones and the edge of learning. Whether it is fully recognized or not, a brave space makes healthy conflict possible. When tension enters the brave space, the educator should coach students to focus on learning from the conflict—either actual or perceived. When the educator recognizes and encourages brave dialogue, students can learn from one another's diverse, lived experiences. Students report feelings of validation when exercising courage and vulnerability to embrace conflict and learn from the engagement with diverse peers.

Establishing the learning environment as a brave space for discussions, debates, and dialogues should begin early in the semester or at the start of a professional program. Educators should help students identify examples of discussions, debates, and dialogues before leading a conversation that requires them to use different forms of communication to engage with their peers. Developing a classroom climate where students engage and recognize conflict's role in learning and growth requires time and practice. However, the return on the time invested in this brave space will be increased sense of student belonging, decreased feelings of marginality, and, finally, inclusion in the form of students seeing ideas through the eyes of their diverse peers.

Commitment to Excellence in Inclusive Teaching by Building Individual Capacity

The work of student belongingness and culturally responsive pedagogies is inherently about supporting student success. Yet, the need to address personal bias is an essential part of inclusive teaching. Increased awareness of self is cited as a best practice for educators to enhance diversity awareness and identity development.

To more closely understand the impact of their social identity and cultural blind spots on their teaching, educators should consider completing a self-assessed diversity audit (Table 3-2). A diversity audit provides educators with valuable information from which they can set goals to address their cultural blind spots or cognitive biases. Although unintentional, when overlooked, cultural blind spots can influence behavior, attitudes, and decisions that impact students.

Diversity audit results can be analyzed through the lenses of:

- Assessing the extent to which an educator has been effective in integrating diversity, equity, and inclusion into course design and policies
- Identifying areas for improvement
- Identifying goals for continued professional development and/or support systems needed to translate audit findings into teaching practices

TABLE 3-2

Sample Questions From Diversity Audit: Self-Assessment

	ALWAYS	SOMETIMES	SELDOM	NEVER
I am conscious of my students' visible and less visible social identities.				
I try not to assume things about my students' group memberships. Instead, I use what students tell me to inform my opinions.				
I recognize my biases and their effect in the learning environment.				
I model conversations where biased comments or actions can be challenged.				

Diversity audits can be especially effective when educators discuss their results with a mentor or peer. It is also a good practice to complete a diversity audit before a class begins and again at the end of the semester to gauge positive changes and where additional efforts are needed.

EXCELLENCE IN INCLUSIVE TEACHING LEADS TO STUDENT AGENCY AND VOICE

Faculty development in the areas of diversity, equity, and inclusion is needed to match the needs of the growing, diverse student populations that characterize college campuses and classrooms. In the absence of organized (or required) faculty development opportunities, educators should self-direct their efforts to build awareness of their cultural blind spots and prioritize student belonging and inclusive teaching. Diversity audits, redesigned syllabus statements, name tents, and intentional conversations about discussion, dialogue, and debate are examples of small shifts in teaching with potential to create measurable outcomes for students, especially students with historically marginalized identities. Students deserve a space where they can engage wholeheartedly—with the content, with each other, and with their own growth as thinkers and leaders (Figure 3-1). "We must be guardians of a space that allows students to breathe and be curious and explore the world and be who they are without suffocation" (Brown, 2018, p. 13). Excellence in inclusive teaching begins in a brave space where educators empower students to discover their agency and, in turn, use their voices to advocate for diversity, equity, and inclusion wherever their personal and professional paths lead.

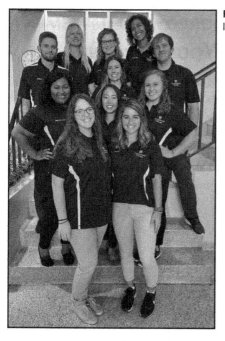

Figure 3-1. Students from diverse backgrounds engage in a leadership role.

RECOMMENDATIONS FOR FUTURE SELF-DIRECTED STUDY: OCCUPATIONAL THERAPY RESEARCH AND TOOLS TO ADVANCE DIVERSITY, EQUITY, AND INCLUSION

As presented in Chapter 1, the occupational therapy education research agenda includes a new category to promote diversity, equity, and inclusion. The goals of the research in this key area are to:

- "Identify best educational practices to recruit and retain a diverse group of students entering professional training
- Identify best educational practices to recruit and retain a diverse roster of faculty
- Identify mechanisms to support underrepresented minorities, both within the educational program and for students entering the occupational therapy workforce
- Identify and develop the best educational practices and coursework within curricula to strengthen students' cultural critical consciousness…." (AOTA, 2018, p. 7212420070p2)

In 2012, the Coalition of Occupational Therapy Advocates for Diversity (COTAD) members undertook efforts to promote diversity and inclusion within the occupational therapy profession. They curated multiple resources, including a student recruitment tool kit for educators, and American Psychological Association resources, blogs, and mentorship for students. In addition, COTAD-ED, a COTAD subcommittee, formed to support current and future educators and their professional development in the areas of diversity, equity, and inclusion. The Multicultural, Diversity, and Inclusion Network created seven tool kits to provide tools and resources to promote diversity in the occupational therapy workforce. Self-directing professional development to include analyzing and synthesizing best teaching practices in diversity, equity, and inclusion reflects the attitudes and behaviors of a lifelong learner. Educators should also prioritize the application of research and tools specific to professional development in the field of occupational therapy. The above research initiatives, coalitions, and tool kits are among the resources recommended for novice and seasoned educators alike.

THREE THINGS YOU CAN DO TOMORROW TO IMPLEMENT INCLUSIVE TEACHING WITH YOUR STUDENTS

The commitment to prioritize diversity, equity, and inclusion in your teaching practice will add value to your students' experiences in and beyond the classroom. The following three examples can transform your teaching practice to underscore the importance of student belonging and mattering:

1. Complete a *Diversity Audit: Self-Assessment* before the start of a new semester; use results to identify blind spots and make specific goals to address those biases in your course materials.

2. Revise your syllabus to include a *Commitment to Inclusion Syllabus Statement*.

3. Designate class time for students to create name plates and communicate your expectation that students will bring their name plates every day.

REFERENCES

American Occupational Therapy Association. (2018). Occupational therapy education research agenda—revised. *American Journal of Occupational Therapy, 72*(Suppl. 2), 7212420070. https://doi.org/10.5014/ajot.2018.72S218

American Occupational Therapy Association. (2019). AOTA unveils vision 2025. http://www.aota.org/ABOUTAOTA/vision-2025.aspx

Brown, B. (2018). *Dare to lead: Brave work. Tough conversations. Whole hearts.* Random House.

Cooper, K. M., Haney, B., Krieg, A., & Brownell, S. E. (2017). What's in a name? The importance of students perceiving that an instructor knows their name in a high-enrollment biology classroom. *Life Sciences Education, 16*(8). https://www.ncbi.nlm.nih.gov/pmc/articles/PMC5332051/pdf/ar8.pdf

Hurtado, S., & Carter, D. E. (1997). Effects of college transition and perceptions of campus racial climate on Latino college students' sense of belonging. *Sociology of Education, 70*(4), 324-345.

Rendon, L. I. (1994) Validating culturally diverse students: Toward a new model of learning and student development. *Innovative Higher Education, 19,* 31-55.

Strayhorn, T. L. (2012). *College students' sense of belonging: A key to educational success for all students.* Routledge.

University of Michigan. (n.d.). The Program on Intergroup Relations. www.igr.umich.edu

University of Missouri. (2018). Inclusive excellence framework. *Inclusion, Diversity, & Equity.* https://diversity.missouri.edu/our-work/inclusive-excellence-framework/

BIBLIOGRAPHY

American Occupational Therapy Association. (2015). Salary & workforce survey. Retrieved from https://www.aota.org/Education-Careers/Advance-Career/Salary-Workforce-Survey.aspx

Baumeister, R. F., & Leary, M. R. (1995). The need to belong: Desire for interpersonal attachment as a fundamental human motivation. *Psychological Bulletin, 117,* 497-529.

Coalition of Occupational Therapy Advocates for Diversity. (2019). Coalition of occupational therapy advocates for diversity. Retrieved from www.cotad.org

Cruz, B. C., Ellerbrock, C. R., Vasquez, A., & Howes, E. V. (Eds). *Talking diversity with teachers and teacher educators: Exercises and critical conversations across the curriculum.* Teachers College Press.

Deci, E. L., & Ryan, R. M. (2000). The "what and "why" of goal pursuits: Human needs and the self-determination of behavior. *Psychological Inquiry, 11,* 227-268.

Evans, N. J., Forney, D. S., & Guido-DiBrito, F. (1998). *Student development in college: Theory, research, and practice.* Jossey-Bass Inc.

Ford, K. (2018, May 5). [Presentation notes on inclusive teaching and self-assessments diversity audits]. MU Faculty Institute for Inclusive Teaching: Building Faculty Capacity and Managing Diversity and Inclusion in the Classroom, University of Missouri.

Institute of Medicine. (2004). *In the nation's compelling interest: Ensuring diversity in the health-care workforce.* National Academies Press.

Kachwaha, T. (2002). Exploring the differences between dialogue, discussion, and debate. [Handout]. MU Faculty Institute for Inclusive Teaching: Building Faculty Capacity and Managing Diversity and Inclusion in the Classroom, University of Missouri.

Ladson-Billings, G. (1994). *The dreamkeepers.* Jossey-Bass Inc.

Rendon, L. I., Jalomo, R. E., & Nora, A. (2000). Theoretical consideration in the study of minority student retention in higher education. In J. M. Braxton (Ed.), *Reworking the student departure puzzle* (pp. 127-156). Vanderbilt University Press.

Saffer, A. (2019). New efforts promoting greater diversity within the profession. Retrieved from https://www.aota.org/Publications-News/otp/Archive/2019/promoting-diversity.aspx

Schlossberg, N. K. (1985). Marginality and mattering: A life span approach. Paper presented at the Annual Meeting of the American Psychological Association, Los Angeles, CA.

Strathman, A., & Spain, J. N. (Eds.). (2015). *The pursuit of teaching excellence: Lessons from the University of Missouri Kemper Teaching Fellows.* University of Missouri Press.

Sue, D. W. (2015). *Race talk and the conspiracy of silence: Understanding and facilitating difficult dialogues on race.* John Wiley & Sons.

CO-CREATION
OF CURRICULUM

Whitney Henderson, OTD, MOT, OTR/L

BASIC TENETS

Higher education develops professionals prepared to meet workforce demands and grows citizens equipped to participate in society. In order to accomplish these goals, educators must produce graduates who can solve real-world problems, work in collaboration, and engage in lifelong learning. Educational literature suggests educators facilitate deep and lifelong learning by engaging in continuous dialogue with their students—not necessarily by effectively planning and delivering course content. Despite its simplicity, educators often forget to ask students about their educational experiences. To foster this dialogue, current literature in higher education advocates that educators encourage students to be active co-creators of their own learning. In *co-creation*, the educator and students work in a collaborative and reciprocal relationship to construct components of the curriculum. In this chapter, we define *curriculum* as course or subject content or the structure of delivery of a module or course.

In most higher education institutions, the educator remains responsible for making the teaching and learning decisions while the students continue to have no voice about their educational process. When educators design a course, they engage in a time-consuming and enduring process. Traditionally, educators research content, develop class structure and policies, determine pace and amount of time devoted to content, select readings and methods of assessment, create assignments and due dates, determine learning activities, launch classes, and receive student feedback following course completion. From the summative feedback and their own observations, educators make a few changes the next time they teach the course. What would happen if educators received feedback before or during the course on these various design aspects? What would you do with this valuable information?

Henderson, W. (Ed.). *Effective Teaching: Instructional Methods and Strategies for Occupational Therapy Education* (pp. 43-71).

In recent years, we note a growth in literature on student engagement calling for educators to explore ways students can fully participate in educational design. Educational research suggests learning is more powerful when educators make changes based on the active involvement of students. However, educators frequently forget students bring unique educational perspectives and experiences to the classroom and often underestimate their ability to contribute meaningfully to curricular conversations. Remember, it is the students who primarily receive and interpret the curriculum. Each student is quite capable of providing valuable insights into how they understand and interact with the curriculum because **they** are the experts in their **own** learning. Students possess direct and recent educational experiences, which provide important resources for teaching. Educators that include students in the course design process challenge conventional notions that students are subordinate to the expert educator in the teaching and learning process.

Involving those we serve in our process is similar to the idea we want our students to understand about their future clients, families, and communities—it is those individuals who are the experts in their own lives. Occupational therapists collaborate with these individuals to actively involve them in dialogue and decision making to guide their own course of action. Furthermore, the health care industry has established the notion of user involvement as best practice. By engaging students in co-creation of curriculum, we (as occupational therapy educators) model the ability to share control in collaborative partnerships.

Co-Creation of Curriculum

In nearly every definition of engaged learning, students take an **active** role in their education. In co-creation of the curriculum, students shift from passive recipients, or consumers of knowledge, to active agents that take authentic responsibility for their own learning. Educators and students form a collaborative partnership in which each have opportunities to equally contribute to the conceptualization of curricular ideas, the decision-making process, delivery of content, and methods of evaluation. In this process, educators share the power because they recognize that students are critical stakeholders in learning. Although the goal is for educators to work with students to clarify and improve educational practices, we want to highlight that this collaborative effort does not replace an educator's expertise or central role of facilitating learning.

In learner-centered environments, educators ask students to participate in either a component of or in all aspects of course design but do not ask them to work beyond their expertise. Students can engage in co-curricular activities ranging from limited involvement of completing satisfaction questionnaires to high involvement of selecting content for a module. Hess (2007) suggests educators afford students opportunities to contribute to decisions in five areas of course design:

1. **Goals:** Decide what the students should learn in the course

2. **Materials:** Determine appropriate resources

3. **Assignments:** Identify readings and assignments completed during and outside of class

4. **Methods:** Select approaches to learning

5. **Evaluation:** Establish the grade mechanism

In addition, educational literature recommends including students in constructing the expectations and policies for a syllabus, prioritizing content, facilitating class periods, and creating peer accountability. When the educator and students work collaboratively in these areas, they each experience significant benefits.

When our professor approached our class about wanting volunteers to be part of course design for a future class, I was immediately interested. The thought of being able to contribute to course design was very appealing because it was an opportunity to share a student's perspective with a teacher in **advance** to a course rather than during midterm or end-of-semester course evaluation. I have typically had great professors who were very knowledgeable and experienced throughout college; however, there were aspects of course design that were lacking due to professors not accurately taking into account the students' perspectives. Every cohort has different learning styles and interests that need to be accounted for when teaching a course. I think it is important for every professor to incorporate student feedback in course design, whether it looks like our group did, or it is something simpler, such as having student liaisons for every class to give feedback from the class to the professor throughout the semester. Although it may initially seem like more work for the professor and the students involved, the benefits outweigh the work.

Having the opportunity to contribute to the design of a course pushed me to be a better peer, allowed me to build a relationship with the professor, and resulted in me being a better professional. By pushing me to be a better peer, I was no longer a part of the group that complained about the course activities because I understood the reasoning behind them. I was then able to explain to my peers to help them understand as well. I also felt responsibility for my peers' learning as a part of the course design group because I was contributing to the development of activities, readings, and other content, and I wanted it to be the best that it could be for my peers.

My favorite part of being involved in course design was the relationship that was built with the professor. Seeing the work that goes into designing a course greatly increases the respect for the amount of work the professor puts into the class. I have always worked hard in school, but after knowing how hard my professor worked on creating content for the course, I wanted to push myself even harder to do my best for her. It also increased my respect for her desire to hear the students' voices. The most important part of a course is what the students learn from it, and when our professor was willing to listen to our input, it maximized our learning so much more.

Each of these positive aspects and results of being involved in course design led to me being a better professional overall. Having course content that was catered to my cohorts' needs allowed for us to be active learners and retain information that I now put into practice today as an occupational therapist. Not only do I put into practice the content that I learned in the course, but I put into practice the confidence I gained in my ability to work on a team and give constructive feedback to leadership because of my experience giving this type of feedback to my professor within this course design group.

Paige Headlee, MOT, OTR/L

Benefits of Co-Creation

When adequately and thoughtfully designed, co-creation provides numerous benefits to the students, educators, and learning context. For meaningful learning to occur, it is critical for educators to actively engage students in and encourage them to take responsibility for their education. When educators include students in the design aspects of curriculum, they catalyze an important shift in responsibility and ownership. In one study, the students stated they began taking accountability for their own learning and started to realize if they were not happy with something in the course, then it was just as much their responsibility as it was the educator. Similarly, students are more likely to participate in a learning activity they do not necessarily enjoy if they felt they had a choice in the decision. Because of this accountability, they feel empowered to contribute ideas, motivated to work hard, engaged with content, and emotionally connected to the course. Students also develop a greater metacognitive awareness about what is being done in the learning context. As they progress and develop in the co-creation process, they consciously analyze what strategies enhance their education, gain a richer study of disciplinary concepts, adopt deeper approaches to learning, and develop critical analysis skills. Students can view the course from the educator's perspective, further developing their metacognitive skills.

In addition, students also develop skills that will undoubtedly boost their transition to professional practice and enhance their ability to meaningfully contribute to their communities. To be successful in practice and society, students must learn to develop and sustain collaborative relationships and effective communication skills as they will work on interdisciplinary teams and develop shared partnerships with clients and families. In co-creation, students have numerous opportunities to sharpen their collaborative and communication skills with peers and educators, as they establish an accountability system to complete tasks, deal with stressors of group work, and attempt to create group cohesion. Students in co-creation gain confidence in expressing their expertise, learn to converse with individuals with different perspectives, and begin to understand how to redirect energy to create a more positive environment. They discover how to solve real-world problems and link learning theories to practice, which becomes critical as they make the shift to the role of educator with the clients, families, and communities they serve. Throughout this entire learning process, students gain significant experiences to perform in educational and practice contexts.

Educators equally profit when they successfully engage students in curricular design. In the design process, educators share learning and workload responsibilities because the students assist in finding and evaluating resources and selecting and implementing instructional methods. Because of this collaboration, educators obtain a broader view of course concepts and often feel less pressure as they shift from the feeling of needing to be a content expert to the role of facilitator. Educators also receive feedback from students during the early stages of design or course implementation when it is easier to make improvements. It is during this communication process in which students further feel a sense of shared ownership because they feel responsible for providing the feedback to make the course successful and to recognize the educator's commitment to learning. As the educator further dialogues with students, they increase confidence and engagement in pedagogy, develop a desire for the scholarship of teaching and learning, boost the classroom experience, and forge a deeper relationship with students. Lastly, educators discover that those students who participate in curricular co-creation share an enthusiasm for the course, convey what the course will entail to their peers, and develop an appreciation for the complexity of the art and science of teaching.

BACKGROUND

In literature, authors note specific requests for active student involvement in higher education curriculum dating back to John Dewey's belief in democracy at the beginning of the 20th century. During the 1960s, advocates further called for active participation as the student movement period spread throughout the United States and Europe. The current higher education landscape continues to call for transformation with the loudest and most common requests for active student participation. In a relatively new strand of scholarship on teaching and learning, educators are beginning to embrace the idea of a democratic community and more authentic forms of co-creation. They are becoming more committed to sharing the responsibility of learning with their students with much of this emerging literature originating within the fields of school education and critical pedagogy. Despite these developments, higher education generally remains educator focused, as institutions and programs face challenges to meet accreditation standards and demonstrate quality assurance.

However, there is a growing body of evidence suggesting students are a valuable and often unrealized resource for addressing these challenges, which provides a strong foundation for what establishes successful educational practices. In addition, many students are favoring the opportunity to participate in co-creation of curriculum.

MODEL

In this section, we highlight two complementary frameworks to guide educators through co-creation of curriculum. We will first discuss the Staged Self-Directed Learning (SSDL) model, which offers educators direction for actively equipping their students to become more self-directed learners. Both higher education and co-creation desire to produce students prepared to enter society as self-directed and lifelong learners. Unfortunately, several educational practices in higher education institutions do more to perpetuate dependency versus creating autonomous learners. Grow (1991) defines *self-direction* as…"the degree of choice that learners have within an institutional situation" (p. 128) and includes the following three features of:

1. Holds a personal quality of autonomy
2. Critically and willingly seeks learning outside of formal instruction (autodidaxy)
3. Student controls learning

In addition, this model operates with the following assumptions:

- Self-direction may be situational—students may not be self-directed in all subjects.
- Self-direction is not entirely situational—it can partly be a personal trait or genetic personality.
- The development of self-direction occurs best in nurturing environments.
- The development of self-direction occurs in stages (or parts).
- Once students develop self-direction, they can transfer this skill to new learning situations.

Students can learn dependency and helplessness, but they can also learn self-direction. Similarly, educators can create dependency or teach self-direction. The SSDL model is built on a strong belief in the value of self-direction and proposes ways educators can empower students to achieve greater autonomy.

In this model, Grow (1991) borrows key concepts from Paul Hersey and Kenneth Blanchard's Situational Leadership Model. According to this leadership model, management is situational or task-specific and corresponds to an employee's *readiness*—the combination of their abilities and motivation. An effective manager employs a mix of directive action and personal interaction to match the employee's current state of readiness and to assist with the advancement of self-directed work. The authors suggest there is no one good way to manage each individual, but everyone can be guided to be more autonomous. Inspired by the phases of situational leadership, Grow (1991) designed four stages in which the educator attempts to match and advance the student's current level of self-direction (Table 4-1).

In stage one, the student is **dependent** and the educator serves as a coach in authority. Students may become temporarily dependent when they encounter a new topic, and some students may challenge the authoritative figure. In this stage, the educator's expertise and effectiveness are important for managing the dependent student. If an educator is lax, students often attempt to take advantage and further develop habits of nonlearning. Educational literature criticizes this stage because of the transmission of knowledge to students. Educators might temporarily need to revisit this stage to build an improved foundation for high levels of learning. An educator should be prepared to meet resistance with attempts to move into more self-directed learning. However, in this stage, educators can begin to require students to design small portions of their learning experiences, so they begin to learn to take responsibility for their own education.

Four Stages of Self-Directed Learning

TABLE 4-1

STAGE	STUDENT	CHARACTERISTICS OF STUDENT	EDUCATOR	CHARACTERISTICS	TEACHING IN THIS STAGE
1	Dependent	Requires an authority figure to provide explicit instruction on what, how, and when to learn Treats educators as the expert or passively progresses through their education by responding to educators that "make" them learn Demonstrates dependency in some or all of the subjects Some students are enduringly dependent; others are temporarily because they lack knowledge, skills, experience, motivation, or confidence Depends on educator to make decision that they will later learn to make on their own	Coach Authority	Learning centers around the educator Serves as the expert Establishes creditability and authority Demonstrates mastery of subject	Clearly organizes and rigorously approaches subject Provides discipline and direction by establishing clear learning objectives and expectations for achievement Establishes clear deadlines Teaches specific, identifiable skills Sets high standards beyond what students believe they can do and creates a reward system for success Keeps communication clear (often one-way) and focused on subject Offers little choice Gives objective grades and offers immediate, frequent, and unbiased feedback Uses lecture, structured drills, very specific assignments, etc.

(continued)

TABLE 4-1 (CONTINUED)

Four Stages of Self-Directed Learning

STAGE	STUDENT	CHARACTERISTICS OF STUDENT	EDUCATOR	CHARACTERISTICS	TEACHING IN THIS STAGE
2	Interested	Demonstrates moderate self-direction Demonstrates interest Responds to motivational techniques Willingly completes assignments and engages in instructional methods when they understand purpose Displays confidence despite lack of knowledge on topic Follows educator if have direction or assistance Responds positively to personal interaction from educator	Motivator Guide	Demonstrates enthusiasm and motivation Makes students excited to learn Implements a directive but highly supported approach Begins to prepare students to become more self-directed Builds confidence	Provides clear explanations of why the subject or skill is important and how assignments will assist students to achieve learning objectives Shows concrete results of what is taught Begins training students in goal setting Transitions from offering praise, which provides extrinsic motivation, to offering encouragement to build intrinsic motivation Helps students start to recognize differences in personalities, goals, and learning styles Sets high standards and provides motivation to achieve Communicates in two-way direction (educator explains and persuades; students give responses and interests) Uses lectures that inspire and have highly interactive drills, leads discussions, and demonstrates and follows with guided practice Provides close supervision and ample positive feedback

(continued)

TABLE 4-1 (CONTINUED)

Four Stages of Self-Directed Learning

STAGE	STUDENT	EDUCATOR	CHARACTERISTICS OF STUDENT	CHARACTERISTICS	TEACHING IN THIS STAGE
3	Involved	Facilitator	Demonstrates intermediate self-direction	Becomes close to being a participant in learning	Provides conscious use of learning strategies
			Possesses skills and knowledge	Shares decision making with students	Offers opportunities to design and implement learning methods
			Views self as active participant in own education	Focuses on facilitation and communication	Offers various tools and learning methods to learn
			Demonstrates readiness to explore a subject with good guidance	Supports students to use skills they possess	Shares experiences and allows others to share own experiences
			Starts to explore some of subject on their own	Assists students to transition to independence	Negotiates goals, standards, and evaluation methods with students in relation to external standard (professional accreditation)
			Potentially needs to develop a deeper sense of self or direction, more confidence, or a greater ability to collaborate with others	Desires to empower learners	Assigns loosely structured and designed group projects
			Benefits from learning more about how they learn		Provides contracts, rubrics, or checklists to allow students to monitor own progress
			Examines self, culture, and contexts		Uses seminars, group projects, or open-ended assignments

(continued)

Four Stages of Self-Directed Learning

TABLE 4-1 (CONTINUED)

STAGE	STUDENT	CHARACTERISTICS OF STUDENT	EDUCATOR	CHARACTERISTICS	TEACHING IN THIS STAGE
		Identifies and values own experiences for learning; learns to identify same characteristics in others' experiences Develops initiative and critical-thinking skills Views self as cocreator Views self as a future professional equal to the educator Desires respect for abilities and opportunities to be involved with other learners and educators Demonstrates strong readiness to collaborate by understanding can accomplish more together			

(continued)

TABLE 4-1 (CONTINUED)

Four Stages of Self-Directed Learning

STAGE	STUDENT	CHARACTERISTICS OF STUDENT	EDUCATOR	CHARACTERISTICS	TEACHING IN THIS STAGE
4	Self-Directed	Demonstrates high level of self-direction Sets own goals and standards (with or without assistance) Uses experts and other resources to achieve goals Takes responsibility for own learning and direction Employs a variety of skills, such as time or project management, self and peer evaluation, resource or information gathering Learns from any kind of educator Thrives in an educational context that provides autonomy Demonstrates psychological maturity	Consultant Delegator	Provides learner-centered education Cultivates learning ability Does not teach subject Encourages students to consult with other students Lessens interaction with students Reduces two-way communication and external motivation and reinforcement; fades back Gradually weans students of being taught Inspires and mentors Provokes learner and fades back Offers concepts or questions or plays devil's advocate	Consults with students to develop tasks (e.g., rubrics, deadlines) Holds meetings to discuss progress and challenges Gives opportunities to work on advanced and meaningful projects Highlights long-term progress for success in professional career or personal life Requires self-evaluation Offers speakers and biographies of role models at various stages of career or life Actively monitors progress; only steps in to offer assistance for self-directing and monitoring skills Uses internships, self-directed experiential (service) learning projects, independent study, thesis projects, student-led discussions

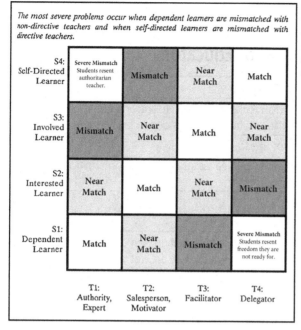

The most severe problems occur when dependent learners are mismatched with non-directive teachers and when self-directed learners are mismatched with directive teachers.

| | T1: | T2: | T3: | T4: |

S4: Self-Directed Learner	**Severe Mismatch** Students resent authoritarian teacher.	Mismatch	Near Match	Match
S3: Involved Learner	Mismatch	Near Match	Match	Near Match
S2: Interested Learner	Near Match	Match	Near Match	Mismatch
S1: Dependent Learner	Match	Near Match	Mismatch	**Severe Mismatch** Students resent freedom they are not ready for.
	T1: Authority, Expert	T2: Salesperson, Motivator	T3: Facilitator	T4: Delegator

Figure 4-1. Grow's matches and mismatches in learning stages and teaching styles. (Reproduced with permission from Grow, G. O. [1991]. Teaching learners to be self-directed. *Adult Education Quarterly, 41*[3], 25. https://doi.org/10.1177/0001848191041003001)

In stage two, students are **interested** in self-directed learning, and the educator plays the role of motivator and guide. In this stage, students become more motivated and encouraged to learn on their own. The educator still provides quite a bit of direction but prepares the students to advance along the continuum by tying the subject to their students' interests and providing strong personal interactions. Educators offer this type of enthusiastic guidance when students are faced with a challenging subject. Their excitement will carry their students until they have adequately learned enough to become more self-motivated. However, the educator must ensure their students do not remain dependent on this extrinsic motivation to learn.

In stage three, students are **involved** in autonomous and adult learning and the educator serves as the facilitator. Students are excited and often do not want to leave this stage and are eager to work with a collegial group. Educators are also excited because students begin to create their own learning situations and develop their own motivation. It is during this phase where the real potential for co-creation occurs, as educators begin to share decision making with students by negotiating course policies and procedures and creating opportunities to design and implement various learning methods.

In stage four, the final stage, students are **self-directed** and the educator functions as a consultant or delegator. Grow (1991) suggests this stage is not fully possible in a higher education setting but remains one of the single most important learning outcomes. Educators remain present in stage four but often fade into the background. They might set a challenge, offer assistance as the students complete the task or ask for support, and empower students to successfully address challenges. There is a shared and pleasant relationship and interaction between the educator and students. The students also have strong relations with the world, task, and peers.

Mismatch Between Learning Stages and Teaching Styles

Everyone experiences challenges when the student's stage of self-direction does not match the educator's teaching style. Grow (1991) provides a grid of 16 potential pairings of teaching styles and learning stages; six are described as mismatches and two of those mismatches are considered severe (Figure 4-1).

TABLE 4-2

Teaching Traps for Educators

STAGE	TEACHING TRAPS FOR EDUCATORS
1	Tendencies to provide instruction in an authoritarian (controlling and punitive) manner; limits students' ability to take initiative and further creates dependency and resistance
2	Tendencies to remain the center of the stage Encourages any student that will listen but leaves students with no additional learning skills or motivation
3	Disappears into the group Accepts and values nearly anything from any student
4	Withdraws too much, which results in losing touch, failing to monitor progress, or allowing students to experience failures for which they are not yet ready

For example, stage four students tend to resent or rebel against the low level and boring demands of the stage one teaching style. The educator attempts to exert control and views these students as uncooperative and unprepared. In turn, the students engage in behaviors in an attempt to get out from under the powerful educator. Similarly, a stage four educator delegates responsibilities that a stage one student is not equipped to successfully handle. The students lack the skills they need to navigate this newfound freedom, feel frustration and anger when expected to make decisions, lack ability to effectively complete tasks, and sense the educator has little personal and professional interest. Some educational literature suggests the method of teaching should match the subject; however, the SSDL model proposes a balance between the educator's direction and students' autonomy—usually set by their ability to participate in self-directed learning.

Educators can progress students by demonstrating a skill, coaching use of the skill, fostering application of the skill, and asking students to work in groups to create new practical situations to perform the skill on each other.

Educators desire for students to be more autonomous in learning but may not have pedagogical methods for advancing them from dependency to self-direction. According to this model, good teaching occurs when the educator balances the level of support with the student's stage of self-direction and empowers them to progress to greater independence in learning. Educators match the stage with the goal to explicitly facilitate the attainment of skills, knowledge, and motivation to help students achieve more autonomous learning in their education and ideally in their personal life. Educators recognize not all students are self-directed and not all will become self-directed when told; however, educators can assume each student possesses the potential to be in control of their own learning (with assistance). Because students can be at any of the four stages, educators may need to approach some students with more direct instruction to better equip them to pursue higher stages. When reviewing Figure 4-1 an additional time, there are 10 areas where the teaching style matches or nearly matches the learning stage. In each of these areas, educators can implement several methods to facilitate self-directed learning (review highlighted areas of Table 4-1). Educators can advance from lectures to directed discussion to loosely structured discussion to student-led discussion within one organized class. They can also use the stages to map the progression of the course or curriculum. The SSDL model describes the advancement, but remember, the progress of the students or class is rarely linear and students will be at different stages at different times. In addition, Grow (1991) highlights common pitfalls educators encounter during each stage (Table 4-2).

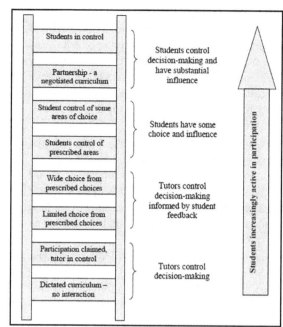

Figure 4-2. Bovill and Bulley's (2011) ladder of student participation. (Reproduced with permission from Bovill, C., & Bulley, C. J. [2011]. A model of active student participation in curriculum design: Exploring desirability and possibility. In C. Rust [Ed.], *Improving student learning [ISL] 18: Global theories and local practices: Institutional, disciplinary and cultural variations.* Series: Improving student learning [18]. Oxford Brookes University: Oxford Centre for Staff and Learning Development.)

Bovill and Bulley (2011) offer a framework for levels and types of student participation in co-creation of curriculum, which aligns well with the previously described SSDL model. As students advance through various stages of self-directed learning, educators can match and implement different types of co-creation strategies to further promote autonomy. The authors created a ladder of student participation in curriculum design based from a model of citizen participation in community planning (Figure 4-2). At the lower steps of the ladder, the educator primarily controls decision making and the students are limited in their active participation in co-creation (similar to stage one of SSDL). Meanwhile, at the higher steps of the ladder, it is the students that have the greatest control of and influence on decisions. They are highly active participants in their own education, suggesting they are stage four, self-directed students. As educators begin to understand where their students reside on the SSDL model, they can use the ladder to identify ways in which to involve students in co-creation. Each step of the ladder is briefly described in the following paragraphs.

The first two steps of the ladder involve the educator controlling the course or curriculum decisions (e.g., teacher-centered learning). In the first step (dictated curriculum—no interaction), the educator delivers the content to the students and does not involve them in any aspect of co-creation. The students simply arrive (or do not arrive) for class. Meanwhile in the second step (participation claimed, tutor in control), the educator claims the students have some control in the educational process but maintains the sole authority over decisions. For example, the educator allows the students to provide feedback but does not implement appropriate changes, so they falsely believe they have a voice. This situation is particularly concerning because the lack of genuine participation can lead students to mistrust the educator, doubt the co-creation process, or leave with feelings of alienation.

In the next two ladder steps, the educator remains in control of co-creation decisions, but their decisions are informed by student feedback. The two ladder steps fit well with stage two or stage three students in the SSDL model. The educator in the third step of the ladder offers students limited choice from a prescribed list of options. In this situation, the educator might allow the students to select what time class will start, a certain instructional method, or the number of lab groups. In the fourth step of the ladder, the educator gives the students a wider range of choices (still from a prescribed set of options). They might allow their students to select the topic of a project or the type of assessment method.

In addition to my passion for occupational therapy, I admire the art of education and find enormous value in mastering the art of teaching. I come from a long line of educators and believe it is naturally ingrained in my being. When presented with the opportunity to collaborate in course design with my peers and professors, I recognized the additional opportunity to take my founding steps into education within the realm of higher education. In addition to my chance to further explore education, this journey enhanced my understanding of academic topics and methods of academic presentation.

My involvement with this experience was humbling and enlightening. I learned that although there are methods of teaching that prove more effective, there is no correct way to learn. Learning is exploratory and unique for each individual. Learning styles can be combined and created to enhance understanding and applicability. I discovered that being an educator is difficult given the requirement to adapt and support students who have an array of learning styles. Respecting and exploring different methods of learning and educating is crucial to our growth as students and our transitional skills into the professional world.

I enjoyed the space this journey allowed to hear from and collaborate with learners who shared and differed in learning experiences. I had the opportunity to build relationships and understand peers within my class who I likely would not have otherwise gotten to know. In a similar manner, I grew closer to faculty, which made them more approachable and relatable through this more intimate setting.

I grew substantially in facilitating and directing my own learning throughout this experience. I will admit, I was a challenger of this idea from the beginning, and my mind was increasingly opened from the start. This process required self-reflection and self-control as I discovered how to transition study habits and alter preparation prior to class in order to gain the full academic benefits of my courses. My transition was not seamless, nor was it for my peers. Negativity surrounded peer conversations at times, but I found pride in being a voice of reason and understanding to my peers to help encourage a more positive learning environment. I found encouragement from my fellow peers involved in course design to continue to grow and influence others. When I hear positivity, I emit and promote positivity, with which this group of collaborators helped substantially.

As I step into the professional world, I am able to pull from my enhanced appreciation and awareness for the quality of education students and peers expect and benefit from. Additionally, I feel responsible for carrying out effective education within my field. As I prepare to take fieldwork students or provide in-services, I prepare with the quality information, research, and hands-on experience necessary to be effective.

Bailey Baucum, MOT, OTR/L

In the last four steps of the ladder, the students begin to influence choices in their education; they take actions to engage in more self-directed learning. On step five, the students control areas in which the educator stipulates. The students might participate in the design of a certain learning module or manage a discussion board. However, in stage six, they possess a higher level of control and choose areas of the course or curriculum they would like to design. The students could choose how they would like to achieve a designated learning objective (e.g., presentation, handout, paper). In the last two steps, the students demonstrate substantial control. The students and the educator form a collaborative partnership to negotiate or create a course or curriculum. They work with each other to co-construct knowledge. Lastly, the students are in control on the eighth step of the ladder and the educator is absent. Such as in stage four of the SSDL model, it is uncommon to view this step

TABLE 4-3

Roles in Co-Creation of Curriculum

ROLE	DESCRIPTION	EXAMPLE
Consultant	Students share and discuss their perspective on the teaching and learning process.	Students review an assignment and rubric. Students as Learners and Teachers: Students not enrolled in course serve as consultant to the educator. (Bovill & Bulley, 2011)
Coresearch	Students meaningfully collaborate with educators on teaching and learning- or subject-based research.	A student works with an educator to explore a research topic. (Butcher & Maunder, 2014)
Pedagogical Codesigner	Students share responsibility with the educator on designing teaching and learning activities.	Students design a course. (Koehler et al., 2004)
Representative	Students express opinions and provide feedback, which contributes to decision in a wide array of institutional activities.	A student serves as a program's representative on the school's student council.

in higher education as the educator traditionally remains present. However, it is possible in some courses as students might design their own learning objectives, a plan to achieve those objectives, complete the experience, and evaluate their own work. In occupational therapy education, this high level of student autonomy and self-direction is more likely to occur during the doctoral capstone experience. The ladder of participation in curriculum design is also similar to the SSDL model in that the higher levels may not always be desirable, as some situations might require lower levels of engagement (with exception of the lower two steps, as those are rarely recommended).

IMPLEMENTATION

Roles in Co-Creation of Curriculum

Educators can engage students in a variety of roles when integrating co-creation of curricula into their educational practices. Bovill and colleagues (2016) identify four roles for student participation (Table 4-3). In order for any of the first three roles to occur, the educator must create the opportunity for co-creation. In addition, these roles are not mutually exclusive, meaning educators can involve students in multiple roles at the same time.

Selection of Students for Participation in Co-Creation of Curriculum

Educators make important decisions when selecting students for participation in any aspect of curricular co-creation. Despite the recognized benefits of co-creation, an educator should not assume sharing power with students is a perfect solution to learning. Some students will lack engagement or motivation to make educational decisions; while other students will resist assuming responsibility because they believe it is the educator's role to complete pedagogical design. Furthermore, a few students might be uncomfortable because they are uncertain about what guidelines and expectations will guide the class at the start of the course. Remember, our students are transitioning to a graduate level of education. They are engaging in a completely new educational experience because they often start their professional education as dependent learners whose educators made the decisions and transmitted knowledge in their undergraduate education.

In order for educators to successfully share power in co-creation, they need to include students that possess intellectual maturity and a certain level of development to assume responsibility. Students across each level of education can gain confidence and capacity when they participate in some form of curricular co-creation. However, educational literature recommends the educator begin with smaller scale involvement with less mature learners and gradually increase their participation as they gain experience and comfort with their own learning. For example, Hess (2007) does not involve first-year students in their first semester in the syllabus creation process. When educators do include students in the small decision-making process early in their education, they should still ensure the students view their role as meaningful and see that it directly relates to or impacts learning. As the students grow as self-directed learners, educators can increase the extent with which they are involved in collaboration. Many first-year students in their second semester become more interested in learning and are ready to participate in syllabus design or other elements of course design. Most upper-level students are willing and able to collaborate with the educator at the start of the course to make design decisions because they have a better understanding of concepts and rigor of courses. Birgbauer (2016) suggests working with advanced and motivated students that demonstrate interest in the topic and ability to engage in self-directed learning.

Educators need to strike a balance between inclusion and selection when including students in a co-creation process. Traditionally, the educator invites students to participate in the opportunity by either extending an offer to the entire class or intentionally seeking out certain students. When considering which students to select, they must consider who has the ability to meaningfully contribute to the partnership and whose voices are heard when chosen or not heard when not chosen. A majority of literature recommends the educator take an inclusive approach and select students whose views, backgrounds, or experiences are diverse or underrepresented. When educators form collaborative relationships with a diverse group of students, they each engage in a deeper and richer learning experience. If a process of selection has to take place (e.g., many students volunteer or there is an application process), it is critical for the educator to establish clear criteria and maintain students' trust in the procedures. The educator must also communicate and ensure the participation in co-creation of curricula is voluntary.

> Some educators secure funds to offer students a stipend.

Specific Methods for Engaging Students in Co-Creation of Curriculum

Co-creation of curriculum is a broad concept that encompasses many diverse approaches to student engagement and several different forms across disciplines and institutions. Educators employ a range of co-creation methods ranging from simple questionnaires to in-depth collaborators on course design. We describe different ways to include students in the co-creation process based on the ladder of student participation moving from lower to higher steps. Several factors influence the selection of these co-creation methods, such as class size, students' development level, educators' experience, time, institutional support, professional accreditation standards, or professional content.

I discovered co-creation of curriculum as I completed the doctoral experiential component of my postprofessional occupational therapy education. At the time, I was an assistant clinical professor and knew I would be significantly redesigning a course. Therefore, I decided to collaborate with five students from our master's degree program to complete this important task. One of my mentors suggested I was crazy, while another mentor said, "Sounds like fun." I am so glad I took the route of involving students in course design because it has been one of the most rewarding experiences in my early career as an occupational therapy educator.

I met weekly with these five students at the start of the summer to prepare for a course taught during the fall semester. Our first meeting was…**interesting**. It became clear the students were accustomed to passive learning and disliked required tasks and skills that required them to become independent and self-directed learners. They were somewhat disappointed with their graduate education because their belief of what occupational therapy education should entail did not match our expectations. The meeting was an eye-opening experience. At the end of the first meeting, I asked the students to read a few articles about and complete their own research on classroom design and instructional methods. During the next meeting, I presented a potential list of topics and goals for the course and they presented what they had learned from their outside research. During this meeting, the students literally transformed before my own eyes. They were excited to learn, discussed what they wanted to learn, and began matching instructional methods with content and learning goals. In fact, they met on their own (unprompted) to further discuss and provided me with a detailed course map the following week. In such a short time, the students had taken **ownership** of their learning. Throughout the rest of the summer, we collaboratively worked to make decisions on readings and resources, course policies, assignments and rubrics, and additional methods of assessment. We also developed a way to systematically collect data to contribute to the scholarship of teaching and learning.

At the start of the fall semester, I explained to the entire cohort the role of the students involved in the co-creation of the course. Based on the findings from a focus group prior to the course, their peers weren't so sure about this process and benefits of co-creation or about the expectations that they would need to be more active learners prepared to engage in self-directed and deep learning. They experienced difficulties and expressed frustrations to the co-creation students during the initial transition period of 4 to 6 weeks. From my experience, this transition was one of the more challenging aspects of the co-creation experience. However, I promise if you stick with it, the rewards will outnumber those challenges. To my own surprise, I give complete credit to the students involved in co-creation for "saving" the course and experience during this trying time. *They strongly advocated for their peers to press on because they knew the benefits and evidence.* Their peers shifted their opinions once they began to recognize their voices were heard as appropriate changes were made to meet their learning needs and understood the benefits when they felt more prepared for and performed well on the first exam. Our postcourse focus group revealed their peers reported everyone in the class can benefit when a few students are included in the design process.

As a result, the students demonstrated excellent learning outcomes and growth in professional reasoning and metacognition. While this is gratifying as an educator, one of the greater rewards is developing deep relationships with students as you navigate the co-creation process. We held each other accountable and grew as both educators and learners.

Whitney Henderson, OTD, MOT, OTR/L

Implementing a Focus Group

Some researchers in co-creation literature believe focus groups are essential to understanding the students' educational experiences. A *focus group* is a simple practice that allows the educator to hear the voice of a small group of students. In regards to co-creation, educators solicit student feedback in a group format to more effectively influence the decisions they make during the teaching and learning process. They use focus groups to engage students in their education, improve interaction in the relationship, make changes to initial course design, and enhance understanding of curriculum viewed through the eyes of students. Brooman and colleagues (2015) implemented a focus group and modified the course based on feedback from the students. As a result, the researcher reported improved grades and pass rates and increased attendance.

Creating a Policy or Grading Scheme

Educators new to co-creation can simply start with one component of course design, such as collaborating with students to create a policy or plan a grading scheme. In a public speaking course, an educator collaborates with students to establish a participation policy for the semester. During the first class, the students discuss in small groups what type of contributions count for credit. The educator drafts a policy based on the consensus of the conversation and presents this version to the students during the next class. The students suggest any additional revisions before adopting a final draft. Weimer (1996) reports initial doubt of the co-creation process, but once the students adopted the policy, the quality and quantity of their participation enriched. In the next example, the educator invited students to contribute to course grading scheme. The educator created a syllabus of the course schedule and reading assignments but left the grading portion blank. As a homework assignment, the students planned the ways in which they would be evaluated throughout the semester. They decided types of assignments and when the assignments would be due. During the next class, the educator and students reached agreement and adopted the grading plan. The educator and students provided positive feedback about this process and demonstrated a high level of engagement and investment in learning. These two collaborative methods provide great examples of ways educators can introduce and scaffold co-creation of curriculum to more novice learners.

Writing the Syllabus

At the start of each semester, the educator often establishes an initial point of contact with the students in the form of a syllabus, which ultimately serves as a learning contract between the two parties. The syllabus gives the students a lasting first impression of the educator and the course. In this document, educators articulate the course goals, recommended materials, class expectations and policies, assigned readings and projects, timelines, instructional methods, and grading mechanisms. Traditionally, they make these important design decisions as they write the syllabus. Educators who include students in the design of some or all aspects of the syllabus engage in a form of co-creation.

Educators can approach student involvement in syllabus construction in a few different ways. One strategy is for the educators to present the students with a list of competencies the course must achieve and a rough draft of the syllabus. The students can elect to adopt the educator-created syllabus or propose changes to various components. In this situation, students often choose to collaborate with the educator to achieve consensus on course decisions reflected in the syllabus. Using a similar strategy, an educator might elect to meet with a group of students before the course begins to assist to structure the course syllabus. Lastly, one educator asked students to interview one another on the first day of class about what they might want to learn in the course. The educator recorded the results, formulated a draft based on this information, allowed students to offer changes based on their own or their peers' learning needs, and devised a final draft. In this strategy, the students believe the educator trusts their judgment and they demonstrate a higher level of motivation as a result.

In educational literature, Hess (2007) offers an example of high student engagement in the fabrication of a syllabus. The author creates a draft syllabus before the start of the course with general information without student input. For the remainder of the syllabus, the educator solicits feedback by providing structure through open-ended questions with blank white spaces for students to write ideas. In addition, he provides a statement reporting they will spend the first day of class formulating collaborative course decisions regarding goals, instructional and evaluation methods, and roles and responsibilities. Hess (2007) emails each student the draft syllabus several days prior to the start of the course, requires the students to review and answer the prompts, and asks they bring their answers to the first class. An educator can also ask students to review syllabi from other courses or institutions to spark ideas and discussion. During the first class, he devotes most of the time to design and explains reasons for including the students in this process. In collaboration, the educator and students brainstorm and discuss ideas for approximately 30 to 50 minutes. The role of the educator is to ensure all voices are heard, clarify comments, document ideas on the board or screen, summarize discussion, reach consensus on decisions, add ideas or respond to questions (as needed), and provide any rationales. Following the first class, Hess (2007) revises the syllabus, suggests solutions to any remaining solutions, emails the students the updated version, and asks to review before the second class. During the second class, they spend 5 to 10 minutes addressing any additional concerns and making revisions before final adoption of the syllabus.

> Educators can also solicit feedback via a survey prior to the start of the course and present themes during the first class.

Hess (2007) strongly believes the value in including the students outweighs the concern with devoting a large amount of time to this process. As a result, he reports students are more invested, work harder, devote more time, complete more research, and feel a great sense of camaraderie and accomplishment. Interestingly, this educator has completed this process in more than 10 courses and identifies common themes related to syllabus construction:

> These expectations are consistent with literature discussing effective educators.

- The students often identify *common goals* but will propose one or two goals the educator had not considered or planned to address in the course. If the educator believes a goal is important, they include in the draft syllabus.
- Students desire *active instructional methods* of discussion, such as small group work, simulations, and experiential learning. They also desire a variety of methods. As they discuss methods, the educator gains insights into the ways the students learn best. In some cases, the students assist with the creation of methods, such as proposing speakers for an expert panel or ideas for service-learning experience.
- The students quickly agree on *their roles and responsibilities* with the most common being prepared for class, actively participating, offering support, and providing mutual respect.
- The students also quickly agree on *the role and responsibility of the educator*. These expectations often include the educator being well prepared for class, facilitating discussion and engagement, treating students with respect, clearly articulating high expectations, showing passion for concepts, providing accurate feedback, and being open to ideas and being accessible.
- Students often demonstrate strong opinions about and preferences for certain *types of evaluation*. Typically, they agree on two to three methods of evaluation, such as exams, participation, and assignments (papers).

Designing a Learning Experience

In several courses, educators allow students to write papers or deliver presentations on topics they select. Educators can further increase student motivation by enabling them to develop their own experiential learning opportunities. In this situation, the students learn the course content, experience the benefits of co-creation, and engage in practical contexts relevant to their future

Figure 4-3. Students meet to participate in the course design process.

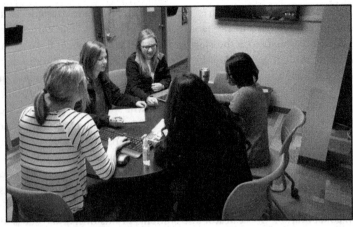

careers. An educator typically meets with a group of students once a week over the course of several weeks to design an experiential-learning experience. Initially, they devote time to form and reach agreement on learning objectives and group goals. Following this important step, the educator and students begin to brainstorm ideas and define and delegate individual responsibilities. It is beneficial for the educator to provide some sort of worksheet that outlines the responsibilities and timelines for tasks to hold everyone (including the educator) accountable. In collaboration with the educator, the students complete many tasks, such as selecting a site, interacting with stakeholders, determining transportation needs, negotiating projects, establishing a contract, creating a timeline, setting a budget, and selecting evaluation methods. Hains and Smith (2012) convey the importance for the students to develop behavioral expectations to hold their peers accountable—it often proves to be a necessary component. It is also important to note that once the students co-create experiential learning, they need to transition back into the traditional role of a student that learns and applies course concepts. In a similar example, an educator asked a group of master's degree students to develop an experiential learning opportunity for geography students in an undergraduate program. The undergraduate students selected which opportunity they wanted to engage in based on their interests and learning needs.

Including Students in the Entire Course Design Process

Educators provide candid descriptions on how to include students in the complexity of course design. We have also involved our occupational therapy students in the redesigning of a graduate level course. In this chapter, we will combine our experiences with educational literature to best navigate this learning experience. Educators establish a design team by inviting students to participate in the co-creation of a course. A course design team typically consists of one to two educators and two to six students. Educators can also include an academic developer as needed. In our experience, one educator collaborated with five students in their second year of an occupational therapy master's degree program. We consulted an experienced educator when needed. Educational literature suggests successful teams meet weekly for 2 to 3 months prior to the course to allow for ample time to redesign the course and to establish true partnerships to hear students' voices (Figure 4-3).

Initially, we met weekly for 3 months prior to the start of the course and reduced to once every other week during the semester. Birgbauer (2016) further recommends scheduling reoccurring meetings on the calendar to demonstrate the work is a priority and to keep the process moving forward. We agree with this recommendation. Although briefly mentioned in educational literature, we strongly encourage educators to explain to the entire group of students at the start of semester

Throughout my undergraduate years, lecture-style learning was the only type of learning I had experienced. Sure, professors would occasionally throw in a video or an interactive project; however, day-to-day learning was presented in a mundane lecture format. Each new lecture started a cycle—giving my full attention for the first quarter of the period, taking notes but not retaining much of the information, and going back to notes several days before the exam to attempt to retain information I hadn't actually learned the first time. After frequently finding myself frustrated with strictly lecture-style courses, I was immediately attracted by the opportunity to be involved in the design of a new course. The opportunity to collaborate with a professor on how I learn material crucial to my career was an intriguing idea in itself.

After immersing myself in the course design process, I quickly became aware of the benefits of being involved. Upon reflection on this experience, I believe these same benefits held true. I felt a sense of ownership for my own learning inside and outside of the classroom and increased comfort and understanding of how the material actually applied to my everyday work as an occupational therapist. I gained a better personal definition of what occupational therapy represents and does as a profession. I experienced improved relationships with my professors and understood how to develop a healthy working/collaborative relationship with an authority figure. Lastly, I had a firsthand perspective of how educators and practitioners put research and literature into action, which brought to light the entire movement behind evidence-based practice.

My involvement in course design facilitated my learning in many ways; mainly the variety of instructional methods throughout the course. We reviewed research, and just as research reported, the instructional methods we selected improved my learning. With this new way of learning, I found that the number of times I reviewed subject material inside the classroom (with my full attention I might add) **increased**, while time spent outside of the classroom continuously studying and reviewing that same subject material significantly **decreased**. I actually learned! In addition, my learning became more thorough in the sense that I began focusing on how the subject matter could be applied to occupational therapy practice rather than just memorizing material for recall on a test. The only challenge I felt I experienced was on the front end of the course; specifically, presenting the initial idea to the rest of our peers. It took our cohort several weeks to stay committed to the different instructional methods simply because lecture style had become our "comfort zone" for learning.

My favorite part of involvement in course design was the incentive to take ownership for my own learning. Additionally, I had a voice in my education, and my experiences mattered. I was truly heard in course design meetings, as professors made immediate and conscious efforts to make changes driven by student feedback. Now as an occupational therapy practitioner, I see two major benefits from this experience: (1) My ability to collaborate with a small group to achieve a common goal that then benefits a larger group (e.g., my day-to-day patients and families) and (2) my ability to review literature and evidence to improve my own practice and patient outcomes. To students and educators looking to use this course design strategy, I say do it! Including students in course design does initially require work on the front end, but the benefits are worth the effort. Additionally, the amount of positive feedback will greatly outnumber any negative feedback or challenges if implemented well.

Lyndi Plattner, MOT, OTR/L

why a small group of their peers are participating in co-creation, the benefits of this process, and what course design includes and does not include. At the end of the semester debrief session, our students highlighted the importance of this conversation. Their peers become less unsettled when they realized students involved in course design were not receiving an advantage in regards to exams and quizzes and began to get "on board" with the idea when they realized beneficial changes were made to the course based on student feedback.

> At some point you must have a pivotal moment where the students understand they have a voice.

After the educator builds a team and designates meeting times, it is time to start the design process. The educator involves students in all aspects of co-creation of a course. As briefly described in Chapter 1, the process begins with a backward design approach in which the educator and students develop the learning goals for the course. We established course goals by collectively reviewing the accreditation standards, the program's curriculum, and a thorough list of potential concepts. We engaged in a lively discussion to clarify any questions, determine which concepts were of greatest interest, and add additional topics the students felt would be useful to include in the course. We came to a consensus on the course concepts and learning goals within two to three meetings.

Educators and students can brainstorm about what concepts are critical to the course and what is essential for the students to know or do as they establish goals. Subsequently, educators and students begin building the instructional and assessment methods that match the learning goals. As educators, we found this portion of the co-creation process exciting and transforming.

We asked the students to evenly divide a list of instructional methods and to research each of these strategies prior to a meeting. Not only did our students research these methods, but they spontaneously met prior to our meeting and started aligning the instructional methods with concepts. During the meeting, they enthusiastically conversed about what they learned and presented their ideas for teaching the various concepts. They began taking ownership of **our** course and understood the evidence behind the ways educators teach. Throughout the semester, we also used meeting times to briefly pilot different instructional methods to highlight potential concerns before implementation and ensure we were meeting our learning goals.

The course design team must contemplate many other decisions, such as course materials, assignments, and evaluation of learning and performance. Using Birgbauer (2016) as a model, we solicited feedback on reading assignments and textbooks. For most of the concepts, we presented textbook readings, articles, and other resources we included in the course in prior years. The students divided and reviewed the concepts and readings. In addition, they searched for any additional resources or articles they found interesting or useful. During meetings, the students provided their opinions and feedback on the readability, appropriateness, and relationship of the learning materials. Together we selected the readings and resources for the course concepts.

Similar to findings discussed above, we elected to include multiple methods of evaluation with a balance between exams and assignments. For the assignments, the course design team initially discussed ideas, such as concept mapping, case studies, or presentations. The educator developed assignment instructions and a rubric and presented them at the following meeting. The students provided feedback and assisted to modify instructions and clarify portions of the rubric. Throughout the semester, the students continued to offer feedback about their learning during the course and recommended changes for future concepts.

Educational literature recognizes challenges in co-creation of a course—even in successful experiences. The course design process is initially taxing on the educator and the students as the students shift from their passive role and educators shift from complete authority and disciplinary expertise in the learning process. In order to be a positive experience, it is crucial that educators and students become comfortable with ambiguity and flexibility. In a typical course, educators and students are accustomed to timelines and due dates. However, in this situation, the educator must trust the students and offer freedom in the decision-making process.

We note it was difficult to deviate from our traditional preparation of having a completely set schedule in place at the start of the course. As we continued to meet with our team throughout the semester, we planned the course 2 to 3 weeks in advance, which offered opportunities to better adapt to the needs and interests of the students as they experienced the course. We encourage educators to complete the course design process in its entirety as the rewards of student development and learning gains, which learner-centered education promises outweigh these challenges. The students become more comfortable in offering constructive and thoughtful feedback and take their role in course design very seriously, as they take ownership for creating an effective course for their educators and their peers.

Creating an Independent Study

In an *independent study*, students create their own course or complete a self-selected project under the guidance of an educator. The students pursue an area of interest with the goal of enhancing their own learning. They become motivated to learn because they select topics that are meaningful and use learning strategies that work best for them. They also prepare for professional practice because they are developing the necessary skills for lifelong engagement in independent and self-directed learning. Although originally created for intellectually talented students, many different students can profit from opportunities that offer greater independence.

Higher education literature provides a dearth of information about an independent study. In this method, the educator serves as the mentor or consultant who guides the students through the educational process. The educator describes the required learning outcomes for the course and clearly develops the expectations in collaboration with the student (e.g., parameters, depth and breadth, good resources, formats). For example, an educator may require students to complete an independent study to meet an objective and Accreditation Council for Occupational Therapy Education standard about implementing the elements of the teaching-learning process. The educator and student negotiate wording and content of learning objectives in an effort to balance the institutional and programmatic requirements with the co-creation process. In addition, they collaboratively determine the amount of time they spend on the project, the learning tasks, number of required references, additional assignments or check-ins, and examples of ways in which they could demonstrate achievement. It will be important for the educator to create an independent study plan template for the students to complete to serve as a contract that outlines the above features (see Appendix).

Following this communication, the students initiate the step of selecting a topic they perceive as new and interesting. In addition, they should choose a topic that is not too easy or too familiar. Students will begin to write the plan for the independent study. They will write their own learning objectives, a variety of learning activities to achieve the objectives, a timeline, the resources they plan to use, and how they plan to demonstrate learning. Literature suggests students experience the most difficulty in this initial step of selecting a topic and outlining the processes to complete the independent study. Before the students submit their independent study plan for approval, the educator can require them to discuss with peers and revise according to feedback. Using the example from above, students could present to a support group on a desired topic, implement a lunch and learn with practitioners, develop a brief speech to educate legislators on a practical concern, or create an educational handout for low-income families served through a community agency. Their learning activities could potentially include interviewing a key informant, reading various articles, creating the presentation or handout, developing a pre and posttest survey, receiving feedback from peers and the target population, writing a community profile, and taking pictures.

In an independent study, educators and students identify a major challenge with implementing clear evaluation and feedback mechanisms. When working with novice students, the educator might need to provide examples to guide the evaluation process, such as a rubric for those students that elect to do a presentation versus those that create a handout. More experienced students can often create their own method for evaluation, which would require an educator's approval. In situations when students complete an entire course for an independent study, the educator and students often agree to the evaluation method of a portfolio in which they include the plan, resources, artifacts, documentation of time, and reflection. Regardless of the method of evaluation, it is important for educators to provide students with formative feedback to monitor progress and offer suggestions for ways to improve their learning. Educators can provide this type of feedback through required check-ins, peer discussion groups, or a seminar.

TIPS AND TRICKS

- Be authentic and open to change as students often doubt they will be taken seriously in the co-creation process.
- Be aware of the language you use to describe co-creation to your students, as you could unintentionally appear as though you will retain some control in the process.
- Be patient, as students need time to develop the language and confidence to clearly articulate their ideas.
- Educators can expose students to a learner-centered assignment to assist with the transition to shared responsibility for learning in larger scale co-creation projects.
- Start small to increase comfort with the idea of co-creation.
- In the early phases of co-creation, develop shared goals with the students.
- It is a learning experience for the educator **and** the students—be comfortable with ambiguity and demonstrate flexibility.
- Be transparent about potential constraints that limit full student involvement in shared decision making.
- Investigate innovative educational practices: Co-creation provides opportunities for educators to engage in the Scholarship of Teaching and Learning.
- Document and reflect on the process to make appropriate changes for future co-creation opportunities.
- Develop a plan and communication to formally end the collaborative partnership.

OPPORTUNITIES FOR REFLECTION AND FEEDBACK

Throughout the co-creation of curriculum, educators can facilitate reflection and feedback using multiple strategies. In alignment with the ideas in this chapter, perhaps the educator should allow the students to select their own methods of reflection and feedback. In many co-creation examples, educators and students elect to complete personal journals to freely showcase their thoughts and emotions in the design experience. The students often discuss their emotional connection to the course and changes in cognitive (metacognitive) levels. Similarly, educators frequently use reflective journaling during student participation in an independent study. The students typically complete one reflective journal per week in which they write a narrative about an interaction they had or something they desire to know more about. The educator provides structure to process and reviews the journal to offer feedback or resources. They may also ask their students to review their journal and write a reflection paper highlighting their growth and learning as a result of engaging in these methods at the conclusion of the semester. Although there is often initial resistance to journaling, students tend to embrace the opportunity to reflect on their personal and professional perspectives. In turn, educators gain a firsthand view of the students' growth.

Educators can also implement a seminar to facilitate the course design process or to enhance an independent study. Throughout a semester, the educator meets with students once a week to engage in deep discussion. They work collaboratively to establish the group norms and expectations (see Chapter 9). In the beginning, the educator facilitates the discussion, but as the semester progresses, the students lead the seminar. Students gain new knowledge and facilitate each other's learning by providing feedback, asking questions, or explaining reasoning or learning based on their experiences. If the seminar is paired with reflective journaling, the educator may also require each student to share two to three journal entries during the seminar throughout the semester.

OVERCOMING CHALLENGES IN CO-CREATION

Many educators express interest in co-creating learning with students, but they struggle with a poor perception of the potential experience or the actual experience as they attempt to move beyond their traditional role. In educational literature, both educators and students identify several challenges in co-creation of curriculum. They typically discuss three types of complex and overlapping challenges: resistance to the co-creation process, navigating institutional constraints, and developing an inclusive approach. We thoroughly describe these areas and offer solutions, so educators and students may experience the multiple benefits co-creation has to offer.

Resistance to the Co-Creation Process

Despite the recognized benefits, educators and students may resist the idea of participation in co-creation of curriculum because of existing habits or perceived risks associated with the process. Typically, educators make decisions influenced by their own experience as a student and teaching traditions, current expectations of students, and inherited practices from their colleagues. Because of these influences, they settle into custom and common educational practices and wonder how students could meaningfully contribute without knowledge of pedagogical design. Educators also question whether students should or should not have a voice in the production of policies and grading schemes. They perceive a potential disruption in the traditional educator-student relationship and express concerns about finding time to participate in co-creation on top of other responsibilities.

Students might also question why they should step out of their traditional passive and comfortable role to participate in co-creation and wonder how they will personally benefit from this process. Many students believe it is the educator's job to determine the learning objectives, course content, assignments, and grading scheme before the start of the course. In this situation, they might hold the view that the educator is attempting to avoid work. When they participate in this process at the start of the course, some students will feel uncomfortable with uncertainty while course design decisions are made. Other students might dislike the use of class time to engage in co-creation because they believe they should instead be addressing course content, while others potentially believe the course is open for negotiation throughout the entire semester.

Educators and students often overcome resistance when they realize their existing habits might not be the most effective learning approach and when they recognize the benefits of co-creation outweigh any apparent risks. One of the simplest solutions is for the educator to clearly articulate the benefits of student participation in co-creation of curriculum and that course design policies (e.g., attendance, grading scheme) made collaboratively at the beginning of the course remain final. In addition, it is important for the educator to give attention to sources of resistance from the start and to actively listen and respond to their concerns. In our experience, we asked our students to read two or three articles on co-creation and allowed time for a brief discussion for any questions or concerns.

> Educators have opportunities to access more information, as the literature on co-creation continues to grow.

In addition, educators need to gradually build the students' confidence in the process to overcome any ongoing resistance. For example, we had five students participate in course design and 39 students that did not participate in this experience. Once the students that did not participate in course design saw the educator incorporating their peers' feedback in and addressing concern about the course, their hesitation quickly decreased. By the end of the semester, both groups of students reported everyone can benefit from co-creation of a course. Lastly, educators and students need opportunities to reflect on their experiences in this process to continue to foster motivation and change.

Navigation of Institutional Constraints

Educators also feel limited to implement co-creation by institutional constraints or professional accreditation. At some institutions, they may feel the institutional structures, norms, cultures, or policies (e.g., workload) present tension with co-creation. It is our hope that administration embraces and supports this process once they are more aware of the literature that supports student voice for learning, retention, and satisfaction. One of the major institutional barriers is a larger class size. Educational literature provides several examples of how to address this barrier by describing different strategies for co-creation in small groups. Meanwhile, other educators might struggle with balancing the specific outcomes of professional standards with student choice into what is and how it is learned. One strategy for overcoming this challenge is presenting the standards to the students and soliciting feedback and ideas for addressing each of these educational requirements. The students will more deeply engage with the content if they have a voice in the process and will also further develop the important skills for lifelong learning.

Creation of an Inclusive Approach

Educators describe challenges in creating a balance between inclusion and selection. As previously stated above, they should be diligent in selecting students for co-creation and reframing perceptions of disadvantaged students. There is a need for educators to recognize the abilities and assets of students from various backgrounds, as their perspectives facilitate benefits for everyone. One immediate solution to this concern is the educator including the entire class or cohort of students in the co-creation process. However, if selection occurs, the educator must clearly establish, maintain, and communicate the criteria.

Provision of Genuine Forms of Co-Creation

Educators that claim participation in co-creation must relinquish control and distribute power to the students. Students experience an empty and frustrating process when educators promise the commitment to co-creation but do not offer authentic forms of participation and continue to treat the students as outsiders. Students distrust the educational process and further resist deviating from their status quo roles and responsibilities.

THREE THINGS YOU CAN DO TOMORROW TO IMPLEMENT CO-CREATION WITH YOUR STUDENTS

1. Conduct a focus group with a small group of students prior to the start of or halfway through the semester.
2. Allow your students to make one course decision, such as a participation policy, how quizzes will be graded, or which readings to assign.
3. Allow your students to select the way they will achieve one of your course learning objectives.

REFERENCES

Birgbauer, E. (2016). Student-assisted course design. *Journal of Undergraduate Neuroscience Education, 15*(1), E3-E5.

Bovill, C., & Bulley, C. J. (2011). A model of active student participation in curriculum design: Exploring desirability and possibility. In C. Rust (Ed.), *Improving student learning (ISL) 18: Global theories and local practices: Institutional, disciplinary and cultural variations. Series: Improving student learning* (pp. 176-188). Oxford Brookes University: Oxford Centre for Staff and Learning Development.

Bovill, C., Cook-Sather, A., Felten, P., Millard, L., & Cheery-Moore, N. (2016). Addressing potential challenges in co-creating learning and teaching: Overcoming resistance, navigating institutional norms and ensuring inclusivity in student-staff partnerships. *Higher Education, 71*, 195-208. http://dx.doi.org/10.1007/s10734-015-9896-4

Brooman, S., Darwent, S., & Pimor, A. (2015). The student voice in higher education curriculum design: Is there value in listening? *Innovations in Education and Teaching International, 52*(6), 633-674. http://dx.doi.org/10.1080/14703297.2014.910128

Butcher, J., & Maunder, R. (2014). Going URB@N: Exploring the impact of undergraduate students as pedagogic researchers. *Innovations in Education and Teaching International, 51*(2), 142-152. http://dx.doi.org/10.1080/14703297.2013.771967

Grow, G. O. (1991). Teaching learners to be self-direction. *Adult Education Quarterly, 41*(3), 125-149.

Hains, B. J., & Smith, B. (2012). Student-centered course design: Empowering students to become self-directed learners. *Journal of Experiential Education, 35*(2), 357-374.

Hess, G. F. (2007). Collaborative course design: Not my course, not their course, but our course. *Washburn Law Journal, 47*, 367-387.

Koehler, M., Mishra, P., Hershey, K., & Peruski, L. (2004). With a little help from your students: A new model for faculty development and online course design. *Journal of Technology and Teacher Education, 12*(1), 25-55.

Weimer, M. E. (1996). *Improving your classroom teaching*. SAGE Publications.

BIBLIOGRAPHY

Bovill, C. (2014). An investigation of co-created curricula within higher education in the UK, Ireland and the USA. *Innovations in Education and Teaching International, 51*(1), 15-25. http://dx.doi.org/10.1080/14703297.2013.770264

Bovill, C., Felten, P., & Cook-Sather, A. (2014, June). Engaging students as partners in learning and teaching: Practical guidance for academic staff and academic developers. In: *International consortium on educational development conference* (pp. 16-18). Stockholm, Sweden.

Carey, P. (2013). Student as co-producer in a marketised higher education system: A case study of students' experience of participation in curriculum design. *Innovations in Education and Teaching International, 50*(3), 250-260. http://dx.doi.org/10.1080/14703297.2013.796714

Cook-Sather, A. (2011). Layered learning: Student consultants deepening classroom and life lessons. *Educational Action Research, 19*(1), 41-57. https://doi.org/10.1080/09650792.2011.547680

Cook-Sather, A. (2015). Dialogue across differences of position, perspective, and identity: Reflective practice in/on student-faculty pedagogical partnership program. *Teachers College Record, 117*, Article 2. http://repository.brynmawr.edu/edu_pubs

Gardebo, J., & Wiggberg, M. (2012). *Students, the university's unspent resource: Revolutionizing higher education through active student participation*. Universitetstryckeriet, Ekonomikum, Uppsala.

Haraldseid, C., Friberg, F., & Aase, K. (2016). How can students contribute? A qualitative study of active student involvement in development of technological learning material for clinical skills training. *BMC Nursing, 15*(2), 1-10. http://dx.doi.org/10.1186/s12912-016-0125-y

Kolomiiets, B. (2018). The roots of independent study in the USA. *Comparative Professional Pedagogy, 8*(4), 85-91. http://dx.doi.org/10.2478/rpp-2018-0059

Mihans, R. J., Long, D. T., & Felten, P. (2008). Power and expertise: Student-faculty collaboration in course design and the scholarship of teaching and learning. *International Journal for the Scholarship of Teaching and Learning, 2*(2), Article 16. https://doi.org/10.20429/ijsotl.2008.020216

Moerkerke, G. (2015). Modern customers and open universities: Can open universities develop a course model in which student become the co-creators of value? *Open Learning, 30*(3), 235-251. http://dx.doi.org/10.1080/02680513.2015.1117969

Rafoth, M. A. (2019). Independent study: Purposes and goals of independent study, independent study and extensiveness in grades K-12. Retrieved from https://education.stateuniversity.com/pages/2080/Independent-Study.html

Turner, T. (2005). *Encouraging self-directed learning by spiraling through a course.* Higher Education Research and Development Society of Australasia Conference.

APPENDIX

INDEPENDENT STUDY PLAN

NAME:

PROJECT/TOPIC:

COURSE OBJECTIVE(S):

Learning Objective	Tasks	Hours Spent	Timeline for Completion	Resources	Outcome to Demonstrate Learning

FLIPPED CLASSROOM

Whitney Henderson, OTD, MOT, OTR/L

Basic Tenets

Educators and researchers are increasingly employing and investigating the use of flipped classroom in higher education. *Flipped classroom* is a relatively new instructional method that requires students to perform a self-directed learning component prior to the classroom instruction component. This blended learning method is different than a typical classroom when students first obtain course content via lecture and assimilate the new knowledge after class. In other words, in a flipped classroom, students complete learning activities that are typically done in class at home and what is traditionally done as homework is completed during class. During the in-class portion, students are active learners compared to passive learners in traditional lecture format.

Additional Names in Literature: reverse instruction, inverted classroom, 24/7 classroom

In the **first** component of flipped classroom, students independently gain exposure to new material prior to class by exercising lower levels of cognitive work to obtain factual knowledge. Frequently, the educator uses a range of technologies to deliver the pre-class content. The students can complete these learning activities at their own pace and on their own time. The educators expect students will take ownership of their learning by completing the pre-class work, so they are prepared to engage in in-class activities.

In the **second** component, educators design a wide range of in-class learning activities that require active engagement, interaction, and higher-level thinking. In this face-to-face interaction, students have opportunities to think critically and apply the knowledge they gained before class to real-world situations or problems. The educator expects students will interact with faculty and peers (Figure 5-1). During class, students receive important and timely feedback and support while they engage in higher cognitive work. In addition, educators can monitor student performance and quickly adjust accordingly during class time.

Henderson, W. (Ed.). *Effective Teaching: Instructional Methods and Strategies for Occupational Therapy Education* (pp. 73-99).
© 2021 Taylor & Francis Group.

Figure 5-1. Students work in a group to complete a case study.

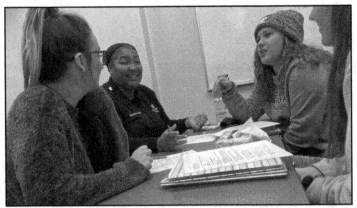

Education literature recognizes numerous benefits for the use of flipped classroom in higher education. Studies suggest students engaged in flipped classroom demonstrate increased communication and teamwork skills. In addition, students develop higher-level thinking skills, such as the ability to problem solve and critically analyze situations to create solutions. They also experience increased motivation for learning and improved performance. We will discuss these findings more in-depth in regard to health professional students throughout this chapter.

Before we move forward, we want to acknowledge the term *flipped learning*. A group of experienced educators created the Flipped Learning Network (FLN), an online community for educators interested in learning about flipped classroom. The FLN provides a formal definition of flipped classroom and flipped learning and does not use these two terms interchangeably. An educator can flip a class, but it does not mean the students will engage in flipped learning. The formal definition of flipped learning is "...a pedagogoical approach in which direct instruction moves from the group learning space to the individual learning space, and the resulting group space is transformed into a dynamic, interactive learning environment where the educator guides students as they apply concepts and engage creatively in the subject matter" (FLN, 2014). They provide four pillars for flipped learning: flexible environment, learning culture, intentional content, and professional educator (FLN, 2014). You can review the FLN website for additional information (https://flippedlearning.org).

> This website also provides a checklist to assess your flipped learning.

BACKGROUND

While some resources argue flipped classroom has been in existence for several years, a majority of educational literature recognizes Jonathan Bergman and Aaron Sams as the pioneers of this model. These two teachers taught high school chemistry at Woodland Park High School in Colorado. In 2006, they realized many students in their classes were missing large amounts of course material because they were traveling to distant, rural areas for sporting events and other school activities. During this time, online videos were in the early stages of development. Sams read about this new technology in a magazine and learned he could record and upload a voiceover PowerPoint presentation. The two educators realized this could be a solution for students that missed class to stay current on course content. A year later, they began recording live lectures using screen capture software. The students who missed class reported enjoying the lectures because they were able to still obtain the information. In addition, the students who were in class reported rewatching the videos and using the videos as a review before a test. Bergman and Sams found they were spending less time ensuring students were caught up with class. Because these videos were posted online, students and teachers across the country found and used the videos for their own chemistry courses.

In addition, Bergman and Sams realized students experienced challenges with transferring information from lectures to homework problems. They recognized the students really needed their assistance when they were stuck on a concept and not when they were talking at them in lecture. Therefore, they asked themselves, "What if we prerecorded all lectures, required the students to view as homework, and used the class time to answer questions and help students understand difficult concepts?" During the 2007 to 2008 school year, these two teachers committed to this method of learning. They realized this model was more efficient because the students were able to conduct experiments and complete problem work during class. They used the same exams from the prior year and had raw data to validate the flipped classroom was better than traditional lecture. A neighboring school asked these two teachers to speak about their model, and a few weeks later, a media outlet produced a short news story. Bergman and Sams began to train educators and speak about flipped classroom around the world.

In addition to Bergman and Sams, we need to recognize a few other pioneers for flipped classroom cited in educational literature. Lage and colleagues (2000) introduced the term *inverted classroom* as a method of teaching an introductory course in economics at Miami University. These educators desired to implement an inverted classroom to better address the different types of learning styles found in their courses. Their description of an inverted classroom mirrors the components of a flipped classroom, and these terms are often used interchangeably. Similarly, Crouch and Mazur (2001) introduced the idea of *peer instruction* after acknowledging students in their physics courses learn little from traditional lecture format. Similar to flipped classroom, students in peer instruction are required to complete readings prior to class. Educators give students credit for answering questions about readings to help identify gaps in knowledge and to provide an incentive to actually complete the readings. During the in-class portion of peer instruction, the students are expected to apply the concepts as they do in flipped classroom. However, educators describe the in-class portion differently than current literature on flipped classroom. In peer instruction, educators provide a short presentation and ask a question. The students think about the answer individually before discussing their answers with their peers. The educator roams the room during the discussion and polls the students for their final answer to ensure understanding before moving to the next concept.

> These educators did not actually coin the term flipped classroom and no one owns the term. Media popularized the term flipped classroom!

Health Professional Education

In January 2012, researchers published the first article about the use of flipped classroom in health professional education. Since this time, educators in various health professions are increasingly using this method in their classrooms. The literature has significantly grown with a majority of the published work cited in pharmacy and nursing education (see Flipped Classroom Evidence Table). One reason for this growth is the well-documented need to prepare health professional students to practice in dynamic and complex health care environments. The strategies we used to teach students in the 20th century are no longer adequate for bridging the education-to-practice gap.

Educators that implement the flipped classroom model have opportunities to facilitate the transition from the classroom to clinical or community-based practice. In the current health care landscape, technology is trending. Therefore, the Department of Health suggested health professionals should incorporate technology to enhance education and training. In a flipped classroom, educators use technology in a variety of ways. In addition, students collaborate with peers and the educator during class, which aids the development of communication and teamwork skills needed to work on interprofessional teams. Lastly, students engage in self-directed and high-level learning in this model. This affords health professional students the opportunity to grow these skills so they can better address the changing needs of clients, families, and communities. For these reasons, flipped classroom and health professional education appear to be a solid match.

THEORY

Educational literature often cites constructivism and behaviorism learning theories to support the use of a flipped classroom in higher education. Flipped classroom applies principles from behavioral learning theory in the portion of learning that occurs outside the classroom. According to the behavioral learning theory, an educator delivers content in the form of lecture, tutorials, or demonstrations (e.g., teacher-centered learning) and students are passive learners. The educator structures and maintains control of the learning context and provides reward structures to reinforce the behavior they desire (e.g., grades). Students engage in lower levels of cognitive learning, such as defining terms, recalling facts, or listing characteristics. In a flipped classroom, educators organize and provide pre-class work. Students complete this foundational learning (e.g., lower cognitive levels) before class in order to participate in class and receive some sort of feedback (reward) via an accountability task.

Meanwhile, educators apply the constructivism learning theory to the portion of flipped classroom that occurs within class. According to constructivist learning theory, students are the primary body of cognition and actively construct their own meaning of knowledge (as discussed in Chapter 1). The past experiences and knowledge of students serve as the basis for learning. In a flipped classroom, they bring new knowledge gained before class and personal experiences to the face-to-face class time. In addition, they construct knowledge by interacting with the world and with other individuals. Therefore, in a flipped classroom, the educator designs active instructional methods that require cooperation and conversation with peers and the educator in order to apply concepts and solve problems. Educators serve as a facilitator and provide students autonomy to freely explore and independently learn the content.

IMPLEMENTATION

As you read the following chapters in this textbook, you will notice a common theme: There is often no one way to deliver an instructional method. A flipped classroom approach to learning is no different, as there are many ways for an educator to flip a class period or course. Despite this information, educational literature does provide a basic structure for implementation of this learning approach.

Preparing for Flipped Classroom

Students in professional programs, such as occupational therapy, are accustomed to traditional forms of passive learning or may not have had exposure to a flipped classroom in their prior educational experiences. For these reasons, it is imperative that educators prepare the students for this shift in learning at the start of the course. **Clear communication and transparency are key factors for successful implementation of a flipped classroom**. Students need to understand what a flipped classroom is, why you are using this teaching-learning strategy, and how this method of learning will benefit them. Students tend to be more accepting of a decision when they understand the reasoning for the change. They should also have a clear understanding of your expectations for the time they will need to devote to complete pre-class activities and the ways you will hold them accountable to the information in class. You can provide this information in a variety of ways, such as a verbal discussion or written handout. Lastly, remember from Chapters 3 and 4, students have a fundamental desire to be heard. You can facilitate discussion so students can provide suggestions or feedback, which you can take into consideration when tweaking or developing course content.

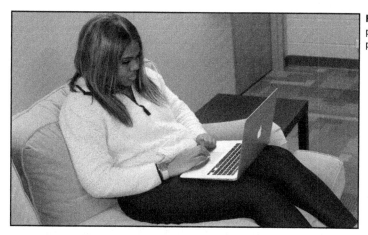

Figure 5-2. A student completes pre-class work at home at their own pace and time.

Pre-Class Work

Students are first exposed to *foundational* content prior to class through an eclectic range of learning activities and technologies. Students complete the pre-class work on their own time and at their own pace (Figure 5-2). Oftentimes, the educator uses various forms of technology to deliver the pre-class content. Examples include videos, audio-video or screen-capture software, voiceover presentations, podcasts, weblinks, automated tutoring systems, case-based presentations, or simulations (see Chapter 14).

However, you can also elect to use low-tech options, such as worksheets, readings, outlines, study guides, discussion boards, or prompting questions. We recommend you implement a combination and variety of low- and high-tech options throughout your course to best meet the needs of different learning styles. No matter which type of learning activities or technologies you select for pre-class work, it is important that you present the content in an organized fashion and provide specific and detailed instructions to avoid student confusion or frustration. You should prepare the learning objectives and develop the pre-class work at least a week or two before the actual class.

> Consider collaborating with an instructional designer at your institution to increase your comfort with available technologies!

Accountability

In order for in-class time to be successful and productive, the students need to arrive prepared to participate by completing the previously described pre-class work. Educators can create some sort of accountability activity to give the students an incentive to prepare for class. Examples include short quizzes, online discussions, submission of questions, worksheets, group work, or short writing assignments. The students appear to be more motivated if you assign a grade to the pre-class activity because they believe it is valuable for their learning. Several educators suggest making the grade for these activities low stake so the students can monitor their own performance without having a heavy effect on their course grade. In several cases, educators simply evaluated accountability activities for completion versus correctness. You could also periodically or randomly collect these activities to reduce the amount of time you spend grading. Not only do students benefit, but you receive valuable information from the accountability activities about what the students do or do not understand. You can further use this information to guide the in-class portion of the flipped classroom model.

> Faculty often describe the initial development of pre-class work as labor intensive!

Write down three additional ways you could hold the students accountable to the pre-class work.

In-Class Time

Despite the focus on the pre-class work, the students and educator experience the greatest benefits during the in-class portion of the flipped classroom model. During this time, you will want to incorporate instructional methods that actively engage students in higher-level cognitive thinking. However, it is important that you still devote time at the start of class to answer questions before transitioning to these in-class activities. Several authors recommend spending the first 10 minutes of each class answering any questions and clarifying any misconceptions or difficult concepts from the pre-class work. When you allow time for this discussion, the students in your course have greater opportunities to correctly practice and apply the concepts during class.

Educators that use a flipped classroom model employ a **myriad** of instructional methods during the in-class time. By using a **range** of methods, you create richer learning opportunities, allow for greater exploration of topics, and meet the needs of various learning styles. Similar to pre-class work, you can use high- and low-tech options or have students work individually or collaboratively in a group. We have provided a short list of instructional methods you could use in your course in Table 5-1. Many of these instructional methods are described in this book. It is our hope that you can incorporate any of the instructional methods in the upcoming chapters into your flipped classroom. In addition to these examples, you can use student response systems, such as iClicker or other applications, to obtain real-time assessment of what the students do and do not understand in class. We will also discuss technology in Chapter 14.

No matter which instructional method you select, we offer a few additional guidelines from literature for successful implementation of the in-class portion of the flipped classroom model:

- Remember, the activity must be active and require higher-level thinking skills, such as application, critical thinking, or professional reasoning.
- Ensure that you are making an explicit connection between the pre-class and in-class content.
- Give clear instructions and guidance.
- Provide enough time to complete the activity or assignment so students can adequately apply the knowledge obtained outside of class.
- Offer prompt feedback.

Educator's Role in the Classroom

Your role in the flipped classroom model is significantly different than your role in a traditional lecture-based model. You no longer deliver the information; you serve as the facilitator of information. As you walk around the room, you help students clarify confusing concepts, provide guiding prompts and feedback, create opportunities for students to connect with one another, and/or moderate discussion (Figure 5-3).

TABLE 5-1

Examples of Instructional Methods Used in Flipped Classroom

- Case studies (Chapter 12)
- Concept mapping (Chapter 11)
- Debate (Chapter 10)
- Discussion panel or expert-led discussion
- Games (Chapter 13)
- Group presentations
- Journal club
- Practical lab activities
- Problem-based learning (Chapter 12)
- Role play or skits (Chapter 7)
- Team-based presentations

After Class

Since the students have completed the harder application work in class, they can review or build on learned content after class. If you recognize students are experiencing challenges with a concept during class, you can provide additional resources, such as readings or a mini-lecture, for students to access after class. Burden and colleagues (2015) created an online folder for each module that offered students optional supplemental resources or learning activities to further enhance their learning. In addition, students can use these optional materials to assess their understanding, clarify areas of confusion, and engage in deeper learning. Similar to the pre-class work, they can complete these learning activities at their own pace, on their own time, and as they see fit.

> When you provide feedback in class, you will not have to provide extensive feedback outside of class.

Reflection

Finally, literature suggests that you engage in self-reflection following the class and course to assess your work and acknowledge feedback. Educators are most effective in implementing a flipped classroom when they are thoughtful about their teaching practices and are continuously modifying their classes (refer to Chapter 2). In a study on the use of flipped classroom in athletic training education, authors reported students provided a large amount of encouraging feedback to the educator and their peers throughout the course. In addition, Galway and colleagues (2015) met as an instructional team and used Gary Rolfe's reflective framework to debrief following each in-class time. Using this structure, educators asked three questions: What, so what, and now what. You might also consider the following questions:

- How did the instructional method I used during class go well? What are areas for improvement?
- How did the students apply the pre-class activities to the in-class activities?
- What gaps in knowledge occurred that need to be better addressed in the pre-class work?
- In what ways did I facilitate learning the best, and in what ways can I improve my facilitation skills during class?
- In what ways did the students demonstrate that they met the learning objectives?
- What feedback did the student provide that could improve this class?

Figure 5-3. Educator roams the room during class to provide feedback.

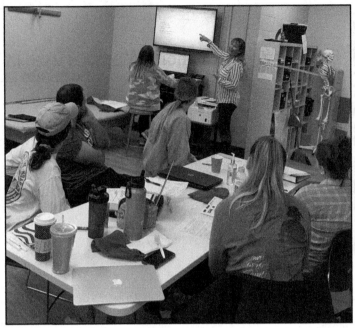

ADDITIONAL IMPLEMENTATION NOTES

Pre-Class Work

- Technologies need to be easy to use and accessible to students.
- Students should have easy access to or awareness of technical support.
- Provide students with a list of the learning objectives, concepts, and pre-class learning activities.
- Attempt to keep recorded lectures short; maximum of 20 minutes.

It generally takes about 30 minutes to create a 10-minute video.

In-Class Time

- Apply learning from pre-class work directly to in-class activities.
- Create a flexible classroom environment.
- Design in-class learning activities so students have enough time to apply the knowledge and skills gained prior to class.
- Serve as a highly supportive and engaged facilitator.
- Be creative and have fun with in-class activities.

After Class

- Engage frequently in reflection throughout the course, so you can modify the learning activities as needed (versus waiting until the end of the course).

TIPS AND TRICKS

General

- A few articles in educational literature suggest not to flip an entire course at once so that you and the students have a gradual introduction to this method of learning. By doing this, authors believe you build expertise in flipping the classroom while also decreasing student resistance. However, from our experience with implementing this instructional method, we support flipping an entire course. We found that student resistance to flipped classroom decreases after a couple of weeks of implementation. We encourage you to be patient and committed to the delivery of flipped classroom as the students take their time to adjust. If you switch between flipped classroom and a traditional classroom, students tend to default to the type of learning they are most comfortable with (traditional lecture) and do not fully adjust to or experience the benefits of flipped classroom.
- If you are new to this instructional method, start with an area of content that you believe can be easily flipped or with content that requires application.
- Using this method of learning takes practice, so stick with it!

Pre-Class Work

- Collaborate with an instructional designer or someone experienced with current technologies to develop pre-class work.
- Educate students to find their personal best way to view and complete the pre-class work.
- Inform the students about and encourage them to use the pause and rewind features of technological activities.
- Teach students about the Cornell method of notetaking (take notes, record questions, and summarize learning; http://lsc.cornell.edu/notes.html).
- Divide the pre-class work into manageable portions.
- Use audiovisuals when possible to provide the content in a multisensory manner.
- Include practice questions in pre-class work so students can apply the new knowledge immediately.

In-Class Time

- Introduce one or two instructional methods per class.

OPPORTUNITIES FOR FEEDBACK AND REFLECTION

Pre-Class Work

Students primarily receive feedback in pre-class work from accountability activities. As stated in the Tips and Tricks section, you can also include reflection and feedback in the pre-class work, so students have the opportunity to apply knowledge. For example, you could ask one or two simple questions about a video or reading. You can begin class with a short discussion of the questions you posed.

Examples of questions:

- How did you see [concept] in action during your fieldwork or in your observation experiences?
- How does [concept] apply to your everyday life?
- How did the reading change your viewpoint of [concept]?
- Do you agree or disagree with [concepts found in article]? Provide your reasoning.
- What additional information do you need to understand [concept]?

In-Class Time

In a flipped classroom, the educator is continuously monitoring student performance and providing immediate feedback during class. In fact, educational literature reports an educator can commit **more** time to the provision of feedback in a flipped classroom. As you roam the classroom, you will constantly observe your students and offer prompt feedback to quickly clarify any misconceptions or gaps in knowledge. You will likely discover that this is a demanding role; however, spending time providing feedback in-class will reduce the need for you to give extensive written feedback after class. As previously mentioned, you will use a variety of instructional methods during the face-to-face portion of a flipped classroom. Each of these instructional methods provide unique opportunities for reflection and feedback, which we will discuss in the following chapters of this book.

APPLICATION TO OCCUPATIONAL THERAPY PRACTICE

The clients we serve in practice are experiencing social changes because of the advent of various forms of technology and participation in more diverse communities. Technology has changed the way our clients work and live, and they are comfortable with its use. In addition, we are noticing shorter lengths of stay and tighter reimbursement in our practice settings. Therefore, it would behoove us to incorporate flipped classroom principles, so our clients can focus on problem solving and applying the ideas to their everyday lives.

Example 1: Implementation of Flipped Classroom Principles During Client Education

Perhaps you are in charge of providing preoperative education to clients scheduled for an elective hip, knee, or shoulder replacement (e.g., "joint camp"). Instead of presenting information to clients and their families in a 2-hour course, you could develop learning materials using various forms of technology. For example, you could create a voiceover presentation or video providing the foundational information. You could also include knowledge checks or a simple worksheet to use in conjunction with the technological component. The client and family can select which option best fits their needs and complete the content at their own pace and on their own time. The client and family would still attend the 2-hour course, but you would ask them to apply the concepts they learned prior to the course to their daily life. Maybe you provide the client with more opportunities to use the adaptive equipment or functional mobility devices, practice bed mobility and tub transfers, or discuss home modification or task adaptations.

Example 2: Implementation of Flipped Classroom When Learning New Techniques

In this second example, we will discuss the use of flipped classroom principles with an individual who has experienced a new injury, such as a spinal cord injury. In this scenario, you are working with this individual in an inpatient rehabilitation setting. Before your next session, you instruct the client to watch several videos or listen to a podcast by clients with similar injuries about how to complete dressing tasks while in long-sitting or at edge of bed with reduced sitting balance. During your session the next day, you answer any of the individual's questions and immediately begin applying what they learned to the actual task of dressing. The individual begins to problem solve while dressing, and you monitor performance and provide feedback.

Advantages

- Increases opportunities for faculty, students, and peer interaction
- Fosters the provision of immediate feedback
- Monitors learning and performance
- Supports a variety of learning styles
- Allows students the opportunity to develop communication skills
- Students can complete the learning activities prior to class at their own pace, at any time, and as many times as they would like
- Increases opportunities for students to apply knowledge
- Invites collaboration, teamwork, and peer interaction
- Allows for more class time for higher-level learning activities
- Allows students experiencing challenges with concepts to receive more assistance to improve understanding
- Expands on what students already know

Challenges

- Students and educators could resist the shift in learning
- Students and educators could experience technical difficulties
- Educators must initially devote significant time, thoughtful planning, and advance preparation to develop pre-class activities and interactive, active in-class activities
- Enrollment may be lower (compared to traditional lecture)
- Information technology department may need to provide support
- Educators must be aware of time students are required to commit to complete learning activities prior to class
- Educators must provide more assessment to ensure students are completing and understanding content (requires extra time to develop and grade)
- Student must find their own answers or wait until class to find the answers

In the space below, list any additional advantages or challenges.

[ ]

Brainstorm strategies for overcoming these challenges when implementing the use of flipped classroom.

[ ]

THREE THINGS YOU CAN DO TOMORROW TO IMPLEMENT FLIPPED CLASSROOM WITH YOUR STUDENTS

1. Ask a colleague or do a quick online search to determine if your institution offers resources for instructional design with technology to help you design pre-class work.
2. Identify one topic you are comfortable with and decide to flip it first. Take a moment to write how you could potentially deliver the content in pre-class work and in-class time.
3. Record one presentation for the students to view prior to class.

Flipped Classroom Evidence Table

Author/Year	Study Objectives	Design and Participants	Intervention and Outcome Measures	Results
Betihavas et al. (2016)	Researchers examined evidence for and outcomes of flipped classroom in nursing education	Design: Systematic review Selected 5 studies Participants: 934 nursing students	4 reviewers participated in selection and data extraction Databases: PubMed, Excerpta Medica, Embase, CINAHL, Education Resources Information Center (ERIC), Scopus Inclusion criteria: • Written in English • Peer-reviewed • Researched use of flipped classroom with nursing students Each study completed in United States between 2012 and 2015	Each study lasted a semester 2 of 5 studies employed quantitative outcome measures, while the other 3 used mixed methods 4 of 5 studies included undergraduate nursing students, while the other focused on postgraduate nursing students • 2 studies examined satisfaction scores; • 1 examined test scores, and 2 used satisfaction and exam scores 3 studies compared student performance in flipped to traditional classrooms; 2 of these studies reported no differences, and 1 study reported significantly higher scores on exams when engaged in flipped classroom approach Of the 4 studies that explored student satisfaction, results were mixed
Chen et al. (2017)	Researchers desired to understand evidence (quality, scope, and effectiveness) of published studies of flipped classroom in medical education	Design: Systematic review Selected 46 articles Participants: Medical students	2 researchers reviewed each article Databases: PubMed, Scopus, Academic Search Premier, Education Full Text, ERIC No date restrictions; written in English	15 of the 46 studies broadly included medical students or were nonspecific; 8 included first- and second-year medical students; 11 included third- and fourth-year medical students; 9 articles included residency; 2 included fellowship Of 46 articles: • 13 commentaries • 9 controlled • 8 postcourse design • 2 pre/post

(continued)

Flipped Classroom Evidence Table (continued)

Author/Year	Study Objectives	Design and Participants	Intervention and Outcome Measures	Results
			Each study completed in United States between 2012 and 2015	• 2 literature reviews • 4 pre/post with postsurvey Themes from 6 controlled studies suggest medical studies were satisfied with flipped classroom, in-class quizzes, and problem-solving practice 3 studies reported positive changes in students' attitudes following participation in flipped classroom Researchers found mixed results of changes in knowledge and skills following flipped classroom
Dombrowski et al. (2018)	Researchers examined the use of a flipped classroom design in an otorhinolaryngology (ORL) course	Design: Quasi-randomized design Participants: 212 medical students enrolled in an ORL course	Intervention: Researchers implemented a flipped classroom design in a practical ORL course by creating an online learning program to be completed before each class session Researchers randomly assigned students to participate in the online program, with about half of the class receiving access to the online program and access being withheld from the other half of the class	Students using the online learning program/flipped classroom felt favorably about both the structure and design of the program Most students using the online learning program felt more prepared and knowledgeable about course topics as a result of the flipped classroom design Nearly two thirds of students enrolled in the online learning program reported frequent use of the program, which was also associated with more positive perceptions of the flipped classroom design Students from both groups expressed interest in ORL topics and using online learning programs more often

(continued)

Flipped Classroom Evidence Table (continued)

Author/Year	Study Objectives	Design and Participants	Intervention and Outcome Measures	Results
			Outcome measures: Evaluation-based questionnaire using 2 different Likert scales completed at the end of the course (4-point Likert scale to evaluate student preparation for class sessions and comprehension of class concepts; 6-point Likert scale to evaluate student perceptions of the online course program)	
Hew & Lo (2018)	Researchers contrasted flipped classroom and traditional classrooms in health professions education	Design: Meta-analysis Included 28 articles Participants: 2,295 participants in flipped classroom and 2,420 participants in traditional classroom	Followed Preferred Reporting Items for Systematic Reviews and Meta-Analyses (PRISMA) guidelines Databases: Academic Search Complete, PubMed, PsycINFO, CINAHL Plus, TOC Premier, British Nursing Index, ERIC Inclusion criteria: • Compared flipped classroom versus traditional classroom • Focused on health professional education • Implemented pre- and in-class activities • Included use of pre-class activities of recorded lectures, instructor voiceover presentation, YouTube videos, TED talks, screencasts, and Khan Academy videos • Had a face-to-face meeting with students • Included a traditional classroom with lecture	Results favor a flipped classroom approach for participants engaged in health professional education Participants in flipped classroom demonstrated greater learning performance 70% of participants reported preference for flipped classroom Use of quizzes at beginning of in-class time makes flipped classroom more effective Participants that preferred the traditional classroom reported pre-class instruction required too much time

(continued)

Flipped Classroom Evidence Table (continued)

Author/Year	Study Objectives	Design and Participants	Intervention and Outcome Measures	Results
			• Randomized controlled trial (RCT), quasi-experimental, or historical cohort-controlled designs • Measured student learning • Written in English • Published in peer-review journal Dates of publication: 2012 to 2017	
Hu et al. (2018)	Researchers examined the efficacy of flipped classroom instructional methods in Chinese nursing educational programs	Design: Meta-analysis Selected 11 studies Participants: 1,484 undergraduate nursing students	2 independent raters evaluated the studies and a third rater was used to resolve any discrepancies Followed PRISMA guidelines Databases: PubMed, Embase, CENTRAL, CINAHL, CNKI, Wanfang Data, VIP Inclusion criteria: • Baccalaureate nursing students in China • Researched the use of flipped classroom as the primary intervention • Comparison methods included traditional in-person lectures • Researched outcomes related to student knowledge and skills • RCTs • Written in English or Chinese Exclusion criteria: • Incomplete data • Conference abstracts	Flipped classroom methods were used in different categories of nursing courses with varying levels of difficulty 8 studies reported an increase in student theoretical knowledge after participation in a flipped classroom design 4 studies reported an increase in nursing skills after participation in a flipped classroom design Evidence presented in each study was graded as low for understanding of content and very low for evaluation of nursing-related skills Sensitivity analysis confirmed findings of meta-analysis

(continued)

Flipped Classroom Evidence Table (continued)

Author/Year	Study Objectives	Design and Participants	Intervention and Outcome Measures	Results
Kim et al. (2019)	Researchers examined the impact of a flipped classroom design on nursing student outcomes in a patient safety course	Design: Quasi-experimental pre/posttest design Participants: 75 nursing students at a university in Seoul, South Korea • Experimental group: 32 students • Control group: 43 students Experimental group inclusion criteria: • Nursing students enrolled in the designated patient safety course in the fall of 2018 • Nursing students who successfully completed the patient safety course • Documented consent to participate	Intervention: Participants in the experimental group participated in a flipped classroom design used to teach World Health Organization concepts related to patient safety in the nursing profession Instructors used a combination of online and in-person sessions over the course of 14 weeks, with each session lasting 2 hours once a week The flipped classroom design included multiple instructional methods, including lectures, group work, group discussions, and online knowledge assessments Control group participants received no intervention and were not enrolled in the patient safety course Outcome measures: • Survey administered to participants, which included questionnaire about student characteristics • PSCSE contains a 5-point Likert scale to assess students' perceptions of attitude, skills, and knowledge related to patient safety competency Experimental group completed the survey at the beginning and end of the semester Control group completed the survey only at the close of the semester	Both groups were similar regarding student characteristics Students who participated in the patient safety course, using a flipped classroom design, demonstrated improvements in all aspects of the Patient Safety Competency Self-Evaluation (PSCSE), including patient safety competency attitudes, skills, and knowledge PSCSE scores, specifically in the patient safety skills and knowledge domains, were significantly higher for those who participated in the patient safety course as opposed to those who did not (control group) when assessed at the end of the semester

(continued)

Flipped Classroom Evidence Table (continued)

Author/Year	Study Objectives	Design and Participants	Intervention and Outcome Measures	Results
McCabe et al. (2017)	Researchers compared the effectiveness of flipped classroom versus traditional didactic course for self-care content Researchers focused on the impact of these teaching methods on student learning	Design: Quasi-experimental design Participants: Pharmacy students; 54 second-year participants in traditional course group (control) and 26 first-year participants in the intervention group (flipped classroom)	Control group: Traditional self-care course with an experiential learning course in community practice Intervention group: Flipped classroom course with online modules in community practice only Outcome measures: Knowledge and confidence scores through a pre/posttest survey (24 items)	Pretest knowledge scores higher in traditional group The traditional group received higher posttest scores than flipped group The traditional course group reported significantly higher confidence than the flipped group in each of the topics
Njie-Carr et al. (2017)	Researchers evaluated evidence of flipped classroom models with nursing students in order to best inform nursing educators	Design: Integrative review Selected 13 studies Participants: Nursing students	4 researchers conducted literature search and reviewed findings Databases: PubMed, Embase, CINAHL, Scopus, Web of Science, Google Scholar; searched additional journals Reviewed national and international studies that used flipped classroom models in nursing education through May 2016 Outcome measures: · Course grades · Student satisfaction	Of the 13 studies, 4 studies were quasi or experimental designs, 5 were descriptive, and 4 were mixed-methods 11 of the 13 studies were completed with undergraduate nursing students; 1 study completed with associate degree nursing students; 1 study with graduate nursing students Variety of content areas Improved course grades and student satisfaction as a result of participation in flipped classroom Studies reported faculty need to dedicate more time for development of course-related activities; need for more technological support Key to success in flipped classroom is student preparation before class

(continued)

Flipped Classroom Evidence Table (continued)

Author/Year	Study Objectives	Design and Participants	Intervention and Outcome Measures	Results
				Vast differences in how educators implemented flipped classroom model
				Students expressed concerns about increased amount of work and ability to manage their time
Ohtake et al. (2018)	Researchers investigated the outcomes of an evidence-based practice (EBP) interprofessional program, using a flipped classroom design, for enhancing EBP-related knowledge and skills in health professions students Researchers aimed to: • Help students develop EBP knowledge and skills • Apply EBP skills to a clinical case • Educate students on the obligations of various health professionals	Design: Cross-sectional posttest Participants: 39 college students in various health professions programs at both the State University of New York College at Buffalo and the University at Buffalo • Students who understood the professional demands of their specific health care field • Students required to have some degree of clinical experience Participating health profession programs: • Dental medicine • Dietetics	Intervention: Faculty members instructed participants to complete 3 modules in preparation for the interprofessional education event: • 2 EBP modules (2 hours in duration) • 1 interprofessional education module about roles and responsibilities (90 minutes in duration) Faculty members facilitated small group discussions amongst participating students Faculty members presented a case study to each small group and instructed group members to collaboratively develop an appropriate response for the patient's health needs Group members contributed their respective health care field's role to the case and supported this contribution with evidence from available literature Faculty members facilitated a final discussion amongst all participants about each group's established plan and the importance of collaboration between health care professionals	Most students scored 75% or greater on the modules assessing knowledge of EBP-related concepts All students demonstrated proficiency (score of 80% or higher) on the modules assessing student understanding of the professional obligations of health care professionals The Comprehensive Readiness for Interprofessional Learning Scale scores significantly improved after completion of both components of the program, including the modules and interprofessional education activity Students reported that knowledge about EBP-related concepts was helpful when working through a patient scenario in a group Students valued the experience of working with other health care professions to solve realistic patient scenarios A majority of students favored the flipped classroom method as compared to less interactive instructional methods, especially in an interprofessional setting

(continued)

Flipped Classroom Evidence Table (continued)

Author/Year	Study Objectives	Design and Participants	Intervention and Outcome Measures	Results
	• Help students learn to collaborate with different professions • Examine the efficacy of a flipped classroom design for implementing an EBP-based interprofessional program	• Medicine • Occupational therapy • Pharmacy • Physical therapy • Social work • Speech-language pathology	Outcome measures: • Student understanding of the EBP process with assessments, which were completed prior to the group activity • Comprehensive Readiness for Interprofessional Learning Scale assessed the students' opinions about and ability to benefit from an interprofessional education experience • Student evaluation of the program in its entirety (5-point Likert scale)	
Park & Park (2018)	Researchers examined the impact of a flipped classroom on nursing student outcomes	Design: Quasi-experimental study with pre/posttest design Participants: 81 nursing students enrolled in an adult health nursing course	Intervention: All students enrolled in an adult health nursing course participated in traditional instructional methods for the first portion of the semester The course instructor implemented a flipped classroom design for students in the experimental group for the remainder of the academic term The flipped classroom structure consisted of a variety of pre-class assignments and in-class activities, such as group work, group discussions, and academic assessments Biweekly, the instructor administered a knowledge check at the end of class Researchers assessed academic performance at the mid-semester mark (pretest) and at the end of the semester (posttest)	Students' critical thinking skills improved after participating in a flipped classroom design Confirmatory factor analysis revealed 2 components of students' critical thinking skills—intellectual integrity and creativity Both of these subcategories of critical thinking also improved after implementation of a flipped classroom design Students' academic performance improved after participating in a flipped classroom design A regression analysis revealed students with greater creative skills and grade point averages were more likely to experience greater academic achievement after participation in a flipped classroom

(continued)

Flipped Classroom Evidence Table (continued)

Author/Year	Study Objectives	Design and Participants	Intervention and Outcome Measures	Results
			Outcome measures: • Critical Thinking Disposition Scale • Self-report measure to assess critical thinking scales (5-point Likert scale) • Student academic performance with evaluation measure developed by study's investigators (4-point Likert scale)	
Pierce & Fox (2012)	Researchers examined the efficacy of a flipped classroom instructional approach for pharmacy students	Design: Cross-sectional, pre/posttest design Participants: 71 pharmacy students enrolled in an 8-week pharmacy integrated therapeutics course; course met 2 times per week for 120 minutes	Intervention: Students took an initial pretest to assess knowledge of course concepts Students reviewed "vodcasts," which are prerecorded lecture videos from a previous academic year, about kidney dialysis prior to attending class Instructors facilitated a process-oriented guided inquiry learning (POGIL) activity in the following class sessions that challenged students to apply the concepts learned in the vodcasts to patient scenarios Outcome measures: • Academic achievement—student knowledge about topics relating to renal pharmacotherapy was assessed by pre/posttest measures occurring before and after the POGIL/flipped classroom activity • Student opinions about the POGIL/flipped classroom activity (10-question survey using a Likert scale to measure student perceptions)	Statistically significant improvement in the students' academic performance after using a flipped classroom model Students who participated in a flipped classroom model in 2012 scored higher on the final examination than students who were not exposed to this method in 2011 The majority of students felt positively about the POGIL activity and flipped classroom structure after implementation of this program Students believed the POGIL activity enhanced student learning and accountability, specifically through watching the vodcasts Over half of the participants (62%) preferred the flipped classroom model to be the dominant model used in the classroom

(continued)

Flipped Classroom Evidence Table (continued)

Author/Year	Study Objectives	Design and Participants	Intervention and Outcome Measures	Results
Presti (2015)	Researchers examined the available literature on flipped classroom instructional methods in higher nursing education	Design: Integrative review Selected 13 studies Participants: Nursing students	Databases: CINAHL, ERIC, PubMed, Medline Industries Search terms: flipped classroom, inverted classroom, nursing education Inclusion criteria: • Researched use of a flipped classroom in the education of nursing students • Undergraduate, graduate, and postgraduate education Articles published between January 2010 and September 2015	Of the 13 studies, 2 studies examined the supporting theories of a flipped classroom approach; the remaining 11 studies reported on the actual experience of using a flipped classroom in nursing education Theoretical frameworks thought to be linked with flipped classrooms include behavioral learning theory, constructivist learning theory, and heutagogy 5 studies reviewed the process of transitioning from a traditional classroom to a flipped classroom, 1 of which reported that a flipped classroom approach was an equally effective teaching strategy as a traditional classroom Student satisfaction was mixed with a flipped classroom approach • Multiple studies reported increase in student involvement and motivation during class activities after implementing flipped classroom format • 1 study mentioned that student satisfaction actually decreased after the use of a flipped classroom, but it is unclear if the flipped classroom was the reason for the lower satisfaction scores Flipped classrooms were associated with higher exam scores in 2 studies

(continued)

Flipped Classroom Evidence Table (continued)

Author/Year	Study Objectives	Design and Participants	Intervention and Outcome Measures	Results
Tan et al. (2017)	Researchers examined the effects of flipped classroom compared to traditional lecture in nursing education Researchers desired to understand the effects of flipped classroom versus traditional classroom on knowledge, skills, and attitudes in nursing education Researchers investigated students' rating of questionnaires about the effectiveness of flipped classroom	Design: Meta-analysis Included 29 studies Participants: Pooled sample size included 1,896 participants in intervention group (flipped classroom) and 1,798 in control group (traditional)	Followed PRISMA guidelines Databases searched: PubMed, EMBASE, Science Direct, CINAHL, Google Scholar, CMKI, WanFang Data, VIP, CMB Inclusion criteria: • Participants in higher education (associate, undergraduate, or postgraduate degree) • RCT design • Intervention group included flipped classroom • Control group included traditional lecture • Measurable outcomes • Written in English or Chinese Exclusion criteria: • Participants from another discipline other than nursing • Non-RCT • Flipped classroom implemented at the same time as another instructional method • Nonextractable outcome data Outcome measures: • Examination scores • Questionnaires	15 studies included undergraduates and 14 studies included associate degree students 16 studies examined theoretical knowledge; of these, 13 demonstrated significant differences between the 2 groups (in support of flipped classroom) 16 studies included scores in skills examination; of these, 13 demonstrated significant differences in favor of flipped classroom 15 studies examined students' self-learning skills; students in these studies agreed flipped classroom improved their learning 19 studies investigated students' self-report of flipped classroom on teaching effectiveness; most students had positive comments about flipped classroom; 87% of students reported preference for flipped classroom

(continued)

Flipped Classroom Evidence Table (continued)

Author/Year	Study Objectives	Design and Participants	Intervention and Outcome Measures	Results
Ward et al. (2018)	Researchers examined the process of implementing a flipped classroom design in nursing classrooms, the perceived efficacy of flipped classrooms, and their impact on student learning	Design: Systematic review

Selected 14 studies

Participants: Nursing students | Databases: CINAHL Complete, Cochrane Library, Lexi-Comp Online, PsychInfo, National Guideline Clearinghouse, Medline Complete, Academic Search Complete

Search terms: flipped classroom and nursing, flipped nursing, flipped classroom and nursing school, nursing course redesign, experiential education methodology, scattered classroom nursing, hybrid nursing class, transformative learning

Inclusion criteria:
- Primary research studies
- Researched the flipped classroom instructional method in post-secondary education programs
- Included either pre/postregistered nursing programs
- Written in English

Exclusion criteria:
- Dissertations, articles, editorials
- Educational programs using a flipped classroom with students other than nursing students
- Research published before 2007 | 7 qualitative, 2 quantitative, 3 quasi-experimental, and 2 mixed methods studies were included in this review

All levels of nursing education (Bachelor of Science in Nursing, doctoral, graduate, associate degree) were represented in this review

Courses utilizing flipped classroom frameworks often assigned material to review prior to each class; specific format of this material ranged from prerecorded lectures to textbook readings

Case studies were commonly implemented during classes (used by 9 of 14 included studies)

Other common in-class activities used in flipped classroom design were group discussions, videos, group projects, and games

Student perceptions of flipped classroom were mixed; majority of studies reported favorable student perceptions of flipped classroom, but many students also reported negative feelings about the time and effort required for flipped classroom design

Results were inconclusive regarding student preference for a flipped classroom over traditional instructional methods |

(continued)

Flipped Classroom Evidence Table (continued)

Author/Year	Study Objectives	Design and Participants	Intervention and Outcome Measures	Results
				Faculty members also reported an increase in time and effort required to successfully implement a flipped classroom design
				Student academic performance increased in nearly all studies that obtained numerical data about flipped classrooms
				Flipped classrooms were found to improve more abstract aspects of student learning, such as judgment and communication skills, in multiple studies

Adapted from American Occupational Therapy Association. (2002). AOTA's evidence-based literature review project: An overview (D. Lieberman & J. Scheer, Eds.). *American Journal of Occupational Therapy, 56*, 344-349. https://doi.org/10.5014/ajot.56.3.344

REFERENCES

American Occupational Therapy Association. (2002). AOTA's evidence-based literature review project: An overview (D. Lieberman & J. Scheer, Eds.). *The American Journal of Occupational Therapy, 56,* 344-349. https://doi.org/10.5014/ajot.56.3.344

Betihavas, V., Bridgman, H., Kornhaber, R., & Cross, M. (2016). The evidence for "flipping out": A systematic review of the flipped classroom in nursing education. *Nurse Education Today, 38,* 15-21. http://dx.doi.org/10.1016/j.nedt.2015.12.010

Burden, M. L., Carlton, K. H., Siktberg, L., & Pavlechko, G. (2015). Flipping the classroom: Strategies for psychiatric-mental health course. *Nurse Educator, 40*(5), 233-236. https://dx.doi.org/10.1097/NNE.0000000000000162

Chen, F., Lui, A. M., & Martinelli, S. M. (2017). A systematic review of the effectiveness of flipped classrooms in medical education. *Medical Education, 51,* 585-597. https://doi.org/10.1111/medu.13272

Crouch, C. H., & Mazur, E. (2001). Peer instruction: Ten years of experience and results. *American Journal of Physics, 69*(9), 970-977. http://dx.doi.org/10.1119/1.1374249

Dombrowski, T., Wrobel, C., Dazert, S., & Volkenstein, S. (2018). Flipped classroom frameworks improve efficacy in undergraduate practical courses – a quasi-randomized pilot study in otorhinolaryngology. *BMC Medical Education, 18*(294), 1-7. https://doi.org/10.1186/s12909-018-1398-5

Flipped Learning Network. (2014). The four pillars of F-L-I-P™ [PDF file]. Retrieved from https://flippedlearning.org/definition-of-flipped-learning/

Galway, L. P., Berry, B., & Takaro, T. K. (2015). Student perceptions and lessons learned from flipping a master's level environmental and occupational health course. *Canadian Journal of Learning and Technology, 41*(2), 1-13.

Hew, K. F., & Lo, C. K. (2018). Flipped classroom improves student learning in health professions education: A meta-analysis. *BMC Medical Education, 18*(38), 1-12. https://doi.org/10.1186/s12909-018-1144-z

Hu, R., Gao, H., Ye, Y., Ni, Z., Jiang, N., & Jiang, X. (2018). Effectiveness of flipped classrooms in Chinese baccalaureate nursing education: A meta-analysis of randomized controlled trials. *International Journal of Nursing Studies, 79,* 94-103. https://doi.org/10.1016/j.ijnurstu.2017.11.012

Kim, Y. M., Yoon, Y. S., Hong, H. C., & Min, A. (2019). Effects of a patient safety course using a flipped classroom approach among undergraduate nursing students: A quasi-experimental study. *Nurse Education Today, 79,* 180-187. https://doi.org/10.1016/j.nedt.2019.05.033

Lage, M. J., Platt, G. J., & Treglia, M. (2000). Inverting the classroom: A gateway to creating an inclusive learning environment. *Journal of Economic Education, 31*(1), 30-43.

McCabe, C., Smith, M. G., & Ferreri, S. P. (2017). Comparison of flipped module to traditional classroom learning in a professional pharmacy course. *Education Science, 7*(73), 1-7. https://dx.doi.org/10.3390/educsci7030073

Njie-Carr, V. P. S., Ludeman, E., Lee, M. C., Dordunoo, D., Trocky, N. M., & Jenkins, L. S. (2017). An integrative review of flipped classroom teaching models in nursing education. *Journal of Professional Nursing, 33*(2), 133-144. http://dx.doi.org/10.1016/j.profnurs.2016.07.001

Ohtake, P. J., Lyons, A., Glogowski, M., Stellrecht, E., Aronoff, N., Grabowski, J., & Zafron, M. L. (2018). Using interprofessional flipped classroom educational strategy for developing evidence-based practice knowledge and skills. *Journal of Interprofessional Education & Practice, 11,* 7-11. http://dx.doi.org/10.1016/j.xjep.2017.12.010

Park, E. O., & Park, J. H. (2018). Quasi-experimental study on the effectiveness of a flipped classroom for teaching adult health nursing. *Japan Journal of Nursing Science, 15,* 125-134.

Pierce, R., & Fox, J. (2012). Vodcasts and active-learning exercises in a "flipped classroom" model of a renal pharmacotherapy module. *American Journal of Pharmaceutical Education, 76*(10), 1-5. https://doi.org/10.5688/ajpe7610196

Presti, C. R. (2015). The flipped learning approach in nursing education: A literature review. *Journal of Nursing Education, 55*(5), 253-257. https://dx.doi.org/10.3928/01484834-20160414-03

Tan, C., Yue, W. G., & Fu, Y. (2017). Effectiveness of flipped classrooms in nursing education: Systematic review and meta-analysis. *Chinese Nursing Research, 4,* 192-200. https://dx.doi.org/10.1016/j.cnre.2017.10.006

Ward, M., Knowlton, M. C., & Laney, C. W. (2018). The flip side of traditional nursing education: A literature review. *Nurse Education in Practice, 29,* 163-171. https://doi.org/10.1016/j.nepr.2018.01.003

BIBLIOGRAPHY

Barbour, C., & Schuessler, J. B. (2019). A preliminary framework to guide implementation of the flipped classroom method in nursing education. *Nurse Education in Practice, 34,* 36-42. https://doi.org/10.1016/j.nepr.2018.11.001

Bergmann, J., & Sams, A. (2012a). Before you flip, consider this. *The Phi Delta Kappan, 94*(2), 25.

Bergmann, J., & Sams, A. (2012b). *Flip your classroom: Reach every student in every class every day.* International Society for Technology in Education.

Boyce, H., Cassilly, H., & Giles, A. K. (2017). Flipping the classroom using interactive mobile applications. *OT Practice, 22*(2), 16-17.

Brame, C. J. (2013). Flipping the classroom. *Vanderbilt University Center for Teaching.* Retrieved from http://cft.vanderbilt.edu/guides-sub-pages/flipping-the-classroom/

Cabi, E. (2018). The impact of the flipped classroom model on students' academic achievement. *International Review of Research in Open and Distributed Learning, 19*(3), 202-221.

Hawks, S. J. (2014). The flipped classroom: Now or never? *AANA Journal, 82*(4), 264-269.

Henderson, W., Coopard, B., & Qi, Y. (2018). Identifying instructional methods for the development of clinical reasoning in entry-level occupational therapy education. *Journal of Occupational Therapy Education, 1*(2), 7211505146.

Hutchings, M., & Quinney, A. (2015). The flipped classroom, disruptive pedagogies, enabling technologies, and wicked problems: Responding to the "bomb in the basement". *The Electronic Journal of e-Learning, 13*(2), 106-119.

Kay, D., & Kiblle, J. (2016). Learning theories 101: Application to everyday teaching and scholarship. *Advanced Physiology Education, 40*, 17-25. https://doi.org/10.1152/advan.00132.2015

Kim, M. K., Kim, S. M., Khera, O., & Getman, J. (2014). The experience of three flipped classrooms in an urban university: An exploration of design principles. *Internet and Higher Education, 22*, 37-50. http://dx.doi.org/10.1016/j.iheduc.2014.04.003

Matsuda, Y., Azaiza, K., & Salani, D. (2017). Flipping the classroom without flipping out the students. *Distance Education, 14*(1), 31-42.

McLaughlin, J. E., Roth, M. T., Glatt, D. M., Gharkholonarehe, N., Davidson, C. A., Griffin, L. M., Esserman, D. A., & Mumper, R. J. (2014). The flipped classroom: A course redesign to foster learning and engagement in a health professions school. *Academic Medicine, 89*(2), 236-243. https://doi.org/10.1097/ACM.0000000000000086

O'Flaherty, J., & Phillips, C. (2015). The use of flipped classrooms in higher education: A scoping review. *Internet and Higher Education, 25*, 85-95. http://dx.doi.org/10.1016/j.iheduc.2015.02.002

Rolfe, G., Freshwater, D., & Jasper, M. (2001). *Critical reflection for nursing and the helping professions: A user's guide.* Palgrave Macmillan.

Telford, M., & Senior, E. (2017). Healthcare students' experiences when integrating e-learning and flipped classroom instructional approaches. *British Journal of Nursing, 26*(11), 617-622.

Thompson, G. A., & Ayers, S. F. (2015). Measuring student engagement in a flipped athletic training classroom. *Journal of Athletic Training Education, 10*(4), 315-322. https://dx.doi.org/10.4085/1004315

Xu, Z., & Shi, Y. (2018). Application of constructivist theory in flipped classroom—take college English teaching as a case study. *Theory and Practice in Language Studies, 8*(7), 880-887. http://dx.doi.org/10.17507/tpls.0807.21

6

EXPERIENTIAL LEARNING INSTRUCTIONAL METHODS

Whitney Henderson, OTD, MOT, OTR/L
Haley Homan, MOT, OTR/L
Kelli Bayne, MOT, OTR/L

BASIC TENETS

Experiential learning instructional methods are high-impact educational practices that afford students opportunities to apply their knowledge and skills to *real-life contexts*. According to the Association for Experiential Education (AEE; 2019), experiential education happens when "… educators purposefully engage with learners in direct **experience** and focused **reflection** in order to increase knowledge, develop skills, clarify values, and develop people's capacity to contribute to their communities." The AEE outlines 12 principles for effective experiential learning practices, while the National Society for Experiential Education identifies eight principles for good practices in experiential learning (Table 6-1). Both groups address similar key points.

In experiential learning methods, students enhance, test, and apply knowledge in an actual practice environment. In addition, they have opportunities to practice skills before entering the demands of professional practice so they can refine critical attributes for effective practice. They need these experiences to be as close to **real life** as possible so they understand the significance and become curious and self-directed (e.g., the difference between simulation and experiential). It is the experience that provides the source for the thoughtful reflection that facilitates learning. They do not simply participate in an experience but engage in an authentic interaction to construct their own meaning to learn deeply. Educational literature provides a great variety of experiential learning opportunities. In this chapter, we will discuss the experiential learning instructional methods of service learning and field experiences. In addition, we will provide several examples of contexts and assignments found in health professional education that provide authenticity.

Similar to our profession's beliefs that our clients and families need to learn skills in the contexts in which they will actually use those skills, our students benefit most when they learn in the actual environments in which they will practice. As discussed in Chapter 1, Schaber (2014) outlined three signature pedagogies unique to occupational therapy education: (1) relational learning, (2) affective

Henderson, W. (Ed.). *Effective Teaching: Instructional Methods and Strategies for Occupational Therapy Education* (pp. 101-127).
© 2021 Taylor & Francis Group.

Table 6-1

Principles for Good Experiential Learning

ASSOCIATION FOR EXPERIENTIAL EDUCATION	NATIONAL SOCIETY FOR EXPERIENTIAL EDUCATION
• Experiential learning occurs when carefully chosen experiences are supported by reflection, critical analysis, and synthesis.	• Intention
• Experiences are structured to require students to take initiative, make decisions, and be accountable for results.	• Preparedness and planning • Acknowledgement
• Throughout the experiential learning process, the students are actively engaged in posing questions, investigating, experimenting, being curious, solving problems, assuming responsibility, being creative, and constructing meaning.	
• Students are engaged intellectually, emotionally, socially, soulfully, and/or physically. This involvement produces a perception that the learning task is authentic.	• Authenticity
• The results of the learning are personal and form the basis for future experience and learning.	• Assessment and evaluation
• Relationships are developed and nurtured: student to self, student to others, and student to the world at large.	
• The educator and students may experience success, failure, adventure, risk-taking, and uncertainty because the outcomes of experience cannot totally be predicted.	
• Opportunities are nurtured for students and educators to explore and examine their own values.	• Reflection
• The educator's primary roles include setting suitable experiences, posing problems, setting boundaries, supporting students, insuring physical and emotional safety, and facilitating the learning process.	• Orientation and training
• The educator recognizes and encourages spontaneous opportunities for learning.	
• Educators strive to be aware of their biases, judgments, and preconceptions and how these influence the learner.	
• The design of the learning experience includes the possibility to learn from natural consequences, mistakes, and successes.	• Monitoring and continuous improvement

TABLE 6-2

Relationship Between Signature Pedagogies and Experiential Learning

SIGNATURE PEDAGOGY	DEFINITION	RELATIONSHIP TO EXPERIENTIAL LEARNING
Relational Learning	Students obtain new knowledge through a human connection.	Students engaged in experiential learning interact with individuals in their communities and reflect on those experiences to develop professional knowledge and personal attributes.
Affective Learning	Students develop a personal identity as they evaluate and alter their attitudes, beliefs, and values.	Students engaged in experiential learning reflect on their attitudes, values, and beliefs, and how their points of view have changed or broadened as a result of participating in the experience.
Highly Contextualized, Active Engagement	Students learn by doing when they actively use their skills and knowledge in a real context.	Students engaged in experiential learning increase and apply their knowledge and skills in a real-life context.

learning, and (3) highly contextualized, active engagement (Table 6-2). In addition, as educators, we have a responsibility to provide our students experience that fosters better understanding of the complex lives of the individuals we serve in practice. When we employ experiential learning in our courses, we promote the characteristics of our professional education.

Occupational therapy evidence in experiential education suggests students are more likely to be prepared for practice. Graduates possess a greater understanding of the link between theory and practice and have improved confidence, professional reasoning, and communication. In addition, our students begin to reconceptualize professional practice and further consider new areas of employment following graduation.

BACKGROUND

The idea of experiential learning has a long history in the field of education. The roots of these instructional methods date back to 4th century B.C. when Aristotle suggested students understand theory after they have the opportunity to apply it to experiences. During the time period between 1910 and 1930, John Dewey produced work challenging educators to create learning opportunities immersed in real-life experiences. In 1938, he published a short book titled, *Experience and Education*, to promote the use of experience to enhance learning, augment learning styles, and develop autonomous learning contexts. In the 1970s, educators recognized and embraced experiential learning. Educators in outdoor and adventure programs were among the early adopters of this method, as they would take their students outside to engage in real-world situations to achieve their desired learning goals. In 1977, the AEE established an international organization "...committed to the practice and promotion of learning through experience" (AEE, 2019). In the following decade, David Kolb further expanded on the work of Dewey to create his experiential learning theory, which provides a framework for this educational practice. Educators in health professional education have commonly included experiential learning as a component of their courses for several decades.

For example, in health professional education literature, we observe more historical information about the experiential learning instructional method of *service learning*. Since the creation of the Health Professions Schools in Service to the Nation program in 1995, educators have widely implemented service learning into their professional curricula. The Corporation for National and Community Service and The Pew Charitable Trusts sponsored this 3-year, 20-institution program to explore how service learning could prepare students in health professions for the ever-changing health delivery system and could foster partnerships between higher education institutions and communities to improve health. As supported by a systematic review, medicine and nursing have been the primary adopters and scholars of service learning to date. In occupational therapy education, we notice the use of service learning around 1997 when scholars reported students gained increase awareness of and insight to diversity and the perspectives of individuals with disabilities. Educators in occupational therapy programs increasingly use service learning. Professional literature provides abundant information for developing these beneficial experiences with much of the research in occupational therapy education composed of qualitative and mixed method designs.

Similarly, since 2003, educators in physical therapy education have integrated service learning into their professional programs. Since that time until 2018, scholars have published approximately 28 studies on the use of this instructional method with physical therapy students. Edison and colleagues (2018) completed a systematic review from 1995 to 2016 on the use of service learning in physical therapy, occupational therapy, and speech therapy programs. During this time frame, the authors included 22 articles for review, which were comprised of service learning experiences at worksites, health and wellness programs, and vocational rehabilitation programs. They found a significant increase in the number of service learning opportunities in work settings. However, many of these studies demonstrated a high risk of bias and did not necessarily translate to an improved ability of students to provide rehabilitation services in these settings (see Experiential Learning Instructional Methods Evidence Table).

THEORY

As previously mentioned, Kolb expanded on Dewey's work to provide a model for experiential learning. Kolb's model of experiential learning is the most widely recognized and used framework for integrating theory and practice. These founding fathers assert learning is richest when students combine their experiences, perceptions, behaviors, and thoughts with reflective practices. Kolb believed students' knowledge occurs as a result of taking in and transforming how they interpret and act on information. During their experiences, students reorganize and restructure course concepts and past experiences to make meaning of their current experiences. They solve problems and make decisions, which necessitates reflection when engaged in experiential learning.

According to this model, they learn through four main phases: (1) concrete experiences, (2) reflective observation, (3) abstract conceptualization, and (4) active experimentation (Figure 6-1). In the concrete experiences and abstract conceptualization phases, students **grasp** (or take in) the information. Whereas in the reflective observation and active experimentation phases, students **transform** the information. This model is often called a *cycle* to more accurately represent the dynamic phases as a spiral of overlapping processes. For learning to occur, students should experience each phase, but where they enter the cycle or the order in which they engage in each phase is less relevant. In fact, students engage in deep learning when they gain some sort of resolution to the tension between the four phases.

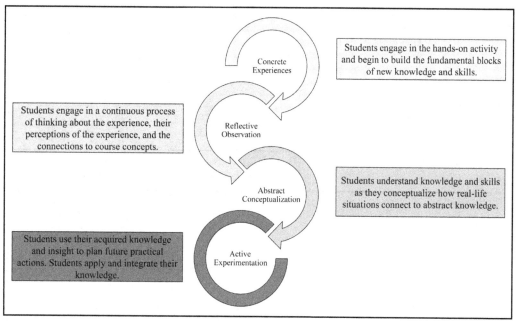

Figure 6-1. Kolb's model of experiential learning.

If applying this model to occupational therapy education, our students would be in the concrete experience phase by simply engaging in the new experiential learning context. In the next phase (reflective observation), we would use various methods to encourage our students to reflect on their observations so they can begin to recognize several perspectives. As we ask our students to reflect, they make sense of this knowledge, understand relationships between concepts, and integrate and refine information into their cognitive structures (abstract conceptualization). Lastly, in active experimentation, we would provide opportunities for our students to take this newly transformed knowledge and apply it to their current and future experiences.

SERVICE LEARNING

Universities, schools, and departments routinely highlight service to the community in their mission statements. When educators implement service learning, they build collaborative relationships between the community and institution. The National Youth Leadership Council (n.d.) describes service learning as an instructional method that integrates meaningful community service with instruction and reflections, with an aim to teach civic responsibilities and strengthen communities. Educational literature identifies three critical elements for authentic and successful implementation of service learning: (1) experiential, (2) reciprocal, and (3) reflection. In this method of instruction, students actively learn by serving their communities in activities related to course concepts (*experiential*). Service learning differs from traditional volunteer and fieldwork experience because there is a mutually beneficial partnership (*reciprocal*). Students gain or refine knowledge and skills related to specified learning objectives, and the community has their identified needs or concerns addressed (Figure 6-2). Lastly, they engage in continuous guided *reflection* to enrich their experiences.

Educators and students can often mistake service learning to be equivalent to volunteer or fieldwork experiences. When students engage in traditional volunteer activities, there is no clear link to learning objectives or professional standards and they do not complete extensive assignments or guided reflections—the cornerstone of service learning. When volunteering, the community (not the student) experiences most of the benefits. Figure 6-3 highlights differences and similarities

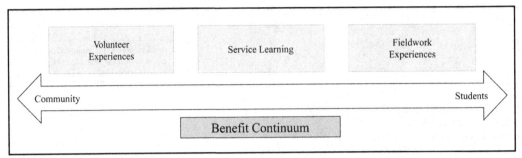

Figure 6-2. Benefit continuum.

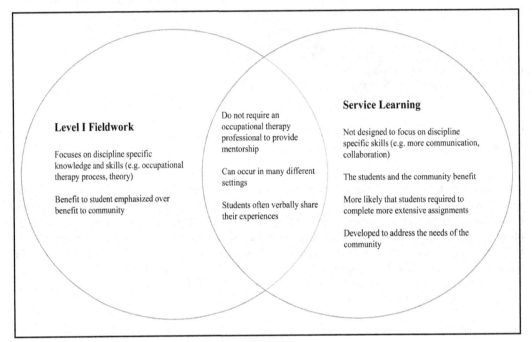

Figure 6-3. Comparison of service learning and Level I fieldwork.

between service learning and Level I fieldwork. In occupational therapy education, fieldwork is often complementary to service learning and not a substitute for an authentic experience. However, educators and fieldwork coordinators can carefully organize service learning as Level I fieldwork when they carefully structure the experience to follow the crucial elements of this instructional method and the requirements for fieldwork accreditation.

IMPLEMENTATION OF SERVICE LEARNING

Educators engage in a complex and tedious process when they develop service learning experiences. Before discussing a series of steps for successful implementation of this instructional method, we want you to consider three different approaches to service learning and contemplate which approach might work best for your course(s) and/or program (Table 6-3). You will want to carefully consider multiple factors when selecting an approach, such as how your program or institution manages the collaborative relationship with the community, how you will provide your students supervision, and how much support or funding your program or institution offers for service learning.

TABLE 6-3	
Approaches to Service Learning	
APPROACH	**DEFINITION**
Integrated	Educators incorporate service learning as a required or elective component of a course. They design the service learning experience to clearly relate to learning objectives and often require more than one visit to the site. In some situations, educators offer service learning for extra credit or students take a course for additional credit hours.
Comprehensive	Educators design a course in which the service learning experience is the central focus of the semester. They design assessments and experiences that are developmentally progressive in nature. Any project the educator designs is also driven by a need identified by the community. In this approach, the educator requires each student to participate in service learning.
Programmatic	Educators in a professional program incorporate service learning at multiple points throughout a curriculum. Educators work together to identify courses appropriate for service learning and to thoughtfully design a sequence of experiences that meet the program's objectives and match the development of their learners.

What other factors would you need to consider when determining how to incorporate service learning in your course?

Educators often develop a partnership with a community site for a "one-time" experience to complete a project rather than creating an ongoing service learning collaboration. However, we want to caution you that educators and the community frequently express frustration with these one-time experiences because they feel pressure to work with each other. In addition, students tend to focus on just completing the assignment and miss the bigger picture of understanding the real needs of the population. In this one-time approach, the students and community are minimally connected.

In educational literature, you will find different frameworks to guide the creation of service learning experiences. We have combined several important steps from various frameworks to provide a broad structure for the implementation of effective service learning.

TABLE 6-4

Examples of Service Learning Partnerships in Literature

- After-school program for at-risk youth
- Adult day center
- Correctional facility
- Domestic abuse shelter
- Drug and alcohol treatment facility
- Facility for individual with HIV
- Group home
- Homeless shelter
- Salvation army
- Sheltered workshop
- Transitional facility

Start With an Idea

Please take a moment to think about your community. In the box below, write down a few potential organizations, businesses, or support groups in your community that could potentially be a community partner for a service learning experience. As you list ideas, remember educators often develop service learning experiences that assist vulnerable populations and communities with health disparities and social injustices. In Table 6-4, we have provided a list of community service partnerships found in health professional educational literature.

Establish a List of Potential Criteria

Before seeking community partners, it is important for educators to establish a list of potential criteria they need in a service learning experience. For example, do you want your students to interact with diverse populations or settings they do not typically encounter in their coursework? What type of contextual issues do you want your students to experience? What types of interaction do you want your students to have with the community? What types of projects or assignments do you think you would want your students to complete? Do your students need opportunities for leadership roles? What learning objectives do you want your students to meet? How much time do you want your students to spend in service learning? What do you want to offer to the community partner?

Take a moment to write down some of your thoughts to these questions in the box on the next page. At this point, your answers to these questions are just solid ideas and not necessarily set in stone. You will need to demonstrate some flexibility with these ideas as you approach your community about a partnership.

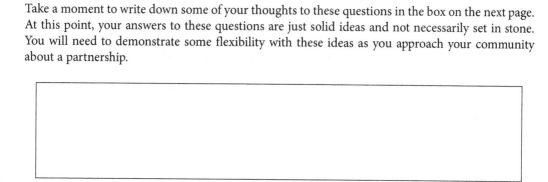

After you have your general list of criteria, you can begin to do your research about potential community partnerships. You can go back to your list in the previous exercise and circle any sites that might be a good match with your criteria or you can meet with your institution's service learning office (if applicable). You can start exploring these partnerships by developing a community profile (e.g., where is the organization, who do they serve, what is the mission and vision, what services do they provide, what types of services might this community need). Oftentimes in service learning, educators ask their students to complete an in-depth community profile and needs assessment in collaboration with their community. In this case, you will need a broad overview of the community partner before further contacting and developing the service learning experience. The community partner might also want to start a new initiative, and students in service learning can provide critical support for development as well.

Create a Partnership and Plan

Once you have an idea and have established criteria, you are ready to explore community partnerships. You will want to locate partnerships whose goals and priorities align with the desired objectives and outcomes you outlined for your course. The relationship between the educator and the community partner is key for successful implementation of service learning. When a strong relationship is present, each group works together effectively to mutually and collaboratively achieve a common goal. The educator and community must develop trust by ensuring comprehensive representation during the entire process, engaging in ongoing dialogue, recognizing each other's unique skills and knowledge, and sharing information about programs (e.g., mission, vision, goals, assets). To establish a win-win relationship, you will need to devote considerable time to meet in person and follow up with a variety of individuals in the community.

> Be aware of how you approach the community—this is critical to the long-term success and sustainability of the service learning relationship!

Before forging forward with a partnership, you and your community partner will want to agree that the experience will be relevant and meaningful to the target population **and** meet the desired learning objectives. You and your community partner will want to engage in detailed planning and mutually agree to several terms prior to your students engaging in service learning to build a sustainable experience. You will need to determine a focus for the service learning experience based on the needs of the community and learning objectives, develop a common vision, define shared outcomes, establish supervision structure and a timeline, decide on an accountability structure, determine assignments and evaluation methods, and understand important policies and procedures. During this step, you will need to have open and ongoing communication with each of the key stakeholders to ensure equal input in the decision-making process. Many educators and/or institutions develop a contract outlining the details described previously. You might also need to

TABLE 6-5

List of Service Learning Assignments and/or Tasks

- Assets map
- Community profile
- Educational materials
- Grant proposal
- Health data
- Historical data
- Key informant or stakeholder interview
- Map of organizational structure
- Marketing and recruitment strategies
- Needs assessment
- Program development
- Program goals and evaluation
- Program implementation
- Strengths, weaknesses, opportunities, and threats analysis
- Walking observation or assessment

meet with the risk management department at your institution and/or the community partnership to discuss any further liability concerns or to establish any risk management policies. After you have reached agreement on many of these areas, you can refine your learning objectives and assignments prior to introducing service learning to your students.

Serve the Community

It is now time for your students to learn from and serve the community. Because many students report feeling anxious or overwhelmed by the demands and newness of the experience, it will be important for you to ensure they are equipped with the prerequisite knowledge and skills before actually engaging in service learning. Similar to other instructional methods discussed in this book, you will clearly outline learning objectives, assignments, expectations, and supervision structures. In Table 6-5, we have provided you with a list of potential assignments. In addition, you or your community partner can provide orientation to the site, which includes discussion of a general overview, the mission and vision, general processes and procedures, traditional programming, tips for working with the population, and the assessment and qualification requirements for services. You will also want to explain to your students that service learning requires flexibility and a willingness to deal with uncertainties and the unexpected.

In this step, your students provide direct community service (Figure 6-4). However, your expectation is that they also learn about the context and make connections between the population/community they are serving and the course concepts. For service learning to be effective, we want our students to develop a passion for the community they are serving, to tackle complex questions and problems, and to move from the idea that they will fix the community to recognizing the community must identify the best methods for change. During service learning, students must allow community members to define the need. You can facilitate this valuable learning experience through assignments, discussions, and reflections. During this step, determine strategies for ongoing monitoring and dialogue during the service learning experience.

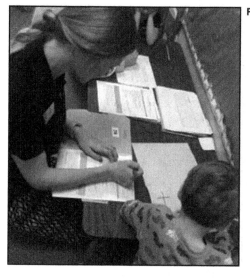

Figure 6-4. A student completes service learning in a preschool.

Reflection and Evaluation

As in many other instructional methods, structured reflection is key to service learning. To maximize outcomes, you will want your students to engage in ongoing reflection and include your community partners in any feedback and evaluation methods. We will further provide ways to achieve these tasks in service learning in the feedback and reflection section of this chapter.

ADDITIONAL IMPLEMENTATION NOTES FOR SERVICE LEARNING

- Ensure that your students understand they are partners invited into the community.
- Create opportunities for your students to truly hear the voice of the community. Your students need to understand what impacts an individual's ability to successfully participate in the community or perform desired occupations.
- Develop a diversity of community partnerships so your students either engage in a variety of experiences and/or have opportunities to hear about other experiences through peers. In the latter, consider setting aside a portion of class for discussion or creating a discussion board, so your students can share with each other.
- Provide training, supervision, and recognition (as needed) to support the community and achieve the learning objectives.
- Be clear on the link of service learning to the course content and/or professional standards.
- Ensure your students are active participants and not passive observers (e.g., completing interviews, facilitating a group, assessing the environment and contexts).

IMPLEMENTATION OF FIELD EXPERIENCES

Educators can also implement the experiential method of a field experience (or a field trip) to develop professional and personal skills for occupational therapy practice. Similar to service learning, students engage in experiences that occur outside the context of the classroom. They demonstrate knowledge from the course within their direct field of study. Typically, students only

Figure 6-5. Students practice completing standardized assessments at a community center.

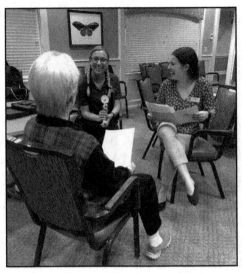

participate in the field experience for a short duration—often one time. For example, they may go to a senior center and collect data on a particular topic (Figure 6-5), observe the disparities and challenges they are learning in class at a local group home, or spend time in an actual intensive care unit to learn about various lines and vital signs. Different than service learning, the only benefit is to the students and not to the setting where they are completing the field experience. The students increase understanding of concepts, learn new behaviors and skills or unlearn old behaviors, and actively move toward levels of independence by being present in a highly contextualized environment.

You can use field experiences to achieve a variety of student competencies in your courses. Although the process will not be as in-depth as the development of service learning, you will want to review each of the steps to implementation outlined in the prior section. Take a moment and return to the list of potential partnerships you created in the earlier exercise. With the idea of field experiences in mind, expand on that list below—what are some additional sites where your students could visit to better understand or practice course concepts?

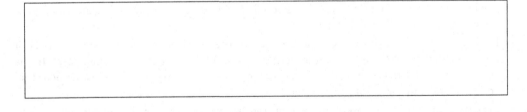

After you have brainstormed ideas, you can ask yourself the same questions about what you need your students to understand or demonstrate in a field experience (see Establish a List of Potential Criteria section). Because there is less focus on benefits to the community in this instructional method, you will spend little to no effort and have minimal necessity for developing a community profile or needs assessment. Next, you will develop a partnership and a plan. Once again, this step will be less daunting than when completed in service learning because your students are in field experiences a very short time and there is not a need to develop shared goals and outcomes. Once you have your plan in place, you build the field experience into your course, and your students complete the task and any associated assignments. Because this is an experiential learning instructional method, you still want to build a reflective component into the field experience.

TABLE 6-6

Reflective Questions for Experiential Learning

1. What thoughts and feelings are you encountering about starting your experience?
2. What areas do you feel most confident and what areas do you feel least confident?
3. How do you plan to use therapeutic use of self during your experience?
4. How can you use experience from a previous encounter with an individual/population to effectively develop rapport or provide information?
5. How has this experience changed the way you think about the population and/or community?
6. How has this experience prepared you for fieldwork and entry-level practice?
7. How has participating in this event enabled you to obtain a deeper understanding of the concepts discussed in class?
8. How has your experience increased your understanding of occupation?
9. How has this experience increased your awareness of the challenges to participation, health, and wellbeing in your community?
10. What similarities do you have with the population/community?

OPPORTUNITIES FOR FEEDBACK AND REFLECTION

As previously mentioned, an essential component of experiential learning instructional methods is students engaging in reflection. Educational literature recognizes numerous benefits of including reflection when implementing this instructional method, such as changing attitudes, skills, and knowledge, promoting lifelong learning, developing professional identity, enhancing civic responsibility, and improving and broadening understanding of course content. As we guide our students through various forms of reflection, they start to think about their community, how their experiences affect them personally, what it might be like to provide occupational therapy services in the community, or how issues or challenges might impact their future practice. Similar to other methods of instruction, you will want to thoughtfully select your type of reflection by considering the setting, community needs, frequency and duration of contact, and the depth of the experience. Because reflection is **cornerstone** to experiential learning, we discuss plenty of examples of rich methods for students to engage in this critical skill.

By reflecting on experiential learning, our students experience personal and professional growth as they recognize and process their own biases, which shapes their attitude and identity. Because many students have preconceived notions about the population or location they will be working with during experiential learning, we can ask our students to describe their assumptions prior to the start of their experience. As they progress through the experience, we can provide journal prompts that ask them to re-examine their values, beliefs, stereotypes, and prejudices and convey their feelings, emotions, thoughts, and observations. Educational literature suggests that by completing this type of reflection, students are more open to new ideas, transform their perspectives, and often notice they are more similar (rather than dissimilar) to the individuals in the community.

Educators commonly employ reflective journaling or essay writing when using experiential learning in their courses. We suggest you generate the questions to ensure the communication is focused on important elements of the experience and is relevant to the learning objectives. You will want to create questions that connect to course content, contextualize their experiences, and challenge them to think critically. In Table 6-6, we have provided a list of 10 questions from experiential education literature for you to consider or adapt. You will find many more questions from the references listed at the end of the chapter.

TABLE 6-7

Additional Reflection Methods for Experiential Learning

- Cultural competence survey or cultural competence assessment
- Exit interview or debriefing
- Focus groups
- Incident journal
- In-class discussion or discussion via online learning system
- Peer-assessment
- Self-assessment and goal setting
- Three-part journal

We want to highlight a few additional methods we found beneficial for engaging students in reflection during experiential learning. One example is the use of *free-fall writing*. With this method, you instruct your students to engage in writing immediately following participation in the experience. Your students set a timer for 8 minutes and spontaneously write and get their uncensored thoughts onto paper. An additional transcription method you can implement is *three-word writing*. As stated in the name, you ask your students to write three words or brief phases that describe their experience. For example, you could ask them to write three words or phrases that describe how they felt when they first interacted with the community or how they felt after they implemented a certain assignment. One final example of a reflection method is *double-entry journal*. Students write down their personal reactions on one side of a piece of paper, and on the other side, you ask them to link one key piece of course content to their reaction and/or experience. While we described several reflection strategies in this section, educational literature provides several other excellent methods (Table 6-7).

While this is beyond the scope of this chapter, you should also consider feedback and reflection methods for the community, faculty, and institution. For example, you might ask the community to complete an exit survey or to participate in a focus group or exit interview. You could require your students to implement some sort of data collection method if they offered education to test the community's new knowledge and skills and satisfaction. As you engage in feedback and evaluation with the community, you understand ways to improve the experience and sustain the partnership. Educators can highlight their participation in experiential learning through number and duration of community partnerships and projects, amount of grants, or total number of presentations or publications. They can reflect on how these experiences influence their educational and professional practices in their dossiers.

APPLICATION TO OCCUPATIONAL THERAPY PRACTICE

Example 1: Use of Service Learning to Facilitate Meaning

Perhaps you are working with a client who has experienced a loss of roles or meaning because of a new disability or life transition. You can use service learning to explore new roles and occupations and to increase your client's sense of meaning and satisfaction. For example, your client is a former nurse and has had a stroke and can no longer work and desires to redefine time and identity. From working in this field, she knows the hospital she previously works at needs blankets for children in the neonatal intensive care unit. Just like in service learning, the relationship is mutually beneficial. Your client regains skills or participation in valued roles and occupations, and the hospital and patients receive needed items and services.

Example 2: Use of Field Experience to Teach a Group of Adolescents About Life Skills

In this scenario, you are working on life skills with a group of adolescents with autism. You are working on social and money management skills and decide to take the group to a restaurant where they can practice ordering from the menu, taking turns engaging in conversation, paying with cash or debit cards, and figuring out tips. After the experience, you can ask the group to reflect by engaging in a group discussion about what went well, what might they do differently, what did they learn, or what strategies were beneficial.

Advantages

- Provides highly contextualized and meaningful experiences
- Allows students to have ample opportunities to practice solving problems
- Enhances students' motivation to learn and have self-confidence
- Develops an understanding of the challenges of fostering therapeutic relationships with diverse populations
- Increases students' understanding of other disciplines if organized as an interprofessional experience
- Facilitates a commitment to lifelong learning
- Suggests students will have higher levels of awareness to community needs and civic engagement following their experiences
- Affords students opportunities to see and make ethical, professional, and culturally sensitive interactions
- Improves skills of professional reasoning, leadership, communication, connection, and touch
- Reports that students experience validation of their choice of profession and develop sense of becoming a professional
- Evidence suggests students demonstrate improved attitudes and broadened perspectives
- Strengthens ties between the program/institution and community
- Increases cultural competence and cross-cultural understanding

---

Challenges

- Requires educator and administration support and resources
- Involves time and effort to develop
- Requires students have transportation or access to transportation to arrive at experiential learning location
- Involves potentially unpredictable situations
- Reports of low methodological quality of studies in some systematic reviews
- Reports that some students feel too much outside the context of the classroom
- Reports that methods for student assessment are potentially ambiguous and uncertain
- Potentially lacks faculty support
- Potential shortages in community partnerships

In the space below, list any additional advantages or challenges.

Brainstorm strategies for overcoming these challenges when implementing the use of experiential learning instructional methods.

THREE THINGS YOU CAN DO TOMORROW TO IMPLEMENT EXPERIENTIAL LEARNING INSTRUCTIONAL METHODS WITH YOUR STUDENTS

1. Make an appointment to meet with your institution's service learning office (if applicable).
2. Ask colleagues for two or three of their connections for potential community partnerships or field experience opportunities.
3. Review your course content and locate one topic that is difficult to teach or challenging for your students to understand in the context of the classroom. Brainstorm about how you could convert that content into a field experience.

Experiential Learning Instructional Methods Evidence Table

SERVICE LEARNING

Author/Year	Study Objectives	Design and Participants	Intervention and Outcome Measures	Results
Bowman (2012)	Researchers examined the impact of a worksite assessment project on occupational therapy students' learning experiences	Design: Posttest survey design Participants: 92 occupational therapy students	Intervention: Students participated in a 1-hour-per-week ergonomics project for a course. They created a project that included a worksite evaluation in a rural area. Students completed projects at a total of 41 different industrial worksites across 10 counties in South Carolina Outcome measures: • Written in English • Community Partner Evaluation of Community-Based Learning Experience Form	93% of students agreed or strongly agreed they learned from being in the community, and 78% reported a desire to keep engaging in community projects Only 48% of students reported a desire to spend more time with their particular setting A large majority of students (86%) rated their learning experience as excellent or very good
Coker (2010)	Researchers investigated the impact of a 1-week experiential learning program on occupational therapy students' critical thinking and clinical reasoning	Design: Quasi-experimental, nonrandomized, pre/posttest; 1 group Participants: 25 master's degree occupational therapy students	Intervention: Students participated in a 1-week day camp for children with hemiplegic cerebral palsy Students received training to provide 1-on-1 constraint-induced movement therapy to their assigned camp participant Students planned daily treatment interventions and wrote daily progress notes Outcome measures: • Self-Assessment of Clinical Reflection and Reasoning (SACRR) • California Critical Thinking Skills Test	Students demonstrated statistically significant improvement from pre to posttest on 22 of the 26 SACRR items (themes of use of theory and frames of reference, ask questions to self, use of protocols, use of decision making and judgment) Students' overall SACRR scores significantly statistically improved from pre to posttest Students' scores improved on the California Critical Thinking Skills Test from pre to posttest; with statistically significant improvements in 3 of the 5 subscales

(continued)

Experiential Learning Instructional Methods Evidence Table (continued)

Author/Year	Study Objectives	Design and Participants	Intervention and Outcome Measures	Results
DeBonis (2016)	Researchers studied the impact of service learning with graduate nursing students	Design: Nonexperimental pre/posttest design Participants: 152 graduate nursing students	Intervention: Students provided 16 to 20 hours of free health care to medically underserved individuals in partnership with Salvation Army Outcome measures: • Centers for Health Communities survey • Preservice questionnaire	Students reported increase intent to volunteer and increase desire to work in an underrepresented setting following their service learning experience Students reported significant increases on each of the 4 items related to civic engagement and 3 of the 6 items related to cultural competence on the Centers for Health Communities survey Students reported significant difference on each item of the questionnaire indicating increased knowledge and understanding of an underserved population
Edison et al. (2018)	Researchers desired to evaluate the rigor of service learning and the scope of these activities related to the occupation of work in the rehabilitation professions	Design: Systematic review Participants: Rehabilitation professional students Researchers included 22 articles	Researchers conducted this systematic review using Preferred Reporting Items for Systematic Reviews and Meta-Analyses (PRISMA) guidelines Researchers searched the following databases: Academic Search Premier, CINAHL, Education Full Text, Education Resources Information Center (ERIC), Embase, Health Source: Nursing/ Academic Edition, PsycINFO, PubMed, Scopus Inclusion criteria: • Published from inception of database to December 2016 • An academic course or program coordinated the service learning experience and linked to specific content	Of the 22 articles, 6 studies included rehabilitation professional students providing services to occupation of work No studies included randomization for group allocation 17 articles used a 1-group, pre/posttest design Each article received a score of weak related to methodological quality

(continued)

Experiential Learning Instructional Methods Evidence Table (continued)

Author/Year	Study Objectives	Design and Participants	Intervention and Outcome Measures	Results
			• Researchers included a student reflection component • Used primary or secondary outcome of evaluation of student service learning experience • Sample included students in 1 or more of trialliance of rehabilitation professionals Exclusion criteria: • Editorials, letters, commentaries, case reports, and review articles • Employed primarily qualitative research methods • Employed 1 group posttest only research design • Not written in English	
Juniarti et al. (2016)	Researchers desired to explore what components of service learning educators can use to develop functional definitions in nursing education	Design: Integrative literature review using a systematic approach Participants: Researchers searched for article with information related to nursing students Researchers included 42 studies in review	Included quantitative and qualitative studies Researchers used a 12-step structured approach Researchers searched the following databases: CINAHL, Medline Industries, ERIC, Scopus, Web of Science Article met the following inclusion criteria: • Published from earliest time of retrieval to June 2015 • Studied nursing students (all levels of education) • Used specific term service learning	No studies demonstrated perfect methodological quality, but 20 studies demonstrated high quality and 22 studies demonstrated moderate quality Most articles were published in the United States A majority of the studies were completed with undergraduate nursing students Of the 42 studies, 15 were qualitative in nature, 5 were descriptive quantitative, 13 were quasi-experimental, 5 were evaluation, 2 were mixed-methods, and 2 were case study designs

(continued)

Experiential Learning Instructional Methods Evidence Table (continued)

Author/Year	Study Objectives	Design and Participants	Intervention and Outcome Measures	Results
			• Employed descriptive studies, qualitative studies, or mixed-method studies in peer-reviewed journal • Used qualitative and quantitative outcomes Exclusion criteria: • Non-English • Online service learning and international service learning	Researchers reported 4 characteristics of service learning following synthesis and analysis: • Structured intracurricular experiential learning • Reflection • Reciprocity • Specific outcomes and benefits
Krout et al. (2010)	Researchers provided data from a 3-year multidisciplinary intergenerational service learning project	Design: Program evaluation with cross sectional pre/posttest design Participants: 225 students (129 completed survey), 8 faculty, 357 older adults (90 completed survey)	Intervention: 4 departments provided students with coursework and 1 interdisciplinary clinical experience; students completed various service learning activities throughout courses and document time spent at various gerontology sites Outcome measures: • Generativity scale for older adults • Civic engagement questions for students • Satisfaction surveys (older adults and students)	Students reported a high degree of satisfaction with service learning Of the 11 statements, students rated 9 of the statements greater than 90% for positive agreement (e.g., more positive attitudes, effectiveness of service learning related to course, communicate with others) Similarly, older adults also expressed a high degree of satisfaction with the experience The older adults also agreed positively (> 90%) toward a majority of the statements (9 out of 11) Students reported larger improvements on 5 of the 9 items on questionnaire, suggesting more positive attitudes toward aging

(continued)

Experiential Learning Instructional Methods Evidence Table (continued)

Author/Year	Study Objectives	Design and Participants	Intervention and Outcome Measures	Results
Leung et al. (2012)	The primary objective of this study was to determine the effects of a service learning project on medical students' knowledge regarding aging	Design: Randomized controlled trial Participants: A total of 124 students from the Bachelor of Medicine, Bachelor of Surgery, or the Bachelor of Nursing programs were recruited for this study; the majority of participants were female	The students were randomly assigned to either the control group, which participated in a 10-week self-directed online learning program regarding aging, or the intervention group, which completed a half-day introductory workshop, a 10-week interaction period, and a half-day intergenerational sharing session 62 students were randomized to the control group and the intervention group respectively Outcome measures: • Students' knowledge regarding aging measured by Palmore's Facts on Aging Quiz • Student disposition toward the aging population measured by Kogan's Attitudes Toward Old People Scale	Students that participated in the intervention group and contributed to the service learning project showed significant increases in knowledge of aging as measured by Palmore's total score The students in the intervention group scored higher than the control group on Palmore's quiz both immediately following the study and 1 month following the study The intervention group also reflected more positive dispositions toward the older adult population as compared to the control group
Short & St. Peters (2017)	Researchers examined the effect of an international service learning on cultural competency with entry-level Doctor of Occupational Therapy students	Design: Cross-sectional pre/posttest design; 1 group Participants: 12 first-year entry-level Doctor of Occupational Therapy students	Intervention: Pretest completed 7 weeks prior to service learning experience Researchers provided instruction on kinesiology, seating and mobility, and Haitian culture, and students participated in several learning activities prior to service learning experience The students and researchers served for Wheel for the World in Haiti; led 5 days of seating and mobility clinics	Students demonstrated large statistically significant difference on metacognitive, motivational, behavioral, and cognitive subscales

(continued)

Experiential Learning Instructional Methods Evidence Table (continued)

Author/Year	Study Objectives	Design and Participants	Intervention and Outcome Measures	Results
			Students completed posttest 1 week after service learning Outcome measure: Cultural Intelligence Scale; 20 items, 4 subscales	
Stetten et al. (2019)	Researchers aimed to provide a literature appraisal to describe interprofessional education service learning	Design: A systematic appraisal Participants: Health professional students (mostly at the graduate level) Researchers included 49 articles in this review	Researchers used PRISMA guidelines to complete study Researchers searched the following databases: CINAHL, PubMed, Education Full Text, Professional Development Collection, PsycINFO, ASSIA, Biotechnology and Bioengineering abstracts, ERIC Inclusion criteria: • Interprofessional group of students with at least 1 health profession • Discuss educational activity that potentially meets service learning definition • Published in peer-review journal • Completed at the graduate level • Written in English	Of the 49 articles, 27 described the interprofessional education service learning as an elective experience, 11 were required, and 5 were unstated 55% of the studies focused on underserved populations Of the health professions, studies featured nursing students the most and physical therapy the least Of the 49 articles, 20 studies focused on participation, attitudes, or knowledge acquisition Researchers employed survey-based attitude assessments the most and focus groups or practice measures the least Researchers only discussed theory in 4 of the studies
Stewart et al. (2012)	Researchers examined the impact of a service learning project on pharmacy students' empathy and to determine predictors of empathy	Design: Cross-sectional pre/posttest survey design Participants: 18 third-, fourth-, and fifth-year pharmacy students	Intervention: Students provided medication therapy management to indigent patients and families at a free primary care clinic 1 time per month Outcome measures: Jefferson Scale of Empathy	Students demonstrated a significant increase in degree of empathy from pre to posttest They did not demonstrate any correlation between demographic factors and empathy change

(continued)

Experiential Learning Instructional Methods Evidence Table (continued)

Author/Year	Study Objectives	Design and Participants	Intervention and Outcome Measures	Results
Watters et al. (2015)	Researchers investigated the effect of participation in a clinic treating individuals with special needs on dentistry, students' ability, comfort, and self-efficacy	Design: Cross-sectional; pre/posttest design Participants: 127 fourth-year dental students	Intervention: Dental students participated in a special needs dentistry clinic in which they provided supervised dental care for individuals with special needs. Each student participated in the clinic for 4 to 6 weeks for half of a day. They provided care in teams of 2 students. They also completed readings and engaged in lecture Outcome measures: Survey	Students agreed less with the following statement after their rotation: People with special needs care less about oral health They reported greater confidence in the treatment of people with cognitive disabilities and medical complexities Students reported greater intention to treat people with special needs in the future and increased interest in this training; they also reported a decreased belief that individuals with special needs should be referred to a specialty clinic/hospital

FIELD EXPERIENCES

Author/Year	Study Objectives	Design and Participants	Intervention and Outcome Measures	Results
Hartman et al. (2018)	Researchers described the integration of 9 field trip experiences into a 4-week radiology clerkship and its effect on learning outcomes and student satisfaction with medical students	Design: Cross-sectional pre/posttest design Participants: 38 third- and fourth-year medical students from 3 institutions	Intervention: Students participated in 9 field trips during a 4-week radiology course to gain exposure to subspecialties and modalities. Researchers created a worksheet and activities for students to complete at each location. Each field trip lasted approximately 1 to 2 hours Outcome measures: A short-answer quiz consisting of 16 questions	Students demonstrated significant improvement on short-answer quiz from pre to posttest Students also provided overwhelmingly positive support for field trips

(continued)

Experiential Learning Instructional Methods Evidence Table (continued)

Author/Year	Study Objectives	Design and Participants	Intervention and Outcome Measures	Results
Scott Stiles et al. (2018)	Researchers evaluated nursing students' cultural competency following completion of a stand-alone culture course that included field activities	Design: Quasi-experimental, nonrandomized 2-group comparison Participants: 72 nursing students; 53 in the intervention group (juniors), 19 in the control group (seniors)	Intervention: Students completed a 15-week, 2-credit-hour course (15 hours of content via lecture and 45 hours of fieldwork experiences [e.g., museums, cemeteries, festivals]). Researchers assigned students to 1 of 4 cultures The control group included graduated seniors that received cultural content via many courses Outcome measures: Transcultural Self-Efficacy Tool	The students in the cultural course improved cognitive subscale scores from 5.10 to 8.07; the control group scored 7.00 The students in the cultural course improved practical subscale scores from 5.56 to 8.27; the control group scored 7.15 The students in the cultural course improved affective subscale scores from 8.27 to 9.41; the control group scored 8.85 All results demonstrated a significant difference

There are a large number of studies related to service learning in occupational therapy education. However, a majority of those studies are qualitative or mixed methods and were not included in this table. We only included high-level studies from health professional education literature due to number of studies.

Adapted from American Occupational Therapy Association. (2002). AOTA's evidence-based literature review project: An overview (D. Lieberman & J. Scheer, Eds.). *American Journal of Occupational Therapy, 56,* 344-349. https://doi.org/10.5014/ajot.56.3.344

REFERENCES

American Occupational Therapy Association. (2002). AOTA's evidence-based literature review project: An overview (D. Lieberman & J. Scheer, Eds.). *The American Journal of Occupational Therapy, 56*, 344-349. https://doi.org/10.5014/ajot.56.3.344

Association for Experiential Education. (2019). https://www.aee.org

Bowman, P. (2012). Ergonomics work assessment in rural industrial settings: A student occupational therapy project. *Work, 43*, 323-329. http://dx.doi.org/10.3233/WOR-2012-1367

Coker, P. (2010). Effects of an experiential learning program on the clinical reasoning and critical thinking skills of occupational therapy students. *Journal of Allied Health, 39*(4), 280-286.

Debonis, R. (2016). Effects of service-learning on graduate nursing students: Care and advocacy for the impoverished. *Journal of Nursing Education, 55*(1), 36-40.

Edison, C., Yuen, H., Vogtle, L., & McCurry, V. (2018). Methodological quality of service learning studies in rehabilitation profession: A systematic review. *Work, 61*, 55-67. https://dx.doi.org/10.3233/WOR-182779

Hartman, M., Thomas, S., & Ayoob, A. (2018). Radiology field trips—a list of "must sees" in the radiology department for medical students: How we do it. *Academic Radiology, 25*(12), 1646-1652.

Juniarti, N., Zannettino, L., Fuller, J., & Grant, J. (2016). Defining service learning in nursing education: An integrative review. *Jurnal Keperawatan Padjadjaran, 4*(2), 200-212.

Krout, J. A., Bergman, E., Bianconi, P., Caldwell, K., Dorsey, J., Durnford, S., Erickson, M. A., Lapp, J., Monroe, J. E., Pogorzala, C., & Valdez Taves, J. (2010). Intergenerational service learning with elders: Multidisciplinary activities and outcomes. *Gerontology & Geriatrics Education, 31*(1), 55-74. http://dx.doi.org/10.1080/02701960903578329

Leung, A. Y. M., Chan, S. S. C., Kwan, C. W., Cheung, M. K. T., Leung, S. S. K., & Fong, D. Y. T. (2012). Service learning in medical and nursing training: A randomized controlled trial. *Advances in Health Sciences Education, 17*(4), 529-545.

National Youth Leadership Council. (n.d.). Retrieved from www.nylc.org

Schaber, P. (2014). Conference proceedings—Keynote address: Searching for and identifying signature pedagogies in occupational therapy education. *American Journal of Occupational Therapy, 68*, S40-S44. https://doi.org/10.5014/ajot.2014.685S08

Scott-Stiles, A., Schuessler, Z., & James, L. (2018). Comparison of two methods of teaching culture to bachelor of science in nursing students. *Journal of Nursing Education, 57*(10), 609-613.

Short, N., & St. Peters, H. Y. Z. (2017). Exploring the impact of service learning in Haiti on the cultural competence of OTD students. *Journal of Occupational Therapy Education, 1*(1), Article 4. https://doi.org/10.26681/jote.2017.010106

Stetten, N. E., Black, E. W., Edwards, M., Schafer, N., & Blue, A. V. (2019). Interprofessional service learning experiences among health professional students: A systematic search and review of learning outcomes. *Journal of Interprofessional Education and Practice, 15*, 60-69.

Stewart, A. L., Tomko, J. R., & Lassila, H. C. (2012). Impact of service learning on pharmacy students' empathy toward patients. *Journal of Community Engagement and Higher Education, 4*(1), 1-5.

Watters, A. L., Stabulas-Savage, J., Toppin, J. D., Janal, M. N., & Robbins, M. R. (2015). Incorporating experiential learning techniques to improve self-efficacy in clinical special care dentistry education. *Journal of Dental Education, 79*(9), 1016-1023.

BIBLIOGRAPHY

Adkins, C., & Simmons, B. (2002). *Outdoor, experiential, and environmental education: Converging or diverging approaches?* ERIC Digest.

Arora, M., Granillo, B., Zepeda, T. K., & Burgess, J. L. (2018). Experiential adult learning: A pathway to enhancing medical countermeasures capabilities. *American Journal of Public Health Perspectives, 108*(S5), S378-S380. http://dx.doi.org/10.2105/AJPH.2018.304703

Babiss, F., Thomas, L., & Fricke, M. (2017). Innovative team training for patient safety: Comparing classroom learning to experiential training. *The Journal of Continuing Education in Nursing, 48*(12), 563-569.

Benson, J. D., & Hansen, A. W. (2007). Moving the classroom to the clinic: The experiences of occupational therapy students during a "living lab". *Occupational Therapy in Health Care, 21*(3), 79-91. http://dx.doi.org/10.1300/J003v21n03_05

Benson, J. D., Provident, I., & Szucs, K. A. (2013). An experiential learning lab embedded in a didactic course: Outcomes from a pediatric intervention course. *Occupational Therapy in Health Care, 27*(1), 46-57. http://dx.doi.org/10.3109/07380577.2012.756599

Bonello, M. (2001). Fieldwork within the context of higher education: A literature review. *British Journal of Occupational Therapy, 62*(2), 93-99.

Cheung, M., & Delavega, E. (2014). Five-way experiential learning model for social work education. *Social Work Education, 33*(8), 1070-1087.

Chorazy, M. L., & Klinedinst, K. S. (2019). Learn by doing: A model for incorporating high-impact experiential learning into an undergraduate public health curriculum. *Curriculum, Instruction, and Pedagogy, 7,* Article 9. http://dx.doi.org/10.3389/fpubh.2019.00031

Dank, Y. H., Nice, F. J., & Truong, H. A. (2017). Academic-community partnership for medical missions: Lessons learned and practical guidance for global health service-learning experiences. *Journal of Health Care for the Poor and Underserved, 28*(1), 8-13. https://doi.org/10.1353/hpu.2017.0002

Digby, C. G., & Pinchin, S. (2019). Using experiential learning to teach health care quality improvement. *Medical Education, 53*(5), 499. http://dx.doi.org/10.1111/medu.13864

Gitlow, L., & Flecky, K. (2005). Integrating disability studies concepts into occupational therapy education using service learning. *American Journal of Occupational Therapy, 59,* 546-553.

Glemon, S. B., Holland, B. A., & Shinnamon, A. F. (1998). Health professions schools in service to the nation. Conference Proceedings, 8. Retrieved from https://digitalcommons.unomaha.edu/cgi/viewcontent.cgi?referer=https://www.google.com/&httpsredir=1&article=1009&context=slceproceedings

Glover, T. L., Narvel, N. R., Schneider, L. A., Horgas, A. L., & Bluck, S. (2018). Nursing students' reactions to an educational experiential immersion in palliative care. *Journal of Nursing Education, 57*(11), 675-679. https://doi.org/10.3928/01484834-20181022-08

Goldbach, W. P., & Stella, T. C. (2017). Experiential learning to advance student readiness for level II fieldwork. *Journal of Occupational Therapy Education, 1*(1), Article 8. https://doi.org/10.26681/jote.2017.010103

Grace, S., Stockhausen, L., Patton, N., & Innes, E. (2018). Experiential learning in nursing and allied health education: Do we need national framework to guide ethical practice? *Nurse Education in Practice, 34,* 56-62.

Gugliucci, M.R., & Weiner, A. (2013). Learning by living: Life-altering medical education through nursing home-based experiential learning. *Gerontology & Geriatrics Education, 34*(1), 60-77. https://dx.doi.org/10.1080/02701960.2013.749254

Hansen, A., Munoz, J., Crist, P., Gupta, J., Ideishi, R., Primeau, L., & Tupe, D. (2007). Service learning: Meaningful, community-centered professional skill development for occupational therapy students. *Occupational Therapy in Health Care, 21*(1/2), 25-49. https://doi.org/10.1080/J003v21n01_03

Hash, K. M., Poole, J., Floyd, M., Moore, C. D., Rogers, A. T., & Tower, L. E. (2017). Innovative experiential learning activities in aging: The experiences of four BEL projects. *Journal of Teaching in Social Work, 37*(2), 156-170.

Henderson, W., Coppard, B., & Qi, Y. (2017). Identifying instructional methods for development of clinical reasoning in entry-level occupational therapy education: A mixed methods design. *Journal of Occupational Therapy Education, 1*(2). https://doi.org/10.26681/jote.2017.010201

Hoppes, S., Bender, D., & DeGrace, B. W. (2005). Service learning is a perfect fit for occupational and physical therapy education. *Journal of Allied Health, 34*(1), 47-50.

Hour, Y. J., Lin, Y. H., Lien, H. Y., & Wong, A. M. K. (2018). A pediatric service-learning program in physical therapy education. *Pediatric Physical Therapy, 30*(2), 148-154. http://dx.doi.org/10.1097/pep.0000000000000498

Knecht-Sabres, L. J. (2010). The use of experiential learning in an occupational therapy program: Can it foster skills for clinical practice? *Occupational Therapy in Health Care, 24*(4), 320-334. http://dx.doi.org/10.3109/07380577.2010.514382

Knecht-Sabres, L. J. (2013). Experiential learning in occupational therapy: Can it enhance readiness for clinical practice? *Journal of Experiential Education, 36*(1), 22-36. http://dx.doi.org/10.1177/1053825913481584

Kwong, K. (2017). Advancing social work practice research education: An innovative, experiential pedagogical approach. *International Journal of Higher Education, 6*(5), 1-13.

Leong, C. (2016). A community outreach blood pressure clinic: Experiential practice site for pharmacy and dental hygiene students trained in physical assessment. *Pharmacy Education, 16*(1), 182-188.

Lewis, L. H., & Williams, C. J. (1994). Experiential learning: Past and present. *New Directions for Adult and Continuing Education, 62,* 5-16.

Lim, S. M., Tan, B. L., Lim, H. B., & Goh, Z. A. (2018). Engaging persons with disabilities as community teachers for experiential learning in occupational therapy education. *Hong Kong Journal of Occupational Therapy, 31*(1), 36-45. http://dx.doi.org/10.1177/1569186118783877

Lorio, A. K., Gore, J. B., Warthen, L., Housley, S. N., & Burgess, E. O. (2016). Teaching dementia care to physical therapy doctoral students: A multimodal experiential learning approach. *Gerontology & Geriatrics Education, 38*(3), 313-324. http://dx.doi.org/10.1080/02701960.2015.1115979

Machin, A. I., & Jones, D. (2014). Interprofessional and service improvement learning and patient safety: A content analysis of pre-registration students' assessments. *Nurse Education Today, 34,* 218-224. http://dx.doi.org/10.1016/j.nedt.2013.06.022

Maloney, S. M., & Griffith, K. (2013). Occupational therapy students' development of therapeutic communication skills during a service-learning experience. *Occupational Therapy in Mental Health, 29*(1), 10-26. http://dx.doi.org/10.1080/0164212X.2013.760288

Maloney, S. M., Myers, C., & Bazyk, J. (2014). The influence of a community-based service-learning experience on the development of occupational therapy students' feelings of civic responsibility. *Occupational Therapy in Mental Health, 30*, 144-161. https://doi.org/10.1080/0164212X.2014.910160

Meiers, J., & Russell, M. J. (2019). An unfolding case study: Supporting contextual psychomotor skill development in novice nursing students. *International Journal of Nursing Education Scholarship, 16*(1). http://dx.doi.org/10.1515/ijnes-2018-0013

Menamin, R. M. C., Grath, M. M. C., Cantillon, P., & Farlane, A. M. (2014). Training socially responsive health care graduates: Is service learning an effective educational approach? *Medical Teacher, 36*, 291-307. http://dx.doi.org/10.3109/0142159X.2013.873118

Milton, L. E., & Otty, R. (2018). Innovations in occupational therapy education: The centralized service learning model. *Journal of Occupational Therapy Education, 2*(1). https://doi.org/10.26681/jote.2018.020108

National Service-Learning Clearing House. (2019). https://community-wealth.org/content/national-service-learning-clearinghouse

National Society for Experiential Education. (2019). Eight principles of good practice for all experiential learning activities. https://www.nsee.org/8-principles

Parmenter, V., & Thomas, H. (2014). WOW! Occupational therapy education and experiential service learning through community volunteering. *British Journal of Occupational Therapy, 78*(4), 241-252.

Perlmutter, M. S., & Tyminski, Q. (2017). A community-based experience to enhance occupational therapy student clinical skills with clients with mental illness. *Journal of Occupational Therapy Education, 1*(2). https://doi.org/10.26681/jote.2017.010203

Pierangleu, L. T., & Lenhart, C. M. (2018). Service-learning: Promoting empathy through the point-in-time count of homeless populations. *Journal of Nursing Education, 57*(7), 436-439. https://doi.org/10.3928/01484834-20180618-10

Revens, K. E., Reynolds, A. D., Suclupe, R. F., Rifkin, C., & Pierce, T. (2018). "You can never understand a culture until you experience it": How an experiential learning course prepared students for practice with Latino communities through learning for advocacy. *Journal of Teaching in Social Work, 38*(3), 277-291.

Schaber, P., Marsh, L., & Wilcox, K. (2012). Relational learning and active engagement in occupational therapy professional education. In R. Gurung, N. Chick, & A. Haynie (Eds.), *Exploring more signature pedagogies: Approaches to teaching disciplinary habits of mind* (pp. 188-202). Stylus.

Simmons, C., & Fisher, A. K. (2014). Promoting cognitive development through field education. *Journal of Social Work Education, 52*(40), 462-472.

Skinner, K., Hyde, S., McPherson, K., & Simpson, M. (2016). Improving students' interpersonal skills through experiential small group learning. *Journal of Learning Design, 9*(1), 21-36.

Talero, P., Kern, S., & Tupe, D. (2015). Culturally responsive care in occupational therapy: An entry-level educational model embedded in service-learning. *Scandinavian Journal of Occupational Therapy, 22*, 95-102. http://dx.doi.org/10.3109/11038128.2014.997287

Thomas, J., & Shane, S. (2012). Preparing future professionals in the field of health promotion: Successful experiential education. *American Journal of Health Education, 43*(3), 185-189.

Tompson, M. M., & Ryan, A. G. (1996). The influence of fieldwork on the professional socialism of occupational therapy students. *British Journal of Occupational Therapy, 59*(2), 65-70.

Wulff, D. H., & Nyquist, J. D. (1988). Using field methods as an instructional tool to improve the academy: Resources for student, faculty, and institutional development. *To Improve the Academy, 7*, 87-98. http://digitalcommons.unl.edu/podimproveacad/163

7

SIMULATION-BASED INSTRUCTIONAL METHODS

Whitney Henderson, OTD, MOT, OTR/L
Bailey Bremser, MOT, OTR/L

BASIC TENETS

Health professional education literature defines *simulation-based instructional methods* as techniques used to replicate important aspects of real-life practice situations in a realistic environment without exposing real clientele to risk or harm. In simulation, students can practice relevant professional experiences in a controlled setting under guidance. They see and feel the potential cost of their actions without experiencing the actual consequences. These methods are immersive, interactive, collaborative, and reflective in nature. Therefore, students can develop the skills to examine and manage situations more effectively before they enter their clinical education or professional practice.

Educators in various health professions are increasingly employing the use of simulation-based instructional methods to achieve professional accreditation standards to bridge the gap between the classroom and practice. In a majority of situations, educators use simulation to supplement their traditional didactic coursework and practicum or internship experiences. Students develop knowledge, skills, and attitudes when engaged in a simulation method that requires them to apply and analyze content (e.g., high-level learning). They become better equipped to deliver client-centered, high-quality services with clients and families with a variety of health care needs. Throughout health professional literature, you will see an assortment of simulation methods ranging from a basic task or concept to a complex and dynamic scenario.

Before moving forward, we want to discuss common terminology under the umbrella term of simulation to ensure consistency and understanding throughout this chapter. In Table 7-1, we describe a variety of simulation-based instructional methods found in literature. We will not discuss each of the methods but will explain the common characteristics and approaches to implementation at a later time.

Henderson, W. (Ed.). *Effective Teaching: Instructional Methods and Strategies for Occupational Therapy Education* (pp. 129-184).
© 2021 Taylor & Francis Group.

TABLE 7-1

Simulation-Based Instructional Methods

TYPE OF METHOD	DESCRIPTION
Human patient simulators (mannequins and part-task trainers)	A computerized full-body mannequin or modelled segment of body (e.g., arm or upper body) that provides realistic physiological and/or pharmacological responses; programed and controlled via computer; often used in nursing and medical education to train clinical skills, such as injections or cardiopulmonary resuscitation.
Laboratory experiences	Educators offer students opportunities to practice skills in contrived environments.
Role play	Students act out practical experiences and psychodynamic processes in a safe environment.
Standardized patient	Educators train individuals to portray real clients, family members, or other team members in a practice situation. They are trained to challenge the students' communication and practical skills.
Virtual immersive reality simulation	Use of computerized technology to immerse the student in an interactive and realistic environment; the student moves to create actual motion and interaction with the game (e.g., use of "Second Life" platform to make home recommendations or ErgoROM to teach ergonomics).

TABLE 7-2

Fidelity Dimensions

DIMENSION	DESCRIPTION
Environmental Fidelity	The degree to which the context replicates the sensory and physical aspects of the practice situation (e.g., space size, auditory cues).
Equipment Fidelity	The degree to which the simulation portrays the objects of the practice situation.
Psychological Fidelity	The degree to which the students perceive the simulation as a real-life practice situation; develops during the simulation.

Another common term you will notice in simulation literature is fidelity. Similar to the different types of methods, simulation includes varying levels of fidelity. *Fidelity* is the extent to which the simulation mimics the actual situation and the degree the students are convinced they would encounter the experience in real life. Literature classifies the level of fidelity based on the amount the method simulates the equipment, environmental, and psychological responses (Table 7-2).

Educators select simulation-based instructional methods with low, medium, and high levels of fidelity (environmental, equipment, and psychological). Their decision about the type of fidelity they use is often influenced by various constraints, such as cost of implementation, the availability of technology, or the time to complete the simulation. Educators select low-fidelity simulation because it is typically more cost effective; however, this type of fidelity offers the lowest form of authenticity and effectiveness. Examples of low fidelity simulation include students completing a basic interview with a simulated patient in a classroom, role playing with a peer, or assessing basic functions, such as heart rate or lung sounds with a static piece of equipment or mannequin. Although high-fidelity simulation often requires more time, cost, technology, and effort, educators select this level of authenticity to engage their students in complex conditions or situations that require them to integrate information to make real-time decisions and actions.

Students engaged in high-fidelity simulation employ higher levels of learning and can demonstrate more complex skills that might reflect demands of fieldwork and practice. Examples of high-fidelity simulation include students completing an evaluation or intervention with a standardized patient in a space designed to mimic an intensive care unit or using high-technology simulators (SimMan 3G or METIman Adult Patient Simulator) that can be designed and controlled by the educator to vocalize or perform responses. Educational literature suggests high-fidelity simulation is more effective for student learning.

Background

Educators have used simulation to teach students engaged in health professions new skills and procedures for at least 1,500 years. Although medical education was the first to employ this method of instruction, nursing education literature widely discusses the prevalent use of simulation. Since its origination, scholars have developed a strong evidence base to support simulation in health professional education (see Simulation-Based Instructional Methods Evidence Table). Health care continues to expand its use of simulation across undergraduate, postgraduate, and professional continuing education and development because of its ability to afford students opportunities to practice decision making, reasoning abilities, and procedural skills in an individual or team-based environment.

During the mid-18th century, health care educators in Europe introduced and commonly used a range of simulation methods. In Paris, Dr. Gregoire was the first obstetrics educator to use simulation to teach students how to use forceps during childbirth. As word spread, his method of instruction became widely known and attractive to current and future students. In London, Sir Richard Manningham established an obstetric teaching hospital and became the first educator to integrate simulation into a clinical teaching program. He created a life-size simulator made with a woman's skeleton and artificial matrix and believed students required supervision and repeated practice with this device to learn to perform various types of deliveries with accuracy. Manningham managed his students' cognitive load by starting with a natural and easy childbirth before advancing to the most difficult deliveries. Later in 1897, Gustav Killen invented the bronchoscopy and demonstrated the technique with a living simulator at a conference in Germany. By the end of the 18th century, educators in Germany, Italy, and the United States were introducing simulation in health care education.

Despite its increase in popularity and spread to other disciplines and countries, the use of simulation during the second half of the 20th century significantly declined for uncited reasons. However, a 1978 report demonstrated higher rates of complications in medicine and attributed these findings to inexperienced trainees performing procedures. Because of this, we began to see a re-emergence of simulation in many health care disciplines over the past 40 years. Health professional education literature highlights a number of additional reasons contributing to a fairly recent growth of simulation, such as:

- An increased number of students entering health professional education but a reduced amount of practice placements to train them
- More restrictive supervision and work-hour (medical residents) guidelines
- The need to implement creative teaching and learning strategies to develop the skills required for professional practice
- The use of technology in curriculums that this generation of students expect during their educational experience
- The increased availability of technology to mimic real-life situations
- Changes in productivity and reimbursement guidelines
- Pressure to reduce orientation times
- The ethical and political policies and need to avoid unnecessary risks
- The need to recreate complex and high-risk health care situations so students can hit the ground running when they enter a fast-paced practice setting

While medicine, nursing, and pharmacy have integrated simulation into their education practices for more than a decade, occupational therapy remains in the early stages of simulation use. We can trace early ideas of simulation in occupational therapy education back to the late 1980s with the instructional method coined *classroom as clinic*. Neistadt (1987, 1992) used classroom as clinic to teach students in a master's degree program the clinical reasoning process during occupational therapy evaluation and treatment. She provided students with information about an adult with a physical disability. In the classroom, the students spent 90 to 120 minutes with the individual to ask questions and perform assessment procedures. The students completed reflection responses and participated in group discussion immediately after the experience. Finally, they completed a presentation in which they role played a team meeting to make discharge recommendations for their individual. In a later publication, Neistadt and Smith (1997) implemented the use of videos during simulation. As you read the Implementation section of this chapter, you will notice similar features in current simulation methods.

Literature considers simulation in occupational therapy education as still emerging due to a lack of studies supporting the use and efficacy of this method in the profession's curricula. As of 2015, there were 57 reports of simulation in occupational therapy education literature (see Simulation-Based Instructional Methods Evidence Table). Educators were using forms of simulation to meet a wide range of competencies (e.g., information gathering, communication, goal setting, professional behavior). Despite this dearth of evidence, a 2010 survey reported every occupational therapy program in Australia was using some form of simulation; all using case studies, role play, and videos but only half using standardized patients. Similarly, Bethea and colleagues (2014) surveyed occupational therapy and occupational therapy assistant programs in the United States during the 2012 to 2013 academic year. Of the 79% of programs that responded, 175 (71%) reported they used some form of simulation, with the most common method being human simulation with students or actors, and the least common method being virtual immersive games with avatar or self-projections. In several articles, occupational therapy students conveyed interest in and preference for high-fidelity simulation. As simulation continues to grow its presence in occupational therapy education, there remains a need for educators to further enhance the evidence of its impact on learning outcomes.

THEORY

Educational literature frequently cites the use of adult learning theory to support the implementation of simulation-based instructional methods. Malcolm Knowles (1980, 1984), the founding father of adult learning theory, widely recognized and adopted the term andragogy (*andra* means "man" and *agogos* means "leader of"). Therefore, *andragogy* is the art and science of helping adults learn. In this type of teaching, the educator serves as a facilitator or a resource and the instructional

TABLE 7-3

Comparison of Pedagogy and Andragogy

PEDAGOGY	CONCEPT	ANDRAGOGY
Learner is dependent; carries out the educator's directions	Concept of the learner	Learner is self-directed
Educator	Responsibility	Learner
Learners have little experience to use as a resource for learning	Role of learner's experience	Learners have experiences and backgrounds that serve as a rich resource for learning
Information is transmitted from educator to learner (lectures, audiovisuals, etc.)	Methodology	Learners are a good resource for one another (group discussions, field experiences, problem-solving projects, etc.)
Learners are ready to learn when told	Readiness to learn	Learners are ready to learn, when they need to know or do something, or to help achieve a goal
Subject-centered orientation	Orientation to learning	Problem-centered orientation
Motivated by external pressures	Motivation to learning	Learners are internally motivated
Postponed	Application of information	Immediate

methods are active, such as simulation and role playing. In contrast, the term *pedagogy* (*paid* means "child" and *agogos* means "leader of") is the art of science of teaching children. From a pedagogy perspective, educators transmit content to the students and the instructional methods are passive, such as lectures, audiovisuals, or readings. These approaches to learning further differ on the foundational principles (Table 7-3). However, we will only highlight the principles of adult learning theory in relation to simulation.

In adult learning theory, the student is self-directed and self-regulated. Adult learners acquire what they want and need to learn and when they want to learn. They develop a readiness to learn when they recognize they need to know the information or they need to perform more effectively in an area of their life. In simulation-based instructional methods, educators discuss the relevance of the experience to their students' professional practice and use the learning objectives to allow the students to make decisions about how to approach the task. Because of this, the students provide their own motivation for participation in simulation and the educator serves as the facilitator.

Adult learners are internally motivated when they believe the outcome is useful, tangible, and immediately applicable to their life. When students engage in these methods, they often experience a sense of community and increased feelings of competency and autonomy. Their *self-efficacy* (the belief that they can execute the task) further contributes to their motivation for learning. Educators design the simulation with a strong understanding of their students' knowledge, so the experience possesses a high probability of success. They also incorporate simulation-based instructional methods into their courses because they have the power to motivate students particularly when they use strategies to promote a respectful and supportive simulation environment.

Another key feature of adult learning is the belief that adult learners have prior knowledge, experiences, backgrounds, and perspectives that serve as a rich resource for learning. Because each student has these unique features, they serve as a great source for each other. As educators, we must create opportunities to elicit and connect new learning to these foundational understandings. In simulation, we accomplish this task in multiple ways. Educators develop simulation so students work side by side to complete the task or observe each other to provide relevant feedback. Educators also use a debriefing phase to guide the students through a reflective process in which they can discuss how their prior knowledge and experiences contributed to their decisions and how new knowledge would change or form new mental models for future situations (e.g., analogical reasoning). During a simulation, students are continuously applying and refining their current mental models. We can further enhance their analogical reasoning by providing opportunities to transfer their knowledge and skills during the deepening phase of the debriefing process (see Implementation section). Not only do adult learning theory principles serve as a guide for developing simulation methods, but it also provides educators with areas to reflect on as they appraise the overall experience.

IMPLEMENTATION

Educators engage in deliberate thought about where and how to use simulation throughout the curriculum. Before reading this section, take a moment to reflect on the following questions in the box below:

- In which areas of my courses do I have some control over the learning objectives?
- What Accreditation Council for Occupational Therapy Education standards are in my courses?
- What simulation methods with characteristics of high environmental or equipment fidelity are appropriate for my courses?
- What level of fidelity can the department reasonably support (e.g., time, costs, resources)?
- Where in the curriculum are my students ready to engage in simulation?

Prior to discussing implementation, we want to provide you with an additional resource for developing simulation experiences in your courses. The National Health Education and Training in Simulation is an international training program for health care professionals and educators designed to improve their simulation practices. They offer online modules and workshops to any individual that uses or intends to use this method of instruction with their students. If you have an interest in improving or incorporating simulation throughout your course or program, we encourage you to access this resource.

Educators employ a variety of approaches for the implementation of simulation-based instructional methods. Nestel and colleagues (2018) offer educators a framework they can apply across a wide range of simulation methods, settings, and professions. We will use the six phases of this framework to outline the implementation of simulation but will also include other valuable sources of information for successful execution in your courses.

Phase 1: Prepare

The preparing phase includes each of the activities that take place before you and your students begin the simulation experience. During this phase, you will need to make several important decisions and perform numerous tasks.

Develop Learning Objectives

As previously discussed, the first step for designing an effective simulation experience is the development of learning objectives. Simply ask yourself, "What do I want my students to achieve or demonstrate during the simulation?" Your learning objectives will guide the remainder of your decisions, such as the level of fidelity, type of case study, progression of events, and design of the debriefing process. As you begin to write the learning objectives, be sure to really consider your students' level of academic and professional preparedness and their needs. It is important the objectives align with your students' knowledge and experiences to provide the "just-right challenge."

For example, you are thinking about simulating an interaction with a patient in an intensive care unit, but your students have not had exposure to the management of lines or leads in their didactic coursework or fieldwork experiences. Therefore, you would not want to write a learning objective about managing lines and leads during activities of daily living. Instead you might simplify the learning objectives, such as establishing rapport with the patient during the development of the occupational profile or explaining the role of occupational therapy.

Educational literature provides additional recommendations for establishing learning objectives for simulation experiences. Remember, learning objectives need to be observable and measurable and should have a range of complexities (e.g., lower-level and higher-level taxonomies). Ideally, you would write three to four broad learning objectives for one simulation, remembering that one objective can address several behaviors. If you create extensive learning objectives, which would likely require a long simulation experience, your students will likely be overwhelmed and you will likely have challenges leading a focused debriefing session. We will reference these learning objectives throughout the remainder of this section, as it is of the greatest importance to determine what specific learning has occurred during the simulation. Gibbs and Dietrich (2017) provide a nice example of learning objectives for an acute care simulation (Figure 7-1).

Design the Scenario

After crafting well-designed learning objectives, you are ready to draft the case scenario. Your learning objectives will drive the decisions you make during this process. Regardless of the type of simulation, you will need to write a case scenario to introduce your students to the experience. We have provided a list of questions for you to consider when writing the case for the simulation experience. As you answer these questions, we recommend you keep your learning objectives in close proximity. Baird and colleagues (2015) provide nice examples of case scenarios if you need a few ideas to get started:

- What does the clinical environment look like?
- What simulation method will help my students achieve the learning objectives?
- What equipment do I need to include in the case scenario?
- What is the client's condition (physical, mental, past medical history, diagnosis, vital signs)?
- What specific events do I need to include so my students have to make decisions and/or achieve the learning objectives (e.g., client experiences orthostatic hypotension during a transfer, family member becomes upset about discharge plan, intracranial pressure increases during bed mobility)?

> Similar to professional practice, the context has a great impact on the quality of learning. You will want to carefully consider the simulated learning environment!

Simulation Scenario	
Scenario	Changes in physiologic factors during transfer
Estimated Scenario Time	15 minute
Estimated Debriefing Time	15 minute
Target Group	OT/PT student

Prerequisite Knowledge

Learners should possess the following competencies prior to participation in this scenario.

Knowledge of tubes and lines and their purpose
Knowledge of precautions
Knowledge of normal HR, O2, and BP values
Basic handling skills
Basic communication skills

Cognitive Skills	Psychomotor Skills
Critical thinking Problem solving	Dependent bed mobility skills Body mechanics

Brief Summary

Students are given the task of getting a patient from supine to sitting on the edge of the bed. They need to be aware of all lines and tubes as well as mobility precautions. Students must be able to monitor physiological changes and respond appropriately to a critical event (drop in O2, spike in HR, or drop in blood pressure). They need to be able to demonstrate appropriate communication skills with the patient and each other throughout the scenario.

Learning Objectives

1.	Demonstrate appropriate infection control (hand washing and gloves).
2.	Demonstrate appropriate communication with patient and team.
3.	Identify all lines and tubes and be able to cite precautions related to each.
4.	Reposition lines and maintain appropriate line position throughout movements of the patient.
5.	Demonstrate proper handling of the patient including maintaining appropriate draping of the patient.
6.	Maintain good body mechanics for all movements.
7.	Recognizes critical event in a timely manner and response appropriately.
8.	Appropriately ending treatment based on clinical reasoning.
9.	Demonstrate appropriate position of patient at end (side rails, call bell, draping).
10.	Demonstrates ability to accurately reflect on performance during debriefing.

Figure 7-1. Example of learning objectives. (Reproduced with permission from Gibbs, D. M., & Dietrich, M. [2017]. Using high fidelity simulation to impact occupational therapy student knowledge, comfort, and confidence in acute care. *Open Journal of Occupational Therapy, 5*[1], Article 10. https://dx.doi.org/10.15453/2168-6408.1225)

- What necessary resources do I need (time, space, and equipment) for each of my students to complete this case scenario?
- How much detail do my students need in order to adequately make decisions?
- How do I create this case scenario to provide my students with a significant challenge?
- What type of fidelity do my students need to meet the learning objectives?
- What additional supporting materials, such as medical images, will my students need?

Your case scenario can include a wide range of content, but you will want the case to proceed in a single direction to avoid overcomplexity that could distract students from the learning objective. However, you will want to include enough details and real-life challenges to promote authenticity.

In many examples, the educator provides a written scenario, but you could also consider the use of video and other various forms of technology to introduce the case to your students. If you need further information on writing a case scenario, please see Chapter 12.

Educational literature highly recommends seeking input from multiple resources, such as clientele, standardized patients, practitioners, and colleagues. By including clients or standardized patients, you ensure their voices are being heard. Current practitioners provide valuable input as they have a good understanding of present practice and the skills and knowledge required to work in a particular setting. They can provide information about the presentation and challenges of a particular client, common methods of assessment, and customary equipment. Your colleagues offer further feedback about clarity of case details and the fit with your students' current knowledge, skills, and experiences. Including these individuals into the design process will no doubt support the success and authenticity of the simulation. However, we caution you that a case study of a real client or family has the potential to be distracting. While a real case study might serve as a great starting point for the simulation, you and the individuals you consult will need to adapt the case to only provide the information necessary to meet your learning objectives to avoid complexity and confusion.

Plan the Logistics

Once you have the case scenario written and a solid idea of what the simulation will entail, you will need to carefully and thoughtfully plan numerous aspects for successful implementation of this method. In the Appendix, we have provided you a checklist to ensure you have considered the important logistics of the simulation. In addition, Shoemaker and colleagues (2011) provide an excellent example of a highly structured simulation schedule called "the Beasley method" that could serve a guide for planning your simulation experiences (Figure 7-2).

As we discussed previously, you can collaborate with other individuals to complete these necessary steps. For example, a practitioner can assist in setting up the environment to look like the desired practice setting, share equipment to complete the simulation, and can help train standardized patients. Occupational therapy or rehabilitation departments in your local area might also allow your department to borrow equipment and devices.

Phase 2: Brief

During this phase, you want to brief your students and your additional facilitators (e.g., faculty, practitioners, and standardized patients as applicable). Your briefing is key for executing a valuable learning experience, as many students initially report feelings of anxiety and stress. Therefore, it is important that you acknowledge and normalize your students' expectations and feelings and establish a safe environment and trustful relationship during this time. We suggest reviewing the following pieces of information with your students:

- Review learning objectives and instructions
- Discuss the environment, equipment, phases, and timeline
- Clarify appropriate attire
- Describe the debrief and feedback process
- Outline their responsibilities and roles as practitioners and observers
- Review evaluation methods and rubrics (e.g., expectations)
- Provide clarity about who is observing and if you are recording the simulation
- Explain how you will secure and archive videos if recording
- Review the confidentiality agreement and have the students sign
- Brief students on the case scenario (potentially provide case scenario during this time depending on schedule)
- Foster an environment of mutual respect and trust

> In order to increase authenticity, ask your students to wear the attire they would be expected to wear in the setting.

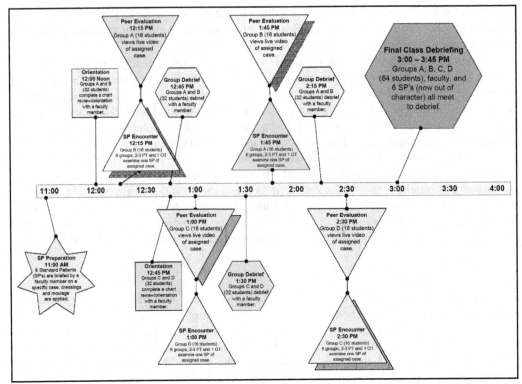

Figure 7-2. Example of simulation schedule. (Reproduced with permission from Shoemaker, M. J., Beasley, J., Cooper, M., Perkins, R., Smith, J., & Swank, C. [2011]. A method for providing high-volume interprofessional simulation encounters in physical and occupational therapy education programs. *Journal of Allied Health, 40*[1], e15-e21.)

You will also want to orient your students by providing a tour of the simulation environment and affording them opportunities to test the equipment. Studies suggest orientation to the equipment and space impact the students' ability to perform. Depending on the time frame, you might choose to complete the brief prior to or on the day of the simulation. Throughout the brief process, allow your students ample time to ask questions. The International Nursing Association for Clinical Simulation and Learning Board of Directors (2011) further outline ways to maintain the professional integrity of the students engaged in simulation, which are applicable to the briefing process.

You will need to brief your additional facilitators on similar matters. Provide these individuals with a list of the learning objectives, a description of your students' characteristics, orientation to the simulator and/or setting, and timeline for the simulation. In addition, any individual assisting you in the actual implementation will need information on how to start, pause, or end the simulation and/or technical equipment, communicate during the simulation, perform the debrief and feedback process, and complete evaluation forms.

Phase 3: Complete the Simulation

After the preparatory work, you and your students are ready to complete the simulation. First, you will introduce the facilitators and students. Remember, your tone during this encounter will set the stage for the simulation experience. During the initial preparation phase, you will have divided your students into small groups. Within these small groups, one set of students will perform the simulation, while the other set of students will observe their performance (Figure 7-3). They will switch roles at some point during the experience. The number of students completing the simulation should most closely resemble professional practice with the option of having them rotate roles.

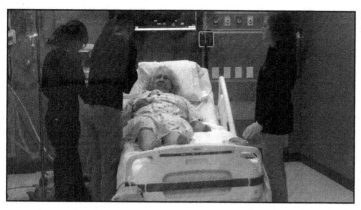

Figure 7-3. Learners engage in simulation.

The designated students participate in the simulation while the facilitator and peers observe their individual performance. You (or another facilitator) will indicate a clear start and begin any audiovisual recording (if applicable). The students actively involved in the simulated environment will determine their course of action in response to the case scenario. The students might experience anxiety; however, this is good and necessary to produce their authentic response to the case. Watch carefully for physical and psychological safety, as they are completing the simulation. In addition, you will immediately observe the students' ability to apply and integrate knowledge.

We would like to draw your attention to one interesting argument in simulation education—the use of a "time out" or temporary pause in action. The literature provides little insight on the use of this strategy. Some scholars believe this strategy could offer an important option for students that experience adverse feelings that could challenge their confidence. However, other scholars cite challenges, such as overuse or increased time to complete the simulation.

Depending on the setup, the observers will watch the simulation on a screen through live video streaming in a different room, through a one-way screen or mirror, or off to side within the actual environment. The observers should talk minimally during the simulation. You will want to encourage them to take notes or complete evaluation materials so they can provide critical feedback during the debriefing process (Figure 7-4).

Traditionally, the debrief and feedback process occurs after the students have completed the simulation. However, some simulation experiences might lend itself to immediate feedback from the facilitator or observers. It will be up to you to decide if the observers can play a supportive role, such as prompting through a radio or "stepping in" during a time out. You can further review the references at the end of the chapter, as there are numerous examples of different ways to implement simulation in health professional education.

Phase 4: Debrief and Feedback

Educational literature frequently cites debriefing as the **most** important element in the learning process and that a majority of the learning occurs after the simulation. *Debriefing* is an educator- or peer-led reflective conversation used to analyze individual and group performance during a simulation experience. It remains a cornerstone of simulation because it serves several key purposes:

- Alters the students' frames of reference and behavior
- Allows them to discuss the rationale for their decisions or indecisions
- Permits the expression of their feelings
- Offers chance to seek others' perspectives
- Affords information about their performance
- Gives opportunities for reflection
- Provides experience for generalization to their future professional practice

Acute Care Simulation Checklist

Student Name:

Satisf	Unsatisf	Task/Skill	Comment
		Follows infection control guidelines:	
		Washes hands before entering room	
		Washes hands on exiting room	
		Gloves to handle patient	
		Communication with patient	
		Confirms patient identify	
		Identifies self name	
		Identifies profession	
		Explains plan for session	
		Responds in professional manner to patient	
		Instructs patient appropriately in treatment process	
		Uses appropriate terms	
		Communication with Team	
		Respectful of team member	
		Collaborates with team member appropriately	
		Communicated effectively during critical event	
		Treatment Session	
		Managing tubes and lines:	
		Identify and trace all lines from patient to origin	
		IV	
		Catheter	
		O2	
		Heart Monitor	
		Rearranges lines in preparation for moving	
		Monitors lines throughout whole movement	
		Positions/handles the patient appropriately	
		Maintain modesty and draping of patient at all times	
		Student maintains good body mechanics	
		Leaves patient in appropriate position (side rails, call bell, draping)	
		Critical Event	
		Recognize critical event in a timely manner	
		Respond appropriately to event	
		Know when event has resolved and is safe to continue or leave patient	

_____   _____
Faculty Observer Signature   Date
Developed by authors with contributions from Renee Brown, PT. PhD

Figure 7-4. Example of checklist. (Reproduced with permission from Gibbs, D. M., & Dietrich, M. [2017]. Using high fidelity simulation to impact occupational therapy student knowledge, comfort, and confidence in acute care. *Open Journal of Occupational Therapy, 5*[1], Article 10. https://dx.doi.org/10.15453/2168-6408.1225)

Scholars agree that debriefing should occur immediately after the simulation rather than delaying to a later date or time. In addition, your debriefing time should equal or double the time your students spend with the simulation.

A debriefing framework outlines several phases with each phase serving a specific function. We suggest adopting a consistent framework to help you structure a debrief and to allow your students to anticipate the flow and form of conversation. It can help novice educators organize the debriefing process and promote their confidence and can also assist more experienced educators with time management and the prioritization of important discussion points. Your role as the facilitator is to guide an active and student-led discussion. Your students should be speaking most of the time and you are simply employing Socratic questions (see Chapter 10). We outline a four-step debriefing process in Table 7-4.

During the discovering phase, you can use objective data to help guide the group discussion, such as checklists, the observer's notes, or the audiovisual material. These methods are particularly useful when you need to increase your students' awareness to their thought processes or behaviors. It would also be beneficial for you to have your learning objectives and observation notes nearby to ensure you are adequately addressing the important ideas. We have also provided additional frameworks for you to explore to determine which best fits your needs (Table 7-5).

If the simulation involves a standardized patient, you can consider adding their input to the debrief and feedback process. Although simulation literature offers little insight into this element, the standardized patient can describe their interaction with the students. The students receive valuable information about their actions and communication that further shape their educational and professional practices.

Phase 5: Reflection

The goal of this phase is to further promote the reflective process that is essential for learning. You will encourage your students to **individually** reflect on their experiences with the simulation. In simulation literature, educators often use a self-assessment or a one-page reflection during this phase. With these methods, students identify their strengths and difficulties, discuss their overall experience, and offer suggestions to improve their learning process. As you design or select methods of reflection, attempt to include an element that compels your students to think about their emotion during the simulation. Similarly, it is just as important that you, your facilitators, and standardized patients reflect on your experiences and contributions. We provide examples of additional reflection methods later in this chapter.

Phase 6: Evaluation

Simulation requires complex evaluation involving multiple methods of assessment and each of the stakeholders. We recommend using qualitative and quantitative methods to assess your students. Remember to review your learning objectives so you can select the best mix of methods to show that your students have demonstrated competency. In Table 7-6, you will find examples of different assessments and assignments. If these examples do not fit your needs, you can modify or develop your own methods. However, we recommend you obtain feedback from your key stakeholders before employing any assessment or assignment. Similar to engaging in reflection, you will also need to evaluate the overall simulation to determine if it met your intended goals.

Table 7-4

Debriefing Phases

PHASE	PURPOSE
1. Prebriefing	Introduces the debrief process: • Outline the timeframe and structure • Establish the goals • Model the ground rules for appropriate behavior and feedback
2. Defusing Remember: Students are psychologically impacted in authentic simulation. They need to vent!	Allows students to freely express their emotional reactions in a safe and open environment: Encourages students to release any stress and anxiety they felt during the simulation to prepare for in-depth analysis and learning Provides the educator insight to the students' perspectives and knowledge gaps: • "What happened during the simulation experience?" • "Why did [X] happen?" • "How did you feel during this experience?"
3. Discovering	Encourages students to identify behaviors and internal frames of references: • "Can you describe your thought process when you did [X]?" • "Can you tell us why you did [X]?" Allows integration of new information for optimal performance in future professional practice: • "How would you handle this situation differently in your future fieldwork?" • "How do these actions reflect [evidence-based practice, occupation-based practice, or current practice guidelines]?" Provides feedback about positive aspects and areas for improvement: • "What went well during the simulation?" • "What behavior or thought process impeded your ability to perform?"
4. Deepening	Builds connections to professional practice: • "What did you learn from this simulation that would improve your future practice?" • "How would you use this new information in the future?" Applies new learning to other similar situations: • Can revisit previous case scenarios • Ask to solve a future case scenario

---

TABLE 7-5

Debriefing Frameworks

- Advocacy-Inquiry Method
- Diamond Debriefing (Barbara Steinwachs)
- Good Judgment Approach
- Promoting Excellence and Reflective Learning in Simulation
- TeamGAINS
- U.S. Military After-Action Review

TABLE 7-6

Examples of Assessments and Assignments in Simulation

QUANTITATIVE METHODS	QUALITATIVE METHODS	ASSIGNMENTS
- Self-evaluation checklist - Peer evaluation - Behavior checklist for performance assessment (Figure 7-5) - Critical Thinking Disposition Inventory - Health Science Reasoning Test - Interdisciplinary Education Perception Scale - Attitudes Toward Mental Illness Questionnaire - Pre/posttest survey - Objective Structured Assessment of Debriefing* - Debriefing Assessment for Simulation in Healthcare*	- Reflective journal - Debriefing logs Qualitative methods allow students to provide open and honest answers. Educators receive valuable information about the learners' feelings and can address issues in a personalized manner.	- Write a subjective, objective, assessment, and plan note - Write goals - Develop interventions based on evaluation findings during simulation - Presentation of case findings - Development of discharge plan with recommendations

* This assessment evaluates the facilitator completing the debrief and feedback phase.

Items for Peer- and Self-Evaluation	
Yes/No	Task
	Patient/Client greeted was greeted appropriately
	Explained role of respective discipline
	Explained the purpose of the therapy session
	Discussed home environment
	Discussed occupations/interests/patient goals
	Discussed family support
	Discussed functional limitations
	Appropriate eye contact
	Appropriate use of body language
	Respectful tone
	Clear and concise language
	Appropriate volume of voice
	Developed rapport
	Professional behavior (absence of inappropriate comments or interactions)
	Demonstrated active listening
	Displayed empathy
	Used open-ended questions appropriately
	Demonstrated correct techniques for psychomotor skills
	Concluded the session appropriately
	Comments:

Figure 7-5. Example of behavioral checklist. (Reproduced with permission from Shoemaker, M. J., Beasley, J., Cooper, M., Perkins, R., Smith, J., & Swank, C. [2011]. A method for providing high-volume interprofessional simulation encounters in physical and occupational therapy education programs. *Journal of Allied Health, 40*[1], e15-e21.)

ADDITIONAL SIMULATION-BASED INSTRUCTIONAL METHODS

Role Play

We would like to highlight another simulation-based instructional method—role playing. *Role playing* is a form of drama that allows the students to simulate practical experiences and psychodynamic processes in a safe environment (Figure 7-6). Moreno (1953) originally developed this instructional method to train individuals on the use of interpersonal relationships when working with clients with mental illnesses. Educators use role playing in a variety of settings and for various purposes. However, we note the most common purpose for and value of the use of role play is to practice elements of human interaction. In role play, students gain experience in dealing with highly charged questions or situations (e.g., "Am I ever going to walk again?" "What did I do to deserve this?" "Am I going to die?"), increasing awareness of their values and attitudes and the feelings of others, and desensitizing their own feelings, so they have confidence working with actual clients in the future.

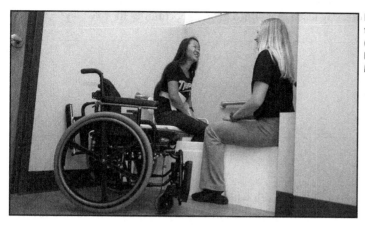

Figure 7-6. Students role play a tub transfer in a home environment. (Reproduced with permission from Keith Borgmeyer/University of Missouri.)

We encourage you to continue to use the phases outlined when developing opportunities for role play in your courses but will also highlight a few additional notes related to this instructional method. Because role play offers lower fidelity, you will find less complexity in each of the implementation phases. Educational literature suggests providing your students with a brief script, so they feel less pressure and more comfort in acting out the situation. However, you would want to explain that your students are not limited to the content in the script. You can develop scripts from actual cases that possess high value (e.g., a case scenario in which a conflict or crisis occurs and the students are forced to make some sort of decision, a scenario that is of interest to students). When you first introduce role play into your courses, ask for volunteers to perform the scenario. At first you will notice many students are reluctant to engage in this method, but you will often find the number of volunteers steadily increases as they realize they are not expected to skillfully act. They are only expected to follow the brief script, provide genuine responses, and ask questions as the situation progresses. Just as previously described, the students who are not engaged in role play observe and offer valuable feedback and analysis during the short debriefing process.

Occupational therapy literature provides numerous examples for the use of role play to develop professional knowledge, attitudes, and skills. Folts and colleagues (1986) used role play to prepare students in an independent study on hospice care. The student played the role of the occupational therapist while the educator played the role of the client and/or family member. In your courses, you could also play the role of client or family member during a laboratory experience or during regular class to enhance the topic of discussion. Bennett and colleagues (2017) asked students to role play a client and the caregiver of that client while another student attempted to teach them how to use various pieces of assistive technology and adaptive equipment. One final example includes the use of role playing to simulate an ethical situation a student might experience in occupational therapy practice. Haddad (1988) assigned each student the role of a multidisciplinary team member so they can determine the best solution for a psychiatrist that is withholding food and hydration from a client in order to modify his behavior. Some occupational therapy educators even suggest the use of role play following Level I fieldwork experiences, so students potentially view additional ways to handle challenging situations.

Although role play is of low fidelity, we recognize advantages to the implementation of this instructional method. Unlike the standardized patient method, you can use role play to provide your students with repeated practice of certain skills because of its simplicity in terms of cost, time, and resources. You can also use this method of instruction in a variety of ways, such as dividing your students into small groups or asking a few students to complete the role play in front of the entire class. Similar to other simulation-based instructional methods, your students are required to flexibly think and appropriately respond to the client, make professional decisions, receive feedback from facilitators and peers, and observe others during role play. When students engage in role play, they become more aware of how a client might feel or behave in that particular situation and often have a change in attitude and behavior as a result.

What areas of content do you currently teach that afford good opportunities for role play?

```


```

Laboratory Experiences

An additional instructional method that can fit within the realm of simulation-based instructional methods includes the use of laboratory experiences. In laboratory experiences, educators offer students opportunities to develop practical skills in a **contrived** context and also provide instant feedback. Some educators and students consider this out-of-context learning to be a negative aspect of this instructional method. However, educational literature cites the primary benefit of laboratory experiences is that students can obtain and practice the necessary and foundational skills without the pressure of working with "real" clients in practical settings. This method affords our students opportunities to master certain skills, so they can later provide safe care for clients and families. When educators combine this hands-on method with feedback and reflection, they assist students to bridge the gap between education and practice.

We suggest using laboratory when your students need opportunities to learn and master basic skills before performing or applying these skills later in their educational or fieldwork experiences (e.g., scaffolding). For example, you might use a laboratory experience when your students are acquiring knowledge about various pieces of adaptive equipment, practicing administration of standardized assessments, learning to perform range of motion or manual muscle testing, palpating various structures of the body, or implementing activity analysis to understand play-based interventions for children. We can elevate learning in traditional laboratory experiences when we use simulation frameworks as a guide. We highlight an adapted framework later.

Our students must acquire many skills in order to be successful during their fieldwork and professional experiences. Skill practice requires educators to find ways to integrate the psychomotor, affective, and cognitive components of skills into the laboratory experiences. When we attend to each of these components, our students engage in meaningful learning, which simulates curiosity, creativity, and critical thinking. For example, our students need opportunities to process their observations and information, develop a mental image for correct completion of skills, practice and receive feedback, and determine if their performance matches the previously created image. By considering the following four phases for the implementation of this instructional method, we can further augment learning.

Designing the Laboratory Experience

As previously discussed throughout this book and this chapter, you will want to carefully consider the learning objectives for the laboratory experience and for the course. It will be critical that you select the most relevant methods to meet the identified learning objectives. Similar to simulation, you will also need to thoughtfully contemplate the flow of the experience, what academic knowledge your students already possess, and what support you will provide about the content you plan to address during the experience. For example, many health professional educators assign readings, require students to watch videos or answer certain questions, or review theory related to a skill in the laboratory.

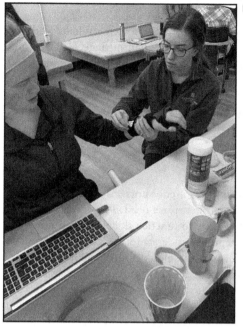

Figure 7-7. Students engage in a laboratory experience.

Conducting the Laboratory Experience

At the start of the laboratory experience (similar to earlier simulation), you will want to complete an initial briefing with your students to clarify instructions, outline expectations, and address any questions or concerns. After the introduction, you may also need to highlight the relevant points for each phase of the experience or demonstrate certain aspects or skills. Your students will divide into pairs or small groups to practice the identified skills during the laboratory experience (Figure 7-7). If your students are rotating between several stations or are completing multiple skills during the duration of the laboratory, you will need to provide them with a reasonable amount of time to practice. During the laboratory experience, you are circulating around the room posing questions, asking to describe thought processes, encouraging peer dialogue and observation, and facilitating understanding and performance of skills.

> It is key that you do not rush your students through the experience—allow 1.5 to 2 times more than you think they will need.

Evaluating Performance

Educational literature provides several options for evaluating your students' performances during and after a laboratory experience. You can use one of these evaluation methods or a combination of methods. Remember to review your objectives and select an evaluation method that best aligns with your learning goals:

- Create a worksheet to guide students through the experience, which asks questions to further develop professional-reasoning and critical-thinking skills, and assign a grade
- Construct a rubric to assign participation points
- Develop a skills checklist that describes successful performance and requires students to demonstrate competency; a peer can also look at the checklist and provide learner feedback

Providing Feedback

As with many other instructional methods, you will need to provide your students feedback during and following participation in the laboratory experience. Your immediate feedback and reinforcement will facilitate your students' ability to master the skill and allow them to understand the rationale behind successful performance. Your feedback works best if it is direct but constructive. After completion of the laboratory, you will likely provide written or verbal feedback using the evaluation method you selected. We will provide other meaningful ways to provide opportunities for feedback and reflection later in this chapter.

Strategies to Elevate Laboratory Experiences

Similar to the ability to respond to changes in simulation, educators can introduce several strategies into laboratory experience to create the element of surprise needed to deepen learning. After your students have had an appropriate amount of time to practice skills, you can present a case study. By including a case study, your students begin to understand the dynamic nature of practice, apply theory and skills to the realistic situations, and develop decision-making, problem-solving, professional-reasoning, and critical-thinking skills in a safe environment. For example, after your students have practiced range of motion or manual muscle testing, provide them with case scenarios in which they have to make decisions about which areas to assess, modify the way they provide the instructions because of a cognitive or language concern, or discuss what they would do if experiencing pain. Similarly, perhaps you are introducing your students to various pieces of adaptive equipment. Following ample practice time, you can present a case study in which they have to teach a client and family how to use the equipment at home or to think about other strategies for completing the task if the client and family cannot afford the adaptive equipment. Lastly, you can role play a particular client and select one to two students to demonstrate the skill at the end of the laboratory experience. Your students are motivated to really learn and practice the concepts because they know they could be required to demonstrate in front of their educator and peers. If you elect to use this strategy, be sure to allow some time for feedback and reflection following the role play. In these situations, our students combine many valuable skills that will later behoove their educational and professional practice.

Potential Issues in Simulation-Based Instructional Methods

Despite increase in popularity and supporting evidence, educators should be aware of potential concerns with the use of simulation-based instructional methods. Many disability communities express concern with use of standardized patients, role play, and/or laboratory experiences because they believe the simulation provides a limited understanding of what an individual actually experiences and reinforces stigmas and negative views. Because of this, students tend to focus their attention to an impairment or condition versus the complexity of challenges to engaging in various occupations, roles, and contexts. Therefore, they develop a false sense of what it is like to live with a particular disability. We note that in a majority of cases, someone who does not have a disability designs the simulation, which further creates an inauthentic experience and feelings of sadness or pity toward the individual. We can overcome this challenge by consulting or hiring individuals with disabilities as we develop simulation methods for our courses. In addition, educators should critically reflect as they design simulation opportunities for occupational therapy education. You can ask yourself a series of questions, such as:

- Can this simulation be harmful to an individual with a disability?
- Does my simulation embody our professional underpinnings?
- Who can I include in the design process to ensure the lived experience is well represented?
- How will my students interpret this experience?

TIPS AND TRICKS

- Allow ample time for the planning phase (some literature recommends a 2-month planning period).
- Invite collaboration within the profession and across professions during the planning phase (e.g., faculty, practitioners, health simulation staff, doctoral candidates).
- Maintain a pool of "clients" from practicum and networking experiences or ask practitioners in your area for potential "clients."
- Consider use of older cohort of students or postprofessional students to serve the standardized patient role.
- Be prepared to frequently evaluate your own personal and professional thought processes.
- Be energetic and flexible during simulation experiences.

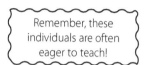
Remember, these individuals are often eager to teach!

- Consider sharing simulation case scenarios (e.g., can you modify a case scenario from the physical therapy or nursing programs?).
- Explore websites that publish information and scenarios (e.g., International Nursing Association for Clinical Simulation and Learning, National League for Nursing Simulation Innovation Resource Center).
- Seek funding for simulation equipment and resources (e.g., grants, foundations, alumni, donors).

OPPORTUNITIES FOR FEEDBACK AND REFLECTION

We have briefly mentioned several examples of feedback and reflection during Phases 4 and 5 in the Implementation section. We will further describe ways you can provide your students with opportunities for engaging in these reflective thought processes. One way to provide students feedback and reflection is through video-reflexivity. In *video-reflexivity*, students review the recorded video of the simulation to engage in verbal or written discussion. You have several options when using this method. First, your students can watch the video alone and write and submit their answers to a series of posited questions.

Secondly, you and your students can watch their video and ask and answer questions on some sort of online platform, such as TORSH Talent (https://www.torsh.co/classroom-observation-tools/torsh-talent/). With this platform, you add time-synced comments via text or audio recording for your students to answer or review. For example, a standardized patient asks the student a challenging question and the student confidently answers this question. You can tag a note to the student that says, "What personal or professional experiences did you rely on to answer this question?" or "In what ways did this question challenge your values or beliefs?" The student can review and respond to each of the comments as they watch the video. You could also have a peer use this platform to provide feedback to the student. Lastly, you and your student can watch the video together (Figure 7-8). In this case, you and your student would engage in a verbal discussion as you ask your students a series of questions about the simulation.

In addition, educational literature provides a series of facilitation strategies during a group process (Table 7-7). We can use these strategies to promote reflection, determine reasons for certain behaviors and decisions, or identify solutions to various problems.

Figure 7-8. The educator and student review video of a simulation.

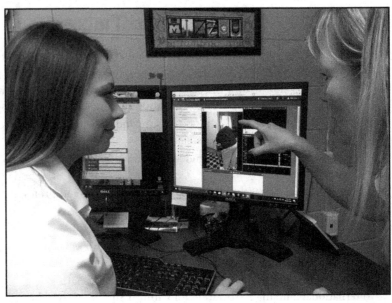

APPLICATION TO OCCUPATIONAL THERAPY PRACTICE

High-quality evidence suggests organizations can substantially improve individual and team performance by properly guiding debriefing processes. We describe two examples of ways you can implement simulation with your clients in professional practice. However, given the strong evidence, we encourage you to consider the inclusion of debriefing processes following departmental, committee, or multidisciplinary team meetings in your professional practice.

Example 1: Use of Driving Simulation With Adolescents

Ratzon and colleagues (2017) provide a nice example of the use of simulation in occupational therapy practice. In this study, they tested the driving skills of 29 teenagers with attention deficit hyperactivity disorder using STISIM Drive—a computer-based driving simulation commonly used for evaluation and treatment. We will expand on this study to further apply the principles of simulation implementation to practice. During the preparation phase, your client's goals would serve as the learning objectives, and their current level of performance and experiences would help guide how you design the simulation. For example, if the client had challenges with divided or selective attention, you could add a variety of tasks (e.g., obstacles, road signs) to the driving simulation to find that just-right challenge. You would brief your client on the simulation, equipment, time, assessment methods, and any other relevant information. The client completes the simulation as you record their performance. You will be observing, but you could also have a parent or peer observe before switching roles. Remember, the debriefing and feedback process is the most important phase of simulation. During this phase, you and the observer could use video, checklists, notes, and quantitative data from the program to debrief with the client. You would finish the simulation by asking the client a few reflective questions and completing any assessment or other data collection methods.

TABLE 7-7

Methods of Reflection and Feedback

REFLECTION METHOD	DESCRIPTION
Circular Questions	The educator invites a student to provide a third-person perspective on the interaction between two people.
Directive Feedback	The educator directly identifies issues and gives specific strategies for improving performance; typically, unidirectional and best suited for situations where there is a clear gap in knowledge and skills.
Focused Facilitation	The educator leads a discussion that encourages self-reflection and identifies reasons for actions and/or decisions (e.g., "I noticed you did [X]. Can you take us through your thought process during that time; what were your greatest successes, what was the biggest challenge, and how did you overcome it?"); the educator is genuinely curious.
Guided Team Self-Correction	The educator asks the students to assess their performance against a defined standard (e.g., teamwork, communication). The students examine and self-correct their actions as a group in which they store for future performance.
Plus-Delta Method	The educator asks an individual or group to discuss areas that went well and areas that require further attention and improvement. If the students identify strengths, but the educator believes those areas are actually in need of improvement, the group further discusses and analyzes the information.

Example 2: Use of Simulation in Caregiver Training Course

Perhaps the home health agency or hospital you work for is hosting a caregiver training course. The participants in this group can learn transfer or bed mobility techniques in a safe environment through use of various simulation methods, such as role play, human patient simulators, or standardized patients. You would want to provide the foundational knowledge before asking the participants to engage in the simulation. In this situation, you would still use the phases outlined in the implementation session to develop and complete the simulation. You will divide the participants into two small groups; one group completes a transfer, while the other group observes before switching roles. The participants have the same responsibilities we previously described with each role. Following the simulation, you complete the debrief and feedback, reflection, and evaluation phases to maximize learning and generalization to home.

Advantages

- Provides authenticity
- Offers a safe environment and low-risk learning experience
- Offers students opportunities to practice skills, develop safe practices, use clinical reasoning and critical thinking, prepare for fieldwork and entry-level practice, and facilitate the integration of professional concepts
- Provides value when in the role of occupational therapist and observer
- Allows educators to assess performance
- Allows students to demonstrate competency
- Affords students opportunities to interact with a real person
- Increases confidence and comfort
- Enables educator to grade or modify the simulation to meet different levels of expectations and diversity of experiences
- Students prefer this method of instruction
- Provides valuable opportunities for interprofessional education

Challenges

- Needs to be able to provide each student with an opportunity to perform the role of the occupational therapy practitioner and the role of observer during simulation
- Challenges with implementation with a large number of students
- Requires time to prepare
- Costs associated with space, technology, and payment of standardized patients
- Requires effort to sustain
- Issues with scheduling and coordination with other disciplines
- Requires educator to learn how to use the technology
- Challenges with allowing students repetitive practice
- Lacks rigorous research that simulation makes a difference; many papers are descriptive in nature
- Practices skills out of context (laboratory experiences)

In the space below, list any additional advantages or challenges.

```
┌──────────────────────────────────────────────────────┐
│                                                        │
│                                                        │
│                                                        │
│                                                        │
│                                                        │
│                                                        │
│                                                        │
└──────────────────────────────────────────────────────┘
```

Brainstorm strategies for overcoming these challenges when implementing the use of simulation-based instructional methods. Jansen and colleagues (2009) discuss challenges and strategies.

```
┌──────────────────────────────────────────────────────┐
│                                                        │
│                                                        │
│                                                        │
│                                                        │
│                                                        │
│                                                        │
└──────────────────────────────────────────────────────┘
```

THREE THINGS YOU CAN DO TOMORROW TO IMPLEMENT SIMULATION-BASED INSTRUCTIONAL METHODS WITH YOUR STUDENTS

1. See if your institution has a clinical simulation specialist to assist in the design of simulation.
2. Pick one topic and sketch a brief 3- to 5-minute role play scenario.
3. Create a worksheet to accompany your lab, which requires your students to use the skills they learn in a simulated scenario.

Simulation-Based Instructional Methods Evidence Table

SIMULATION*

Author/Year	Study Objectives	Design and Participants	Intervention and Outcome Measures	Results
Adib-Hajbaghery & Sharifi (2017)	Researchers evaluated evidence of simulation and its effect on critical thinking in nurses and nursing students	Design: Systematic literature review Selected 16 research studies Participants: 1,399 participants	2 independent reviewers participated in article selection and data extraction and review Dates of publication: January 1975 to June 2015 Databases: PubMed, Science Direct, ProQuest, Education Resources Information Center (ERIC), Google Scholar, Ovid, MagIran, SID Inclusion criteria: • Researched use of simulation in nursing and nursing education • Compared simulation with standard teaching practices • Reflected on simulation's effect on critical thinking • Written in English or Farsi • Original publication • Primary outcome measure was critical thinking	Of the 16 studies, 9 were experimental and 7 were quasi-experimental Of the 16 studies, 12 used high-fidelity patient simulation, 1 used electronic interaction, 2 used standardized patients, and 1 used video scenario 8 studies found that learning through simulation improves and promotes critical thinking in nurses and nursing students 8 studies reported that simulations were ineffective in enhancing critical thinking skills Learning through simulation can promote clinical judgment and self-efficacy
Bennett et al. (2017)	Researchers examined evidence for and outcomes of simulation to develop professional competencies in occupational therapy education	Design: Literature review Included 57 articles Participants: Occupational therapy students	Databases: MedLine, CINAHL, ERIC Inclusion criteria: • Written in English • Published and researched use of simulation in undergraduate or graduate-entry occupational therapy education	Of the 57 studies, 22 used written case studies, 13 used standardized patients, 15 used video case studies, 7 used computer-based and virtual reality cases, 8 used role-play, and 4 used mannequins

(continued)

Simulation-Based Instructional Methods Evidence Table (continued)

Author/Year	Study Objectives	Design and Participants	Intervention and Outcome Measures	Results
			• Interprofessional activities involved occupational therapy students All study designs were included in the literature review	Use of video case studies in interprofessional education are beneficial in increasing empathy and knowledge of professional roles Use of role play and problem-based learning written case studies increases achievement of learning objectives Standardized patients provide an authentic experience that allow students to develop skills needed to provide client-centered and culturally competent care Simulation activities provide a safe and flexible learning environment for students Simulation can be delivered in varying levels of fidelity All modalities of stimulation should include feedback, clear expectations, controlled environment, and active participation Modalities should be evaluated for cost-effectiveness, appropriateness, and level of authenticity
Brydges et al. (2015)	Researchers evaluated the effectiveness of simulation-based learning on self-regulated learning	Design: Systematic review and meta-analysis Included 32 research studies Participants: 2,482 health professional trainees	Databases: MedLine, Embase, CINAHL, ERIC, Web of Science, Scopus Inclusion criteria: • Quantitative study designs • Compared simulation-based interventions with other types of simulation-based interventions or no intervention	Approximately 34% of the studies investigated medical students and 34% investigated nursing students Of the 32 studies, 5 implemented a single group pre/posttest design and 22 were randomized trials

(continued)

Simulation-Based Instructional Methods Evidence Table (continued)

Author/Year	Study Objectives	Design and Participants	Intervention and Outcome Measures	Results
				Of the 32 studies, 59% included evidence that supported the validity of an outcome measure
				26 studies blinded assessment to learning outcomes
				Of the 32 studies, 11 studies included an outcome measure of learning retention
				This review included 5 comparisons between unsupervised training, unsupported training, and no intervention; pooled effect size small, but statistically significant for unsupervised training
				Researchers reported comparison of pooled results found significant support for training with educational supports (supported training) over unsupported training
				Unsupervised training resulted in lower immediate posttest outcomes than instructor-supervised training
Cant & Cooper (2017)	Researchers aimed to identify the effectiveness of simulation in prelicensure nursing programs	Design: Umbrella review (reviews of reviews) Participants: Undergraduate nursing students Researchers included 25 studies in this review	Databases: CINAHL, PubMed, Google Scholar Searched for articles 2010 to 2015 Inclusion criteria: • Described impact of simulation on nursing students	Researchers include 12 integrative reviews and 13 systematic reviews
				A majority of studies included a mix of experimental and quasi-experimental designs
				Studies included a diverse variety of simulation topics
				Most studies used a mannequin or patient actor

(continued)

Simulation-Based Instructional Methods Evidence Table (continued)

Author/Year	Study Objectives	Design and Participants	Intervention and Outcome Measures	Results
			Excluded studies: • Reviewed simulation prebrief, debrief, theory, qualitative reviews of student or faculty experience, interprofessional staff • Not available in English	A majority of reviews reported improved knowledge and critical thinking following simulation experience Many studies report simulation lacking high-quality research, particularly for transfer of skills to practice Simulation improves students' self-efficacy Studies commonly report student satisfaction with simulation with mixed results on confidence
Cook et al. (2011)	Researchers desired to summarize evidence of technology-related simulation in health professional students	Design: Systematic review and meta-analysis Participants: Total of 35,226 health professional students Researchers included 609 articles	Researchers used Preferred Reporting Items for Systematic Reviews and Meta-Analyses (PRISMA) guidelines to complete the review Databases: MedLine, Embase, CINAHL, PsycINFO, ERIC, Web of Science, Scopus Inclusion criteria: • Published in any language • Investigated use of technology-enhanced simulation to teach health professional students • Any educational level • Simulation compared to no intervention • Used outcome measure that assessed learning, behaviors, or effects on patients Excluded use of computer-based virtual patients due to recent review	Of the 609 studies, researchers completed 564 at a simulation center Of the 609 studies, 426 assessed process skills Researchers reported simulation training demonstrated moderate to large, statistically significant positive results (however, high inconsistencies) The pooled effect size suggesting large gains in knowledge as a result of simulation The pooled effect size for process skills reflects positive gains, but large inconsistencies Large effect size for behavior When compared to no intervention, simulation enhanced with technology consistently associated with large effect on knowledge, skills, and behaviors and moderate effects on outcomes related to patients

(continued)

Simulation-Based Instructional Methods Evidence Table (continued)

Author/Year	Study Objectives	Design and Participants	Intervention and Outcome Measures	Results
Doolen et al. (2016)	Researchers appraised evidence of high-fidelity simulation (HFS) in nursing education to provide educators with areas for further exploration	Design: Review of simulation reviews; systematic literature search Participants: Undergraduate nursing students Researchers included 7 studies in this review	Researchers appraised literature with Critical Appraisal Skills Programme guidelines Databases: PubMed, Academic Search Premier, CINAHL, Scopus, MedLine, ProQuest nursing journals, Excerpta Medica, PsycINFO	Researchers reported vast differences in design and assessment methods Of the 7 included articles, 5 were integrative reviews and 2 were literature reviews Researchers found no systematic reviews or meta-analysis met inclusion criteria Researchers reported a need for more methodologically sound research for translation to practice The studies reported a wide variety of challenges to completing HFS 3 of the 5 integrative reviews suggest simulation is an effective instructional method 1 major theme was the use of debriefing
Haddeland et al. (2018)	Researchers summarized evidence of the effect of HFS in nursing education, particularly in content area of deteriorating patients	Design: Systematic review and meta-analysis Participants: Undergraduate nursing students Researchers included 12 studies across 14 articles	Researchers searched the following databases: CINAHL, Medline, Embase, PsycINFO, ERIC, the Cochrane Library, and SveMed+ Inclusion criteria: • Included a pre/posttest design • Intervention of HFS • Intervention compared to traditional lecture methods or traditional clinical training • Written in English	Of the 12 studies, 8 were quasi-experimental designs 2 of the 12 studies were high quality, while the remaining 10 studies were medium quality All studies included debriefing Outcome measures included knowledge, skill performance, and self-confidence In 4 studies that included an outcome of satisfaction, all reported students were very satisfied with HFS experience

(continued)

Simulation-Based Instructional Methods Evidence Table (continued)

Author/Year	Study Objectives	Design and Participants	Intervention and Outcome Measures	Results
			• Intervention targeted ability to recognize and respond to a deteriorating adult patient • Sample included undergraduate nursing students • Level II Kirkpatrick's framework Exclusion criteria: • Studies that tested HFS against other forms of simulation or clinical practice (real patients) • If HFS was included in a course over a long period of time	Researchers reported the pooled effect sizes between groups favored HFS on skill performance 1 study demonstrated improvement in self-confidence; 2 studies did not In HFS experience, students need briefing, clear objectives, support, feedback, and debriefing
Harder (2010)	Researchers examined existing literature on the use and effectiveness of HFS in health care education	Design: Systematic review Included 23 articles Participants: Health science students	Databases: MedLine, PubMed, CINAHL, Cochrane Collaboration Dates of publication: 2003 to 2007 Inclusion criteria: • Participant performance was evaluated through the use of HFS • Included assessment of simulation intervention • Involved health science education • Utilized quantitative or comparative methods, or both Exclusion criteria: • Published earlier than 2003 • Descriptive in nature • Low-fidelity and mid-fidelity simulations	Of the 23 studies, researchers completed 16 in nursing, 6 in medicine, and 1 interdisciplinary Of the 23 studies, 10 were pre/posttest design Simulation-based learning can improve student performance and clinical skills Participation in simulated learning experiences can significantly increase students' clinical confidence and perceived competence

(continued)

Simulation-Based Instructional Methods Evidence Table (continued)

Author/Year	Study Objectives	Design and Participants	Intervention and Outcome Measures	Results
Hasan et al. (2017)	Researchers examined current evidence on efficacy of simulation instructional methods for improving clinical skills in pharmacy students	Design: Systematic review Picked 12 studies Participants: Undergraduate pharmacy students	1 researcher evaluated titles of relevant studies and 2 other researchers evaluated both abstracts and entire papers for relevance; 2 more researchers participated in data extraction Databases: MedLine, CINAHL Inclusion criteria: • Written in English • Researched use of simulation methods and skills • Published between January 1, 2000 and December 31, 2015 • Outcome measures were skill- or performance-based • Longitudinal, pre/posttest, and posttest-only designs Exclusion criteria: • Outcome measures assessed cognition and student knowledge	Included studies utilized a variety of research designs, including pre/posttest, descriptive with posttest only, descriptive with repeated measures, and longitudinal design Variety of instructional methods were used within the studies, including simulation experiences with human patients, standardized patients, real patients, and electronic medical records All simulation-based instructional methods produced positive student outcomes Participants demonstrated improved skills related to medication management, medication knowledge, and patient interaction about medication Participants were better able to recognize physical distress in patients and evaluate patient's physical health through vital signs Human patient simulation was an effective method of simulation-based instruction with pharmacy students
Kaplonyi et al. (2017)	Researchers evaluated current research to determine the influence of simulation-based learning on communication skills	Design: Systematic review Reviewed 60 studies Participants: Allied health professional students	2 independent investigators screened and reviewed articles using PRISMA guidelines Databases: Ovid, MedLine, ProQuest, CINAHL, ERIC Inclusion criteria: • Studies reported outcome measures	Of the 60 studies, 42 studies included outcomes with medical students, 11 with nursing students, and 10 with allied health students Only 2 studies reported patient outcomes; mixed results

(continued)

Simulation-Based Instructional Methods Evidence Table (continued)

Author/Year	Study Objectives	Design and Participants	Intervention and Outcome Measures	Results
			• At least 1 outcome measure focused on person-centered communication skills • Students participated in intervention • Written in English • Peer-reviewed • Included a trained simulated patient • Intervention included direct feedback from simulated patient	A majority of studies assessed a form of behavior change in students' communication skills; several studies reported improved communication as a result of simulation with a third-party rater; standardized patients also reported higher communication effectiveness Of the 60 studies, 25 reported an outcome measure of change in knowledge; study design varied 34 reported on response to use of standardized patients for communication skill development; a majority of studies reported satisfaction (but did not look forward to the experience) Overall, students reported statistically significant improvements in communication skills and confidence following learning with standardized patients
Labrague et al. (2018)	Researchers evaluated the current literature on the use of interprofessional simulation instructional methods on nursing students' academic performance	Design: Integrative review Included 30 studies Participants: Health professional students from academic programs including: • Nursing • Radiography • Physiotherapy	Databases: CINAHL, Scopus, PubMed, PsycINFO, MedLine Inclusion criteria: • Peer-reviewed • Written in English • Research published no earlier than 2010	Majority of studies included in the review were quantitative 27 studies were graded as moderate for quality of evidence 15 studies reported an increase in students' ability to communicate with others after participation in an interprofessional education–based simulation program

(continued)

Simulation-Based Instructional Methods Evidence Table (continued)

Author/Year	Study Objectives	Design and Participants	Intervention and Outcome Measures	Results
		• Pharmacy • Physical therapy • Nutrition • Social work • Respiratory therapy • Health administration • Occupational therapy		Interprofessional simulation experiences positively impacted students' knowledge of other health professionals' roles on interdisciplinary teams in 17 studies 17 articles discussed the increase in collaborative skills after students participated in interprofessional simulation activities Interprofessional simulation experiences positively impacted the confidence of students in clinical settings in 10 studies 7 studies discussed students' increased desire to participate in interprofessional education activities after participating in interprofessional simulation activities
Labrague et al. (2019)	Researchers explored evidence related to the use of HFS on nursing students' anxiety and self-confidence	Design: Systematic review Participants: Nursing studies Researchers included 35 studies	Databases: ProQuest, Scopus, MedLine, PubMed Central, CINAHL, PsycINFO Inclusion criteria: • Evaluated HFS on student anxiety and confidence • Peer-reviewed • Written in English • Published between 2007 and 2017 Exclusion criteria: • Studied other forms of simulation • Used other outcome measures	7 of the 35 studies were randomized controlled trials (RCTs), and 11 used a pre/posttest design without a control group 29 of the 35 studies examined effects of HFS on confidence with majority improving increased confidence; 3 studies demonstrated no significant changes 7 studies explored HFS on anxiety with a majority of studies suggesting HFS reduced anxiety

(continued)

Simulation-Based Instructional Methods Evidence Table (continued)

Author/Year	Study Objectives	Design and Participants	Intervention and Outcome Measures	Results
Levett-Jones & Lapkin (2013)	Researchers examined and synthesized best current evidence on the effectiveness of debriefing in simulation learning experiences	Design: Systematic review Included 10 research papers Participants (all identified through convenience sampling): • Anesthetists and anesthesia residents • Nursing students • Medical students • Nurses	Dates of publication: January 2000 to September 2011 Inclusion criteria: • Evaluated the use of debriefing in simulated learning experiences • Involved health professionals and/or health professional students • Outcome measures were objectively measured 2 reviewers completed appraisal following Joanna Briggs Institute guidelines	All 10 studies were RCTs Studies primarily included outcomes related to technical and nontechnical skills Size studies compared video-facilitated debriefing with other types of debriefing methods Studies demonstrated statistically significant improvements from pre to posttest on skills regardless of type of debrief
Mori et al. (2015)	Researchers analyzed existing literature on the impact of simulation in physical therapy education	Design: Systematic literature search Reviewed 23 articles Participants: Physical therapy students	1 reviewer participated in data extraction; another reviewer analyzed data for quality and accuracy Databases: MedLine, CINAHL, Embase, Scopus, Web of Science Inclusion criteria: • Study participants were physical therapy students • Intervention included a simulated learning experience • Included, at minimum, a posttest study design to assess the effectiveness of intervention	Feedback provided by simulators enhances skill development, increases accuracy, and decreases variability; however, many studies reported poor long-term retention Low-fidelity simulations (such as computer games) can contribute to student learning Students reported high satisfaction with human simulation experiences and indicated an increase in confidence and decrease in anxiety Human simulation experiences are beneficial to student learning but can be costly and time-consuming

(continued)

Simulation-Based Instructional Methods Evidence Table (continued)

Author/Year	Study Objectives	Design and Participants	Intervention and Outcome Measures	Results
			Primary outcomes included student satisfaction with simulated learning experience, behavior changes, and standardized educational measures Researchers rated article quality with the MERSQI instrument	HFS learning experiences have the potential to replace and/or augment clinical time Role play aids in development of communication skills and provides an opportunity for hands-on learning; however, it lacks realism Simulation is most effective when it presents a just-right challenge
Ogard-Repal et al. (2018)	Researchers examined the current evidence on student outcomes in mental health nursing when using simulation-based methods with standardized patients	Design: Integrative literature review Selected 6 studies Participants: Undergraduate nursing students	2 researchers evaluated the articles for inclusion in the review; another researcher participated in data extraction and another evaluated the quality of the evidence Databases: CINAHL, Embase, MedLine, PsycINFO, SveMed+ Dates of publication: 2013 to 2016 Inclusion criteria: • Primary research • Written in English • Use of standardized patients in mental health nursing education • Undergraduate nursing students • Researched use of standardized patients in simulation experiences to prepare for patient interaction • Peer-reviewed	5 studies demonstrated an enhanced sense of students' self-confidence in various aspects of clinical performance after a simulation experience with standardized patients 3 studies discussed improvements in skills necessary for clinical practice, such as the development of empathy In 6 studies, students experienced less worry related to nursing in the mental health setting after participation in the standardized patient simulation 1 study discussed the changes in student perceptions of mental health care 3 studies described an increase in self-awareness, specifically of one's performance and skill level, after participating in a standardized patient simulation

(continued)

Simulation-Based Instructional Methods Evidence Table (continued)

Author/Year	Study Objectives	Design and Participants	Intervention and Outcome Measures	Results
Palominos et al. (2019)	Researchers examined the current evidence on simulation-based activities and students' experiences of making mistakes during these learning experiences	Design: Integrative literature review Selected 11 studies Participants: 609 students • Nursing students • Medical students • Midwifery students • Medical imaging students	Researchers followed Whittemore and Knafl's framework Databases: MedLine, CINAHL, PsycINFO, ProQuest, Scopus, Google Scholar Inclusion criteria: • Written in English • Published from 2000 to 2018 • Primary research articles • Researched student perceptions of making errors during simulation experiences	7 studies used a qualitative approach; 4 studies used a mixed methods design Many students felt some degree of negativity, such as disappointment, about errors made during simulation-based activities Simulation activities provided a safe environment for student learners to make errors and learn from decisions that resulted in negative clinical outcomes Students often acknowledged mistakes made during simulation activities as opportunities to grow as a student through meaningful feedback provided by instructors Students realized the serious relationship between mistakes made in a simulated clinical environment and potential impacts on patient health status Simulation-based activities had many positive impacts over time, such as increasing student confidence and deepening their understanding of the patient care process
Pritchard et al. (2016)	Researchers desired to synthesize and appraise evidence related to the use of standardized patients in physical therapy education	Design: Systematic review and meta-analysis Participants: Physical therapy students	Researchers used 2 tools to assess risk of bias Researchers searched the following databases: Ovid, MedLine, PubMed, Allied and Complementary Medicine database, ERIC, CINAHL Plus	Only 5 of 13 studies that reported quantitative data placed participants in a control and experimental group Majority (n = 7) of the studies included in this review were case series; single cohort designs 3 articles reported on 5 randomized controlled studies

(continued)

Simulation-Based Instructional Methods Evidence Table (continued)

Author/Year	Study Objectives	Design and Participants	Intervention and Outcome Measures	Results
		Researchers included 16 studies across 14 articles	Inclusion criteria: • An empirical study that reported qualitative and quantitative data on use of standardized patients with any learning outcome • Included undergraduate or graduate physical therapy students • Simulation patients portrayed the role of a patient • Written in English • Published in a peer-reviewed journal Exclusion criteria: • Lacked data specific to physical therapy students • If role of patient played by students	Standardized patient simulation focused on advancing students' knowledge/skills/behaviors/attitudes (wide variety of targets) 2 randomized studies replaced clinical experiences with simulation Most studies provided training to the standardized patient Researchers reported pooled analysis of the 4 studies replaced 25% of clinical experiences with simulation; demonstrated no significant differences No significant differences were found between role play and standardized patients in competency or satisfaction; students in standardized patient experience reported statistically significant differences for the value of experience and in anxiety 1 study demonstrated no significant difference between the experimental group (standardized patients) and the control group (no intervention) Students demonstrated a significantly higher postinteraction score following participation in the standardized patient method In thematic analysis, researchers reported 1 major theme—learning with standardized patients was a valuable experience; reported 1 minor theme—learning with standardized patients can be challenging

(continued)

Simulation-Based Instructional Methods Evidence Table (continued)

Author/Year	Study Objectives	Design and Participants	Intervention and Outcome Measures	Results
Shin et al. (2015)	Researchers examined the current literature on the efficacy of simulation-based activities in nursing education	Design: Meta-analysis Selected 20 studies Participants: Nursing students	2 researchers independently participated in data extraction Databases: EBSCO, MedLine, ScienceDirect, ERIC Inclusion criteria: • Research including the use of partial-task trainers, standardized patients, full-body task trainers, high-fidelity mannequins • Research obtained quantitative data • Researched nursing student learning as the primary outcome measure • Used experimental and quasi-experimental research designs • Nursing students or nurses in nursing education • Written in English Exclusion criteria: • No control group • No comparison between simulation teaching and other instructional methods • Literature reviews • Nonempirical studies • Qualitative studies • Data about effect size	Only one fourth of the included studies used randomization methods Within the simulation experience, 12 studies used high-fidelity mannequins, 3 used low-fidelity mannequins, and 3 more used standardized patients Medium-to-large effect size for overall impact of simulation experiences on nursing student outcomes (pooled random effects standardized mean difference of 0.71) Simulation learning produced the largest effect sizes for graduate students and nurse practitioners Performance-based assessment of skills had the largest effect sizes, especially when the outcome of interest was psychomotor ability Simulation-based experiences that used high-fidelity mannequins and occurred in clinical practice–related courses also demonstrated large effect sizes Randomization of participants produced smaller effect sizes than nonrandomization methods

(continued)

Simulation-Based Instructional Methods Evidence Table (continued)

Author/Year	Study Objectives	Design and Participants	Intervention and Outcome Measures	Results
Smith et al. (2018)	Researchers evaluated the efficacy of simulation-based learning experiences (SBLEs) on improving communication skills in palliative care nursing education	Design: Systematic review Included 30 studies Participants: Nursing students and practicing nurses	Followed PRISMA guidelines 2 reviewers screened abstracts; 2 additional reviewers assessed articles in their entirety Databases: CINAHL, MedLine, PsycINFO, ERIC, Web of Science Researchers also searched ProQuest Dissertations & Theses Global, Worldcat Dissertations and Theses, NLM Gateway Inclusion criteria: • Researched simulated learning instructional methods • Used technology • Nursing students and nurses • Emphasized patient interactions occurring at the end of life • Included evaluation Exclusion criteria: • Letters, commentaries, news articles • Not written in English • Research with insufficient details about study procedures and participants Researchers used the Kirkpatrick Model to rank the level of assessment used in each study: • Reaction: Participants' reaction to SBLE	Undergraduate nursing students were most commonly using SBLEs Conversations within SBLEs was either based or based on palliative care principles Nearly half of the time, communication was limited to nurses, patients, and the families; other scenarios included input from other health care professionals 28 studies included a debriefing session, most often led by nursing instructors Technology was included in nearly each SBLE, often including HFS or video recordings The most common way to participate in SBLEs was through various methods of role play, but other methods of scenario enactment were also used 20 of the studies reported the content in their SBLE scenarios were created from members of their own team, while 8 other studies reported using outside sources The Nursing Education Simulation Framework by Jefferies, the Simulation Learning Pyramid, and the End-of-Life Nursing Education Consortium curriculum were utilized by multiple studies to aid in forming the SBLE program

(continued)

Simulation-Based Instructional Methods Evidence Table (continued)

Author/Year	Study Objectives	Design and Participants	Intervention and Outcome Measures	Results
			• Learning: Participants' knowledge obtained from SBLE • Behavior: Participants' actions learned from SBLE being used • Results: Participants' behaviors impacting patient outcomes in clinical practice	The majority of studies included communication with adult patients in hospital, hospice, or home health settings Pediatric patients were less common in this review Kirkpatrick's level of evaluation: • Level I (Reaction) assessments were used in 16 studies • Level II (Learning) assessments were used in 12 studies • Level III (Behavior) assessments were used in 2 articles • Level IV (Results) assessments were not utilized in this review
Zhang et al. (2019)	Researchers evaluated effectiveness of video-assisted debriefing following simulation in health professional education	Design: Systematic review Researchers included 23 studies in this review Participants: Health professional students (total of 1,145 participants)	Researchers followed PRISMA guidelines Researchers searched following databases: PubMed, MedLine, CINAHL, ScienceDirect, Scopus, Web of Science, PsycINFO Inclusion criteria: • Experimental studies of quasi-experimental and RCT designs that used video-assisted debriefing in simulation • Published 2000 to present Exclusion criteria: • Study completed in a clinic or other setting	Of the 23 studies, 14 were RCTs The methodological quality of studies averaged 9.5 indicating moderate to high quality 4 studies examined students' response to video-assisted debriefing using a survey; studies reported high satisfaction with perception the method was helpful for learning and an effective teaching method

(continued)

Simulation-Based Instructional Methods Evidence Table (continued)

Author/Year	Study Objectives	Design and Participants	Intervention and Outcome Measures	Results
			• Study included non–health care participants • Study evaluated effects other than simulation components • Written in non-English	In 3 studies reviewing the learning experience of video-assisted debriefing, studies reported this method facilitated connections between theory and practice, increased self-awareness, and encouraged and motivated to engage in reflection and critique 2 of the studies reported finding that the use of video-assisted debriefing on knowledge and attitude; the results are mixed, as 1 study reported no significant differences between 2 groups of medical students and 1 nursing study reported a decrease in knowledge in the video-assisted debriefing group 14 studies evaluated students' skills with technical skills significantly improving in video-assisted debriefing groups; in nontechnical skills, students performed better with communication, clinical judgment, situational awareness, decision making, task management, and team function Of the 8 studies that measured performance, students improved performance after video-assisted debriefing

(continued)

Simulation-Based Instructional Methods Evidence Table (continued)

LABORATORY EXPERIENCES

Author/Year	Study Objectives	Design and Participants	Intervention and Outcome Measures	Results
Anderson (2018)	Researchers measured effectiveness of a lab experience to teach effective body mechanics to massage therapists	Design: Cross-sectional pre/posttest design Participants: 4 cohorts of 17 students in a kinesiology course for massage students	Intervention: Throughout the semester, students participated in periodic laboratory sessions on proper body mechanics and filled out reflection journals on their experiences Outcome measures: Researchers administered 2 ergonomics risk factor assessments at the beginning and end of the semester	Students experienced a statistically significant reduction in ergonomics risk factors
Iorio et al. (2017)	Researchers investigated a 12-hour experiential learning module (primary laboratory experiences) on physical therapy students' knowledge and confidence	Design: Cross-sectional pre/posttest design Participants: 31 Doctor of Physical Therapy students (third-year)	Intervention: Students participated in a 12-hour multimodal experiential module Students completed: • 4 hours of traditional didactic lecture • 2 hours of online video lecture • Virtual Dementia Tour lab (8-minute activity) and debrief • 2-hour clinical lab at a memory care unit • Book club Outcome measures: • Confidence in Dementia Scale: 9 items • Knowledge in Dementia Scale: 16 items	Following the Virtual Dementia Tour, students reported an improved understanding of the challenges and needs of someone with dementia They also reported a significant greater appreciation for people with dementia with inappropriate behaviors Students also demonstrated significant increase on the Confidence in Dementia Scale outcome measure; after the module, the students reported an average confidence score of 36.97, suggesting students felt very confident On the Knowledge in Dementia Scale, there was no significant change in overall score (ceiling effect)
Shahsavari et al. (2017)	Researchers studied the impact of a clinical skills lab refresher course on nursing students' anxiety, self-efficacy, and clinical performance	Design: Nonrandomized controlled trial (pre/posttest design)	Intervention: The intervention group enrolled in a 3-day course to practice 10 basic nursing procedures in the clinical skill lab under the supervision of instructors The control group did not attend this course	As a result of a lab, students experienced decreased anxiety, increased self-efficacy, and improved clinical skills prior to beginning their internships

(continued)

Simulation-Based Instructional Methods Evidence Table (continued)

Author/Year	Study Objectives	Design and Participants	Intervention and Outcome Measures	Results
		Participants: 160 undergraduate nursing students	Outcome measures: • Students' anxiety • Clinical self-efficacy • Clinical skills practice	

Smithson et al. (2015)	Researchers examined the evidence on the use of standardized patients with pharmacy students	Design: Integrative review
		
		Participants: Pharmacy students
		
		Researchers included 28 articles
			Researchers searched the following databases: Scopus, CINAHL, PubMed, ProQuest, Science Direct, MedLine, A+ Education, ERIC
			
			Inclusion criteria:
			• Peer-reviewed articles
			• Written in English
			• Published between January 2000 and December 2013
				Researchers identified 4 main themes from the articles
				• Students' preference for type of standardized patient:
				  ○ Demonstrate preference for standardized patient
				  ○ Rate the experience positively
				  ○ Prefer nonpharmacy participants play the standardized patients
				• Application and efficacy
				  ○ Beneficial for knowledge transfer, but not more beneficial than other methods of simulation
				  ○ Acquire a wide range of skills
				• Student assessment
				  ○ Use of formative and summative assessment
				  ○ Standardized patients performing assessment is beneficial
				  ○ Feedback improves student performance

(continued)

Simulation-Based Instructional Methods Evidence Table (continued)

Author/Year	Study Objectives	Design and Participants	Intervention and Outcome Measures	Results
				Cost ◦ Can be cost effective, but is expensive ◦ Resources are a common barrier ◦ Need more evidence to ensure return on investment

ROLE PLAY**

Author/Year	Study Objectives	Design and Participants	Intervention and Outcome Measures	Results
Alfes (2015)	Researchers compared impact of role play and standardized patients on nursing students' knowledge, attitudes, and self-efficacy	Design: Experimental crossover design Participants: 2 cohorts; 77 nursing students total	Intervention: Researchers randomly assigned students to group A (participated in standardized patient first) or group B (role play experience first) In role play, the students play roles of patient or nurse; in the standardized patient method, they only played the role of nurse Students switched groups and experienced other intervention. Outcome measures: • Mental Health Nursing Clinical Confidence Scale (self-efficacy) • Test (8 items; knowledge) • Attitudes toward mental illness questionnaire (attitudes) (Completed 3 times)	Students demonstrated increases in self-efficacy over time, but no significant differences found between groups Each group demonstrated improvement in knowledge over time, but no significant differences found between groups Each group demonstrated improvement in attitude over time, but no significant differences found between groups

(continued)

Simulation-Based Instructional Methods Evidence Table (continued)

Author/Year	Study Objectives	Design and Participants	Intervention and Outcome Measures	Results
Bosse et al. (2012)	Researchers determined effects of role play and standardized patients on communication competencies of medical students	Design: Randomized controlled Participants: 103 fifth-year medical students; pediatric rotation	Intervention: Researchers randomly assigned students to 1 of 3 groups • Communication training and role play with course content • Communication training and standardized patient with course content • Couse content only (control) Course content included seminars, problem-based learning, virtual patients, bedside teaching, etc. Researchers developed 9 cases that fit role play and standardized patient scenarios Outcome measures: • Questionnaire • Organization for Security and Co-operation in Europe (OSCE) • Self-efficacy rating of communication skills • Calgary-Cambridge Referenced Observation Guide	No significant differences between groups at pretest on self-efficacy; following intervention the role play and standardized patient groups demonstrated significantly higher scores on self-efficacy than control group; role play and standardized patients did not differ OSCE scores demonstrated differences in the 3 groups on communication; both role play and standardized patient groups demonstrated higher scores than control; however, even higher ratings noted in role play over standardized patients with a medium- to high-effect size Role play and standardized patient groups revealed significantly higher scores on understanding parents' perspective; role play highest In building relationships, there were not significant differences between the 3 groups In regards to exploration or problems and providing structure, both intervention groups showed higher scores than control group; no differences between 2 intervention groups

(continued)

Simulation-Based Instructional Methods Evidence Table (continued)

Author/Year	Study Objectives	Design and Participants	Intervention and Outcome Measures	Results
Delbert & Schrader (2019)	Researchers explored effectiveness of drama approach in promotion of learning and self-perceived acquisition of skills and comfort/confidence in conflict management with occupational therapy students	Design: Cross-section pre/posttest design Participants: 40 occupational therapy students in master's degree program	Intervention: Students enrolled in a fieldwork seminar course; met weekly Students engaged in 2 1-hour classes on consecutive weeks with focus on drama sessions for conflict management Researchers introduced conflict management via presentation. Next, they introduced process drama and asked the students to perform the settings and characters on various fieldwork scenarios. During the following class period, students reported on scenarios and engaged in a warm-up activity before role playing additional scenarios (students wrote these scenarios the prior week) Outcome measures: Survey (questions about confidence, comfort, and competence)	Researchers reported significant difference in 2 questions; 1 related to confidence, 1 related to comfort; the competence questions did show significant difference from pre to posttest The effect size for confidence demonstrated medium effect—students reported higher level of confidence following experience The size effect for comfort demonstrated large effect—students reported higher levels of comfort Students reported enjoying the experience and reported anxiety about acting
Lewis et al. (2018)	Researchers evaluated the impact of interprofessional simulation role play tutorial with DVD on students' perception	Design: Posttest survey design Participants: 111 speech and occupational therapy students across 4 years	Intervention: Students watched introductory model prior to video. Researchers divided students from each profession into groups of 5 to 7 members. Researchers recorded a child with autism and students watched the video In their groups, they developed and assessed an evaluation plan, assessed results, and planned intervention. They engaged in discussion and participated in role play throughout the activity Outcome measures: Survey (13 questions)	Of the 13 items on the questionnaire, 88.5% of participants either positively agreed or strongly agreed with each statement Students reported highest mean agreement with the organization and value of interprofessional collaboration, and reported lowest mean agreement with the statement that it was clear what would take place during tutorial

(continued)

Simulation-Based Instructional Methods Evidence Table (continued)

Author/Year	Study Objectives	Design and Participants	Intervention and Outcome Measures	Results
McIvor & Karnes (2019)	Researchers explored the use of role play to facilitate occupational therapy students' ability to develop a therapeutic relationship via telehealth	Design: Cross-section pre/posttest design Participants: 16 students from 3 programs of occupational therapy, physical therapy, and exercise and sport science Students excluded if they have previously engaged in a fieldwork experience	Intervention: Students participated in 3 modules over the course of 2 sessions; module 1 reviewed information related to telehealth via lecture; module 2 provided information on developing a therapeutic relationship using the Intentional Relationship Model with mindful skill development; students role played in module 3 with a standardized patient via phone, face-to-face, and video conference A graduate student and faculty served as the actors The researcher also facilitated a debrief session following role play Outcome measures: Survey	50% of students were from the physical therapy program Students reported significant change in confidence in ability to maintain a therapeutic relationship with clients via telehealth Students indicated role play was an effective method for teaching therapeutic relationship skills They also agreed lecture was an effective method
Ronning & Bjorkly (2019)	Researchers completed an integrative literature review to understand role play and reflection on students' development of therapeutic skills	Design: Integrative review Researchers included 4 articles in the review	Databases: Ovid, CINAHL, Cochrane, Science Direct, Swemed, Norart, ProQuest, Google Scholar Inclusion criteria: • Implemented educational use of role play with reflection • Trained therapeutic communication skills • Studied mental health at least on bachelor's level • Written in English and Scandinavian	2 studies were qualitative, and 2 studies were quantitative in nature; 3 used surveys or questionnaires, and 1 used a focus group Students reported role play increased understanding and awareness of suicide Results from surveys and questionnaires demonstrated role play enhanced therapeutic and communication skills Lack of data on generalizability to professional practice Supervision and reflection in role play facilitates professional and interpersonal competence

(continued)

Simulation-Based Instructional Methods Evidence Table (continued)

Author/Year	Study Objectives	Design and Participants	Intervention and Outcome Measures	Results
			Exclusion criteria: • Not empirical research articles • Investigated use of standardized patients, mannequins, or avatars • Did not address teaching mental health; only physical health symptoms • Did not investigate clinical role play • Investigated just reflection • Did not use role play and reflection	
Taylor et al. (2018)	Researchers examined differences in standardized patient and role play instructional methods on communication skills training in undergraduate medical students	Design: Randomized, crossover trial Participants: First- and second-year undergraduate medical students; analyzed 610 recordings—303 role play and 307 standardized patients	Intervention: Researchers assigned students to 1 or 2 groups. In the first course, a group of students participated in role play and the second group participated with standardized patients for communication skills training. In the next course, the 2 groups switched methods. Researchers recorded various observations and rated using an objective scale Outcome measures: • Calgary-Cambridge Referenced Observation Guide • Online survey	For each task in the Calgary-Cambridge Referenced Observation Guide, students did not demonstrate any statistical significance between the 2 groups on any of the 4 tasks In all comparisons between the 2 groups, there were no statistically significant differences between the standardized patients and role play
Wiskin et al. (2011)	Researchers aimed to identify if simulations (role play) impacted students' attitudes toward individuals needing sexually transmitted infection testing	Design: RCT	Intervention: Researchers divided students into groups of 8 to 9 members for the role play. Student role played a scenario about a young man needing sexually transmitted infection testing	Results demonstrated no significant differences between the experimental and control groups on questionnaire Researchers found no significant differences between age groups

(continued)

Simulation-Based Instructional Methods Evidence Table (continued)

Author/Year	Study Objectives	Design and Participants	Intervention and Outcome Measures	Results
		Participants: 229 second-year Bachelor of Medicine, Bachelor of Surgery students; 175 in control group and 124 in experimental group	The experimental group completed the questionnaire after engaging in role play. The control group completed the questionnaire prior to role play. Outcome measures: Questionnaire (25 questions)	Students of White British ethnic groups demonstrated a significantly more positive attitude than other groups
Xiong et al. (2017)	Researchers examined how mixed media education (lectures, videos, role play, feedback) improved nursing students' knowledge, attitudes, and compliance with standard precautions	Design: RCT; 2-arm; pre/posttest. Participants: 80 nursing students	Intervention: The experimental group engaged in 3 mixed media sessions biweekly (lectures, videos, role play, feedback). The control group completed a self-study to learn about standard precautions. Outcome measures: • Knowledge with standard precautions questionnaire • Attitude with Standard Precautions Scale • Compliance with Standard Precautions Scale • Bacterial colony measurement	Students in the experimental group demonstrated significantly increased scores on knowledge, attitude, and compliance scales. There was no significant change in the control group. Each group performed better for hand hygiene from pre to posttest. For group comparison, the experimental group demonstrated significantly higher scores than the control group in the areas of knowledge, attitudes, and compliance. They also performed significantly higher on hand hygiene than the control group

* Due to the large volume of studies on simulation, the authors only included systematic reviews, literature reviews, and meta-analyses across health care disciplines. We also recognize there are additional high-level reviews throughout health professional literature. However, because of the scope of and resources for this project, we were unable to include each finding from the vast amount of simulation reviews. It is our hope the included reviews still assist your implementation of simulation into your courses.

** Due to the large number of studies on role play in medical and nursing education, we limited our search to systematic reviews, literature reviews, meta-analyses, and randomized controlled trials in health professional education. We also included quantitative designs in occupational therapy education.

Adapted from American Occupational Therapy Association. (2002). AOTA's evidence-based literature review project: An overview (D. Lieberman & J. Scheer, Eds.). *American Journal of Occupational Therapy, 56,* 344-349. https://doi.org/10.5014/ajot.56.3.344

REFERENCES

Adib-Hajbaghery, M., & Sharifi, N. (2017). Effect of simulation training on the development of nurses and nursing students' critical thinking: A systematic literature review. *Nurse Education Today, 50,* 17-24. http://dx.doi.org/10.1016/j.nedt.2016.12.011

Alfes, C. M. (2015). Standardized patient versus role-play strategies: A comparative study measuring patient-centered care and safety in psychiatric mental health nursing. *Nursing Education Perspectives, 36*(6), 403-405. http://dx.doi.org/10.5480/14-1535

American Occupational Therapy Association. (2002). AOTA's evidence-based literature review project: An overview (D. Lieberman & J. Scheer, Eds.). *The American Journal of Occupational Therapy, 56,* 344-349. https://doi.org/10.5014/ajot.56.3.344

Anderson, R. B. (2018). Improving body mechanics using experiential learning and ergonomic tools in massage therapy education. *International Journal of Therapeutic Massage and Bodywork, 11*(4), 23-31.

Baird, J. M., Raina, K. D., Rogers, J. C., O'Donnell, J., & Holm, M. B. (2015). Wheelchair transfer simulations to enhance procedural skills and clinical reasoning. *American Journal of Occupational Therapy, 69*(Suppl. 2), 6912185020. http://dx.doi.org/10.5014/ajot.2015.018697

Bennett, S., Rodger, S., Fitzgerald, C., & Gibson, L. (2017). Simulation in occupational therapy curricula: A literature review. *Australian Occupational Therapy Journal, 64,* 314-327.

Bethea, D. P., Castillo, D. C., & Harvison, N. (2014). Use of simulation in occupational therapy education: Way of the future? *American Journal of Occupational Therapy, 68,* S32-S39. http://dx.doi.org/10.5014/ajot.2014.012716

Bosse, H. M., Schultz, J. H., Nickel, M., Lutz, T., Junger, J., Huwendiek, S., & Nikendei, C. (2012). The effect of using standardized patients or peer role play on ratings of undergraduate communication training: A randomized controlled trial. *Patient Education and Counseling, 87,* 300-306. http://dx.doi.org/10.1016/j.pec.2011.10.007

Brydges, R., Manzone, J., Shanks, D., Hatala, R., Hamstra, S. J., Zendejas, B., & Cook, D. A. (2015). Self-regulated learning in simulation-based training: A systematic review and meta-analysis. *Medical Education, 49,* 368-378. http://dx.doi.org/10.1111/medu.12649

Cant, R. P., & Cooper, S. J. (2017). Use of simulation-based learning in undergraduate nurse education: An umbrella systematic review. *Nurse Education Today, 49,* 63-71. http://dx.doi.org/10.1016/j.nedt.2016.11.015

Cook, D. A., Hatala, R., Brydges, R., Zendejas, B., Szostek, J. H., Wang, A. T., Erwin, P. J., & Hamstra, S. J. (2011). Technology-enhanced simulation for health professional education: A systematic review and meta-analysis. *JAMA, 306*(9), 978-988.

Delbert, T., & Schrader, T. (2019). Conflict management in occupational therapy education: Process drama as a teaching strategy. *Journal of Occupational Therapy Education, 3*(2), Article 9. https://doi.org/10.26681/jote.2019.030209

Doolen, J., Mariani, B., Ata, T., Horsley, T. L., O'Rourke, J., McAfee, K., Cross, C. L. (2016). High-fidelity simulation in undergraduate nursing education: A review of simulation reviews. *Clinical Simulation in Nursing, 12,* 290-302. http://dx.doi.org/10.1016/j.ecns.2016.01.009

Folts, D., Tigges, K., & Weisman, T. (1986). Occupational therapy in hospice home care: A student tutorial. *American Journal of Occupational Therapy, 40*(9), 623-628.

Gibbs, D. M., & Dietrich, M. (2017). Using high fidelity simulation to impact occupational therapy student knowledge, comfort, and confidence in acute care. *The Open Journal of Occupational Therapy, 5*(1), Article 10. https://dx.doi.org/10.15453/2168-6408.1225

Haddad, A. M. (1988). Teaching ethical analysis in occupational therapy. *American Journal of Occupational Therapy, 42*(5), 300-304.

Haddeland, K., Slettebo, A., Carstens, P., & Fossum, M. (2018). Nursing students managing deteriorating patients: A systematic review and meta-analysis. *Clinical Simulation in Nursing, 21,* 1-15. https://doi.org/10.1016/j.ecns.2018.05.001

Harder, B. N. (2010). Use of simulation in teaching and learning in health sciences: A systematic review. *Journal of Nursing Education, 49,* 23-28. http://dx.doi.org/10.3928/01484834-20090828-08

Hasan, S. S., Chong, D. W. K., Se, W. P., Kumar, S., Ahmed, S. I., & Mittal, P. (2017). Simulation-based instruction for pharmacy practice skill development: A review of the literature. *Archives of Pharmacy Practice, 8,* 43-50.

International Nursing Association for Clinical Simulation and Learning Board of Directors. (2011). Standard II: Professional integrity of the participant. *Clinical Simulation in Nursing, 7*(45), s8-s9.

Jansen, D. A., Johnson, N., Larnson, G., Berry, C., & Brenner, G. H. (2009). Nursing faculty perceptions of obstacles to utilizing manikin-based simulations and proposed solutions. *Clinical Simulation in Nursing, 5*(1), e9-e16. http://dx.doi.org/10.1016/j.ecns.2008.09.004

Kaplonyi, J., Bowles, K., Nestel, D., Kiegaldie, D., Maloney, S., Haines, T., & Williams, C. (2017). Understanding the impact of simulated patients on health care learners' communication skills: A systematic review. *Medical Education, 51,* 1209-1219.

Knowles, M. S. (1980). *The modern practice of adult education: From pedagogy to andragogy.* Follett Publishing Company.

Knowles, M. S. (1984). Introduction: The art and science of helping adults learn. In M. S. Knowles (Ed.), *Andragogy in action: Applying modern principles of adult learning* (pp. 1-21). Jossey-Bass.

Labrague, L. J., McEnroe-Petitte, D. M., Bowling, A. M., Nwafor, C. E., & Tsaras, K. (2019). High-fidelity simulation and nursing students' anxiety and self-confidence: A systematic review. *Nursing Forum, 54*, 358-368.

Labrague, L. J., McEnroe-Petitte, D. M., Fronda, D. C., & Obeidat, A. A. (2018). Interprofessional simulation in undergraduate nursing program: An integrative review. *Nurse Education Today, 67*, 46-55. https://doi.org/10.1016/j.nedt.2018.05.001

Levett-Jones, T., & Lapkin, S. (2013). A systematic review of the effectiveness of simulation debriefing in health professional education. *Nurse Education Today, 34*, e58-e63. http://dx.doi.org/10.1016/j.nedt.2013.09.020

Lewis, A., Rudd, C. J., & Mills, B. (2018). Working with children with autism: An interprofessional simulation-based tutorial for speech pathology and occupational therapy students. *Journal of Interprofessional Care, 32*(2), 242-244. https://doi.org/10.1080/13561820.2017.1388221

Lorio, A. K., Gore, J. B., Warthen, L., Housley, S. N., & Burgessm, E. O. (2017). Teaching dementia care to physical therapy doctoral students: A multimodal experiential learning approach. *Gerontology & Geriatrics Education, 38*(3), 313-324. http://doi.org/10.1080/02701960.2015.1115979

McIvor, L., & Karnes, M. (2019). Role-play as an effective way to teach relationship building with Telehealth. *The Open Journal of Occupational Therapy, 7*(2), Article 10. https://doi.org/10.15453/2168-6408.1527

Moreno, J. L. (1953). *Who shall survive?* Beacon House.

Mori, B., Carnahan, H., & Herold, J. (2015). Use of simulation learning experiences in physical therapy entry-to-practice curricula: A systematic review. *Physiotherapy Canada, 67*(2), 194-202. http://dx.doi.org/10.3138/ptc.2014-40E

Neistadt, M. E. (1987). Classroom as clinic: A model for teaching clinical reasoning in occupational therapy education. *American Journal of Occupational Therapy, 41*(10), 631-637.

Neistadt, M. E. (1992). The classroom as clinic: Applications for a method of teaching clinical reasoning. *American Journal of Occupational Therapy, 46*(9), 814-819.

Neistadt, M. E., & Smith, R. E. (1997). Teaching diagnostic reasoning: Using a classroom-as-clinic methodology with videotapes. *American Journal of Occupational Therapy, 51*(5), 360-368.

Nestel, D., Kelly, M., Jolly, B., & Watson, M. (2018). *Healthcare simulation education: Evidence, theory and practice.* John Wiley & Sons.

Ogard-Repal, A., Knutson De Presno, A., & Fossum, M. (2018). Simulation with standardized patients to prepare undergraduate nursing students for mental health clinical practice: An integrative literature review. *Nurse Education Today, 66*, 149-157. https://doi.org/10.1016/j.nedt.2018.04.018

Palominos, E., Levett-Jones, T., Power, T., & Martinez-Maldonado, R. (2019). Healthcare students' perceptions and experiences of making errors in simulation: An integrative review. *Nurse Education Today, 77*, 32-39. https://doi.org/10.1016/j.nedt.2019.02.013

Pritchard, S. A., Blackstock, F. C., Nestel, D., & Keating, J. L. (2016). Simulated patients in physical therapy education: Systematic review and meta-analysis. *Physical Therapy, 96*(9), 1342-1353.

Ratzon, N. Z., Lunievsky, E. K., Ashkenasi, A., Laks, J., & Cohen, H. (2017). Simulated driving skills evaluation of teenagers with attention deficit hyperactivity disorder before driving lessons. *American Journal of Occupational Therapy, 71*, 7103220010. https://doi.org/10.5014/ajot.2017.020164

Ronning, S. B., & Bjorkly, S. (2019). The use of clinical role-play and reflection in learning therapeutic communication skills in mental health education: An integrative review. *Advances in Medical Education and Practice, 10*, 415-425. http://doi.org/10.2147/AMEP.S202115

Shahsasvari, H., Ghiyasvandian, S., Houser, M. L., Zakerimoghadam, M., Kermanshahi, S. S. N., & Torabi, S. (2017). Effect of a clinical skills refresher course on the clinical performance, anxiety, and self-efficacy of the final year undergraduate nursing students. *Nurse Education in Practice, 27*, 151-156. http://dx.doi.org/10.1016/j.nepr.2017.08.006

Shin, S., Park, J. H., & Kim, J. H. (2015). Effectiveness of patient simulation in nursing education: Meta-analysis. *Nurse Education Today, 35*, 176-182. http://dx.doi.org/10.1016/j.nedt.2014.09.009

Shoemaker, M. J., Beasley, J., Cooper, M., Perkins, R., Smith, J., & Swank, C. (2011). A method for providing high-volume interprofessional simulation encounters in physical and occupational therapy education programs. *Journal of Allied Health, 40*(1), 15-21.

Smith, M. B., Macieira, T. G. R., Bumbach, M. D., Garbutt, S. J., Citty, S. W., Stephen, A., Ansell, M., Glover, T. L., & Keenan, G. (2018). The use of simulation to teach nursing students and clinicians palliative care and end-of-life communication: A systematic review. *American Journal of Hospice & Palliative Medicine, 35*(8), 1140-1154.

Smithson, J., Bellingan, M., Glass, B., & Mills, J. (2015). Standardized patients in pharmacy education: An integrative literature review. *Currents in Pharmacy Teaching and Learning, 7*, 851-863. http://dx.doi.org/10.1016/j.cptl.2015.08.002

Taylor, S., Bobba, S., Roome, S., Ahmadzai, M., Tran, D., Vickers, D., Bhatti, M., De Silva, D., Dunstan, L., Falconer, R., Kaur, H., Kitson, J., Patel, J., & Shulruf, B. (2018). Simulated patient and role play methodologies for communication skills training in an undergraduate medical program: Randomized, crossover trial. *Education for Health, 31*(1), 10-16. http://dx.doi.org/10.4103/1357-6283.239040

Wiskin, C., Roberts, L., & Roalfe, A. (2011). The impact of discussing a sexual history in role-play simulation teaching on pre-clinical student attitudes towards people who submit for STI testing. *Medical Teacher, 33,* e324-e332. http://dx.doi.org/10.3109/0142159X.2011.575902

Xiong, P., Zhang, J., Wang, X., Wu, T. L., & Hall, B. J. (2017). Effects of mixed media education intervention program on increasing knowledge, attitude, and compliance with standard precautions among nursing students: A randomized controlled trial. *American Journal of Infection Control, 45,* 389-395. http://dx.doi.org/10.1016/j.ajic.2016.11.006

Zhang, H., Morelius, E., Goh, S. H. L., & Wang, W. (2019). Effectiveness of video-assisted debriefing in simulation-based health professional education: A systematic review of quantitative evidence. *Nurse Educator, 44*(3), E1-E6. http://dx.doi.org/10.1097/NNE.0000000000000562

BIBLIOGRAPHY

Baird, J. M., Raina, K. D., Rogers, J. C., O'Donnell, J., Terhorst, L., & Holm, M. B. (2015). Simulation strategies to teach patient transfers: Self-efficacy by strategy. *American Journal of Occupational Therapy Education, 69*(Suppl. 2), 6912185030. http://dx.doi.org/10.5014/ajot.2015.018705

Benson, J. D., Provident, I., & Szucs, K. A. (2013). An experiential learning lab embedded in a didactic course: Outcomes from a pediatric intervention course. *Occupational Therapy in Health Care, 27*(1), 46-57. http://dx.doi.org/10.3109/07380577.2012.756599

Bradley, G., Whittington, S., & Mottram, P. (2013). Enhancing occupational therapy education through simulation. *British Journal of Occupational Therapy, 76*(1), 43-46. http://dx.doi.org/10.4276/030802213X13576469254775

Chown, G., & Horn, L. (2017). Simulating experiences: Using interprofessional lab simulation in occupational therapy. *OT Practice, 22*(20), 13-15.

Fu, C. P., Yeh, J. H., Su, C. T., Liu, C. H., Chang, W. Y., Chen Y. L., Yang, A. L., & Wang, C. C. (2017). Using children as standardized patients in OSCE in pediatric occupational therapy. *Medical Teacher, 39*(8), 851-858. https://doi.org/10.1080/0142159X.2017.1320540

Giles, A. K., Carson, N. E., Breland, H. L., Coker-Bolt, P., & Bowman, P. J. (2014). Conference proceedings—Use of simulated patients and reflective video analysis to assess occupational therapy students' preparedness for fieldwork. *American Journal of Occupational Therapy, 68,* S57-S66. http://dx.doi.org/10.5014/ajot.2014.685S03

Jacobs, R., Beyer, E., & Carter, K. (2017). Interprofessional simulation education designed to teach occupational therapy and nursing students complex patient transfers. *Journal of Interprofessional Education and Practice, 6,* 67-70. http://dx.doi.org/10.1016/j.xjep.2016.12.002

Jensen, G. M., & Mostrom, E. (2013). *Handbook of teaching and learning for physical therapists* (3rd ed.). Elsevier.

Knecht-Sabres, L. J., Kovic, M., Wallingford, M., & St. Amand, L. E. (2013). Preparing occupational therapy students for the complexities of clinical practice. *The Open Journal of Occupational Therapy, 1*(3), Article 4. http://doi.org/10.15453/2168-6408.1047

Lowenstein, A. J., & Bradsaw, M. J. (2001). *Fuszard's innovatie teaching strategies in nursing* (3rd ed.). ASPEN.

Meiers, J., & Russell, M. J. (2019). An unfolding case study: Supporting contextual psychomotor skill development in novice nursing students. *International Journal of Nursing Education Scholarship, 16*(1), 1-9.

Merryman, B. M. (2010). Effects of simulated learning and facilitated debriefing on student understanding of mental illness. *Occupational Therapy in Mental Health, 26*(1), 18-31. https://doi.org/10.1080/01642120903513933

Monash University. (2019). NHET-SIM: National health education and training in simulation. https://www.monash.edu/medicine/nhet-sim/home

Ozelie, R., Both, C., Fricke, E., & Maddock, C. (2016). High-fidelity simulation in occupational therapy curriculum: Impact on level II fieldwork performance. *The Open Journal of Occupational Therapy, 4*(4), Article 9. https://doi.org/10.15453/2168-6408.1242

Pront, L., & NcNeill, L. (2019). Nursing students' perception of a clinical learning assessment activity: "Linking the puzzle pieces of theory to practice." *Nurse Education in Practice, 36,* 85-90. https://doi.org/10.1016/j.nepr.2019.03.008

Shea, C. (2015). High-fidelity simulation: A tool for occupational therapy education. *The Open Journal of Occupational Therapy, 3*(4), Article 8. https://doi.org/10.15453/2168-6408.1155

Silverman, F. (2010). Teaching qualitative research methods using a simulation exercise. *Education Special Interest Section Quarterly, 20*(2), 1-4.

Smallfield, S., & Anderson, A. J. (2012). Using active learning to teach assistive technology. *Education Special Interest Section Quarterly, 22*(3), 1-4.

Snyder, M. D., Fitzloff, B. M., Fiedler, R., & Lambke, M. R. (2000). Preparing nursing students for contemporary practice: Restructuring the psychomotor skills laboratory. *Educational Innovation, 39*(5), 229-230.

Steinwachs, B. (1992). How to facilitate a debriefing. *Simulation and Gaming, 23*(2), 186-195.

Thomas, E. M., Rybski, M. F., Apke, T. L., Kegelmeyer, D. A., & Kloos, A. D. (2017). An acute interprofessional simulation experience for occupational and physical therapy students: Key findings from a survey study. *Journal of Interprofessional Care, 31*(3), 317-324. http://dx.doi.org/10.1080/13561820.2017.1280006

VanLeit, B. (1995). Using the case method to develop clinical reasoning skills in problem-based learning. *American Journal of Occupational Therapy, 49*(4), 349-353.

VanPuymbrouck, L., Heffrom, J. L., Sheth, A. J., The, K. J., Lee, D. (2017). Experiential learning: Critical analysis of standardized patient and disability simulation. *Journal of Occupational Therapy Education, 1*(3), Article 5. https://doi.org/10.26681/jote.2017.010305

Winkelmann, Z. K., Eberman, L. E., Edler, J. R., Livingston, L. B., Games, K. E. (2018). Curation of a simulation experience by the clinical scholar: An educational technique in postprofessional athletic training. *Athletic Training Education Journal, 13*(2), 185-193. http://dx.doi.org/10.4085/1302185

Wu, R., & Shea, C. K. (2009). Using simulations to prepare OT students for ICU practice. *Education Special Interest Section Quarterly, 19*(4), 1-4.

Zigmont, J. J., Kappus, L. J., & Sudikoff, S. N. (2011). Theoretical foundations of learning through simulation. *Seminars in Perinatology, 35*(2), 47-51.

APPENDIX

SIMULATION PLANNING CHECKLIST

METHOD OF SIMULATION:	
LEARNING OBJECTIVES:	
1.	
2.	
3.	
BRIEF DESCRIPTION OF CASE:	

Logistic	*Notes/Ideas*
Date of simulation	
Schedule space for simulation	
Location of simulation	
Develop timeline for simulation events (e.g., briefing, simulation time, debriefing)	
List of simulation equipment needed	
List who will secure information	
Medical equipment needed	
Identify and recruit standardized patients (if applicable)	
Write scripts for standardized patients or role play and obtain feedback on scripts (if applicable)	
Determine and develop method of training standardized patients (if applicable)	
Train standardized patients (if applicable)	
Check to make sure simulation and medical equipment work	
Determine if technical support is needed	
Secure assistance for simulation experiences (faculty, staff, doctoral students, practitioners)	
Divide students into groups (simulation and debriefing)	

continued

SIMULATION PLANNING CHECKLIST (CONTINUED)

Create a schedule for students and other individuals involved in simulation experience	
Determine and/or develop methods of assessment	
Determine observation methods (e.g., video, class, checklist)	
Select debriefing procedures	
Develop confidentiality agreement to protect students' performances and/or issues that might arise during debriefing process	

COOPERATIVE LEARNING INSTRUCTIONAL METHODS

Whitney Henderson, OTD, MOT, OTR/L

BASIC TENETS

Cooperative learning is an instructional method in which students actively engage in a small group to achieve a common educational or social goal. The students are responsible for governing the group dynamics to share and acquire the professional knowledge and skills they need for practice. Successful cooperative learning requires

> Additional Names in Literature: collaborative learning, small group learning

important group work skills (soft skills), such as communication, time management, leadership, problem solving, and role sharing. Employers across a variety of disciplines report group work skills are the most sought-after attributes in graduates entering and succeeding in the 21st century workforce. Therefore, we need to consider pedagogical approaches that facilitate the development of these critical soft skills. In addition to these skills, cooperative learning promotes interaction, requires accountability, improves the ability to view other's perspectives, and develops higher critical-thinking and professional-reasoning skills.

Before moving forward, we want to highlight differences between cooperative learning and peer learning (also called peer teaching or peer mentoring). Peer learning is similar to cooperative learning because students work together in a small group to maximize their own and each other's learning. However, in peer learning, students are in a similar social group but are **not** necessarily in the same course or year of study. Examples of peer learning include a teaching or laboratory assistant or a more **advanced** learner providing one-on-one or group tutoring or advising. In this method of learning, the students share a similar base of knowledge and experiences. Therefore, the advanced student possesses the ability to explain important concepts to the novice student at a level they can understand. Despite similar benefits and outcomes between the two instructional methods, we will not use these terms interchangeably and will only discuss instructional methods reflective of cooperative learning in this chapter.

Henderson, W. (Ed.). *Effective Teaching: Instructional Methods and Strategies for Occupational Therapy Education* (pp. 185-215).

Later in this chapter, we will discuss the implementation of three cooperative learning instructional methods: (1) fishbowl discussion, (2) jigsaw classroom, and (3) team-based learning.

BACKGROUND

Educators have successfully implemented and investigated cooperative learning methods for more than 60 years. We can trace the roots of cooperative learning back to the 1960s when David Johnson at the University of Minnesota began training educators on the effective use of small groups. Later in the decade, Roger Johnson joined David Johnson, and they extensively trained educators in science courses on the use of cooperative learning instructional methods. However, this method of instruction remained relatively unknown or unused for 20 years because society promoted interpersonal competition and rugged individualism. During this time, educators believed students learned best alone and became "strong" through isolation. In the 1980s, social scientists started to challenge this notion and described the essential role peer interaction and relationships play in learning. Since this decade, educators in higher education and professional training programs have widely accepted and successfully implemented cooperative learning instructional methods into their classrooms (see Cooperative Learning Instructional Methods Evidence Table). In fact, many educators consider cooperative learning a dominant instructional method throughout schools and universities across the world. Nursing educators have employed collaborative learning methods in their programs for several decades. According to literature, near the end of the 1990s, nursing education in the United States was the first to implement a study on cooperative learning in this professional field.

THEORY

Social interdependence theory best guides the implementation of cooperative learning in higher education settings. This theory is considered one of the most successful applications of social and educational psychology due to its lengthy history and rich evidence supporting the value of cooperative learning. Since the 1800s, researchers have conducted more than 750 studies on the use of social interdependence theory to guide the development and implementation of this instructional method. They have researched this theory in a variety of settings with diverse backgrounds and a wide range of ages. In addition, researchers have investigated the theoretical underpinnings in several different countries and over various time periods. Because of these efforts, social interdependence theory has strong external validity and generalizability. Literature provides us with examples of effective educational practices that integrate theory and research into our everyday teaching approaches.

We can trace the roots of social interdependence theory to the gestalt psychology movement at the University of Berlin. When studying perception and behavior, Kurt Koffka, a founding father of the Gestalt School of Psychology, focused on the whole unit versus the parts of the unit. He believed humans acquire meaningful views of the world by perceiving experiences as a whole versus a summary of the individual components. Therefore, groups were dynamic wholes, and the individuals who comprise the group experience various levels of interdependence. Kurt Lewin further expanded these ideas suggesting group members are made interdependent through their common goal. As each member recognizes the objective, they experience a state of tension that motivates them to achieve their common goal. The group is continuously fluctuating as one member or subgroup influences any other member or subgroup. Morton Deutsch further added to these notions by exploring the two different types of tension or social interdependence: positive and negative (Table 8-1).

TABLE 8-1		
Interdependence		
TYPE OF INTERDEPENDENCE	**DESCRIPTION**	**OUTCOME**
Positive	The group members perceive they have the ability to achieve the goal if the other members in the cooperative relationship attain their goals.	Creates a productive interaction in which group members encourage and assist other members' efforts to reach the common goal (promotive interaction).
Negative	Group members perceive the ability to obtain their goals only when other members fail to obtain their goals, creating a competitive relationship.	Creates a conflicting interaction in which group members discourage or obstruct other members' efforts to reach the common goal (contrient interaction).

If the group member(s) does not recognize a relationship between their goal and other members' ability to achieve a goal, no interdependence exists. Therefore, the way in which the members structure their goal (*interdependence*) influences how they interact (*interaction*), and the pattern of interaction determines the outcome of the group process (*outcome*). These three variables serve as the basic theoretical premises of social interdependence theory.

Individuals experience three psychological processes through social interdependence (Table 8-2). If group members sense the positive interdependence processes, they are more likely to put effort and time on tasks, provide greater personal and task-oriented support, and feel a greater sense of self-esteem and psychological health (outcome). In order to achieve positive outcomes, social interdependence theory highlights five essential elements for cooperative learning, which we will discuss in-depth in the Implementation section of this chapter.

IMPLEMENTATION

It is important to note that cooperative learning is different than group work traditionally found during class. In cooperative learning, each student has a role or responsibility to fulfill, which makes the interaction more complex than simple group work. Educators can organize students into small groups and ask them to work together, but this action alone does not necessarily constitute or produce cooperative learning. In order to use this method of instruction, we must understand what is and what is not a cooperative learning group (Figure 8-1).

In addition, educators should not assume the students in their courses know how to effectively interact with each other or that these soft skills will magically appear when they place their students in groups. Therefore, there is a need for educators to teach students group work skills, so they are motivated to grow and use these essential practice attributes.

TABLE 8-2

Psychological Processes

POSITIVE INTERDEPENDENCE	THREE PSYCHOLOGICAL PROCESSES	NEGATIVE INTERDEPENDENCE
Substitutability	The extent to which one member's actions substitute for another member's actions so they do not duplicate efforts.	Nonsubstitutability
Positive Cathexis	The degree to which a member invests psychological energy outside of oneself.	Negative Cathexis
Inducibility	The member's openness to being influenced and to influencing other members.	Resistance

	Pseudo Learning Group	Traditional Classroom Learning Group	Cooperative Learning Group	High-Performance Learning Group
Level of Engagement	Students have no interest in working together	Students accept that they have to work together	Students work together to accomplish a common goal	Students in the group meets criteria for demonstrating cooperative learning and outperforms reasonable expectations
Evaluation	Students believe they will be evaluated by a ranking system of lowest to highest performance	Educators evaluate students as individuals, but not as group members	Students seek outcomes that benefit all group members	
Behavior	Students hide information from one another; attempt to mislead or confuse each other; lack trust	Students pursue other group member's information, but are not motivated to teach them; some students seek a free ride while others feel exploited	Students discuss material with other members, help each other understand, and encourage each other to perform well	Students are highly committed to the group
Outcome	The overall sum of the finished product is less that the potential of each individual student	The overall sum of the finished product is more than some student's potential, but less than some student's potential	The overall product is more than the sum of each student's portion; each student performs higher than would have if worked individually	The group's success is greater than most cooperative groups; few groups achieve this level of performance

Cooperation →

Figure 8-1. Types of groups.

Teaching Group Work Skills

In order for your students to achieve a mutual learning goal, they must get to know, trust, accept, and support each other; communicate with clarity and accuracy; and resolve conflicts effectively. Therefore, for your cooperative learning instructional methods to be successful, we recommend you devote time to teach your students group work skills and strategies for resolving issues. Educational

T-Chart	
Encouraging Participation	
Looks Like	**Sounds Like**
Smiles	What is your idea?
Eye contact	Awesome!
Thumbs up	Good idea!
Pat on back	That's interesting!

Figure 8-2. Example of a T-chart. (Reproduced with permission from Johnson, D. W., & Johnson, R. T. [1990]. Social skills for successful group work. *Educational Leadership, 47*[4], 29-33.)

literature provides several approaches for completing this phase of implementation. First, students must recognize the need to use these skills. Students are motivated to learn when they believe they will be better if they know or possess these skills. We recommend the following strategies:

- Explain why these skills are important for their current education and future professional careers
- Demonstrate good group work skills
- Inform students they will be rewarded for using these soft skills (further taps into the learners' motivation)

David Johnson and Roger Johnson (1990) recommend educators use a T-chart to help learners understand a particular group work skill (Figure 8-2). After drawing a chart, you will select a group work skill and ask the students, "What does this skill look like?" and "What does this skill sound like?" As a group, you will discuss and model until your students have a clear idea of the skills you desire in cooperative learning.

We know students master skills through practice. When we teach our students the important psychomotor skills of our profession (e.g., transfers, range of motion), we often provide them with opportunities for practice until they demonstrate competency. Mastering a social skill is no different, as our students need opportunities to perform group work skills again and again. We provide a couple of examples of ways you can give your students more experience with these skills. One method is to have your students divide into groups of two or three to role play particular skills. You could also divide them into small groups and assign each student the role of a certain type of group member (e.g., the encourager, the summarizer, the recorder, the reader). Every student in your course needs opportunities to develop group work skills and to fulfill different group roles. As they are completing any of these activities or any other cooperative learning tasks in your courses, it is important for you to consistently cue or reinforce group work skills for a period of time. In fact, 30 years ago, David Johnson and Roger Johnson (1990) encouraged educators to "be relentless" in emphasizing the use of cooperative skills.

Lastly, our students need to process how well and how frequently they are using group work skills. You will want to provide your students with time to discuss, describe, or reflect on their use of these skills to improve their own and their group's performance. We will provide strategies for group processing later in this chapter. In summary, it is essential that our students persevere in practicing these skills. They have to practice long enough to move from an awkward stage to a stage in which the use of these skills becomes routine and automatic. We encourage you to continue to use cooperative learning methods, provide continuous feedback, and reward the use of strong group work skills.

TABLE 8-3

Essential Elements of Cooperative Learning

ESSENTIAL ELEMENT	DEFINITION
Positive Interdependence	The students in the group share a common goal and complete the tasks together; they understand they cannot succeed unless the group succeeds.
Individual Accountability	The students hold each other accountable for achievement of group goals.
Promotive Interaction	The variety of strategies students use to encourage and facilitate teamwork, trust, and communication among the group members.
Appropriate Use of Social Skills	The students understand and use proper group work skills.
Group Processing	The students have opportunities to reflect on the group experience and what they have learned from one another.

Essential Elements of Cooperative Learning

In educational literature, David Johnson and Roger Johnson (1990, 1999, 2005, 2009) describe the five essential elements of cooperative learning (Table 8-3). Scholars believe these five elements must be executed at the same time for cooperative learning to truly and effectively occur. If these interrelated elements occur in the learning context, you can anticipate cooperative learning to improve your students' efforts and achievements, the quality of their relationships, and their psychological health. It will be important for you to have a sound understanding of these elements, so you can structure a well-designed cooperative learning activity.

We have provided you with examples of each element. Take a moment to list additional strategies you can use to achieve the five essential elements (Table 8-4).

Structuring a Cooperative Learning Group

You can implement cooperative learning instructional methods in a variety of ways. For example, your students can collaborate for a class period or for several weeks to achieve a particular learning outcome. They can also complete a variety of assignments (e.g., conduct a survey, write a report, give a presentation, or create an educational program). However, the way you structure your groups or activities will influence how well the groups perform. Before discussing how to implement the specific instructional methods, we will provide a few basic elements to consider as you are carefully designing your cooperative learning activities.

Make Several Pre-Instructional Decisions

In order to provide clarity and reduce strain, you can make a number of pre-instructional decisions, such as determining the learning objectives, selecting the size of the groups, deciding how the students will be divided into groups, assigning roles, suggesting materials or resources, or choosing the room arrangement. You can use three different methods to group your students: (1) Allow your students to select, (2) randomly assign the students, or (3) assign the students based on their abilities

TABLE 8-4

Examples of Essential Elements

ESSENTIAL ELEMENT	EXAMPLE OF ELEMENT IN ACTION	ADDITIONAL EXAMPLES
Positive Interdependence	The students in the group discuss or write their learning goal; plan roles and topics (Figure 8-3). The students review the learning objectives and develop a plan for the assignment. The educator offers a joint reward (if every group member achieves a certain score on a quiz, each individual receives 2 bonus points).	
Individual Accountability	The educator randomly selects one student's work to represent the entire group. Peer evaluation.	
Promotive Interaction	The educator encourages students to share resources and information. Students provide each other feedback to improve their portion of the task.	
Appropriate Use of Social Skills	The educator teaches and rewards group work skills. The educator encourages the students to resolve conflicts in a constructive manner.	
Group Processing	The students identify three strengths and three areas for improvement following cooperative learning. The students use a checklist to rate the group's performance.	

and experiences. While each grouping method has advantages and disadvantages, the literature on the specific instructional methods we outline later suggest the third option of assigning students based on abilities and experiences, so groups possess diverse views and skills.

Provide Explanations

Prior to working in groups, you will need to give explicit instruction of the cooperative learning activities, which includes defining the assignment, discussing how you will grade the individual student and the group, and explaining certain criteria the students need to meet to achieve success. It is during this time that you should revisit the five essential elements of collaborative learning (e.g., reviewing the common goal, explaining social skills).

Watch for passive group members during this time!

GROUP MEMBERS

Name	Phone	e-mail

**Indicate Group Coordinator

Preferred Topic

1. _____

2. _____

3. _____

Final Topic Assignment

_____

Meeting w/Dr. Stewart   1) _____

2) _____

Presentation Date   _____

Figure 8-3. Example of a group planning form. (Reproduced with permission from Stewart, S. R., & Gonzalez, L. S. [2006]. Instruction in professional issues using a cooperative learning, case study approach. *Communication Disorders Quarterly, 27*[3], 14. https://doi.org/10.1177/15257401060270030401)

Monitor Learning

You will want to determine a strategy for monitoring learning and be prepared to intervene to ensure your students are adequately applying knowledge and using appropriate group work skills. Your sound observation and data collection skills will serve you well as you facilitate them during cooperative learning activities.

Write three strategies you can employ to monitor learning during cooperative learning tasks.

Assess Student Learning

As previously mentioned, you will need to provide your students with opportunities to evaluate their individual and their group's performance. In addition, you will also assess your students according to the method you discussed prior to the start of the cooperative learning task. It is important that you design cooperative learning activities that hold your students accountable as individuals and as group members (e.g., individual grade **and** group grade). We offer several strategies:

- Complete peer and self evaluation
- Give individual quizzes or tests
- Randomly select one student's assignment or quiz to represent the group
- Ask students to explain what they have learned
- Complete a group processing sheet

SPECIFIC COOPERATIVE LEARNING INSTRUCTIONAL METHODS

Fishbowl Discussion

In this cooperative learning instructional method, a portion of your students sit in a circle in the center of the room, while the remainder of your students sit around the circle, similar to fish in a fishbowl. The students inside the bowl engage in discussion, while the students outside the bowl listen, observe, and provide ongoing feedback (Figure 8-4). In this dynamic and interactive method of instruction, students must be prepared and actively participate and share and build their experiences and knowledge with others. Because there are variations in the description of a fishbowl discussion, we will provide a general overview of the most common procedures for implementation found in educational literature.

For a fishbowl discussion, you will divide your students into small groups. In most of the educational literature about this topic, you will see range in size from three to nine students with five to six students per group being the most common. You want the groups large enough so there are diverse points of view but small enough so that every student can adequately participate in the discussion. After you have formed the groups, you will determine what content will be researched or discussed. You might assign the content or provide the group with guidelines to select their own content. Each student should demonstrate interest if the group is choosing their own area of content (e.g., positive interdependence). When selecting topics, you want to consider content that is complex enough for multiple viewpoints and answers but also relevant to their professional context. A few examples include questions related to productivity requirements, end-of-life care, evidence-based practice, or client confidentiality. In occupational therapy education literature, educators have used this method to apply various theories or models to the evaluation and intervention of a practical scenario.

After the content is determined, each student works independently to learn as much as possible in preparation for the discussion (e.g., readings, videos, evidence). The group meets an additional time to develop a list of eight to 10 questions they believe are most important to address during the discussion. You will want to collect these questions prior to the date of their fishbowl discussion to ensure the group is adequately prepared and to guide them to any additional resources or thoughts if needed. We would like to note that in some references, the educator actually selects the discussion questions to guide their students' understanding of the content. However, we believe your students will have more motivation and a richer learning experience if they select the questions and construct meaning in their own way. Remember, you can review these questions prior to class to ensure they are on the right track. You could also require each group briefly meet with you prior to their assigned implementation date.

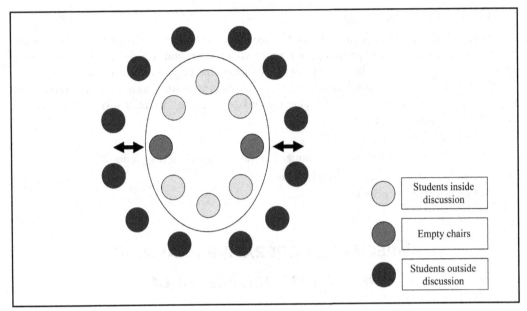

Figure 8-4. Fishbowl discussion.

You might elect to do several fishbowl discussions in one class period or one per class period. Regardless of the method you choose, you will set up the room in the same manner. The inner circle will contain one or two additional seats than the number of students in the group (e.g., if the group has five students, you will place six to seven chairs in the inner circle). The remainder of the class surrounds the outside of the inner circle. Many educators will demonstrate this instructional method and review behaviors for positive group performance prior to the start of the fishbowl discussion. As the group prepares for their discussion prior to class, they will need to select a facilitator. The facilitator will be responsible for providing the class with a brief introduction to the content and organization of the discussion, which is typically no more than 2 minutes in length. After this introduction, the students in the fishbowl are responsible for beginning and executing the discussion. The students talk with other group members about the content and each student is expected to contribute to this learning process. You should allow approximately 20 to 25 minutes for discussion, and the facilitator keeps the group on track to ensure important points are conversed in the allotted time.

While the inner circle is engaged in discussion, the students outside the fishbowl actively listen and observe. You will also find some variation about entering and leaving the fishbowl. In some literature, students on the outside of the fishbowl are allowed to enter the inner circle at any time and sit in one of the empty chairs if they wish to further contribute to, clarify, or question content in the discussion. In addition, you can enter the fishbowl to serve various roles, such as the prodder or devil's advocate. You might even join the discussion for a brief period of evaluation, but a majority of your time is spent on the outside. Once you or the outside student has contributed to the discussion, they immediately leave the inner circle so other students can join. In a "high-powered" discussion, these two seats become of the most popular and integral positions. However, other pieces of literature do not discuss allowing outside students in the inner circle because the fishbowl is a protected space that allows your students to develop rapport. In this situation, you would not need the extra chairs as previously discussed. Regardless of which way you select, the outside students are responsible for taking notes, evaluating, and providing feedback to each student and the group as a whole using the method of assessment you selected prior to class. You should also review this information with your students prior to the start of the fishbowl discussion.

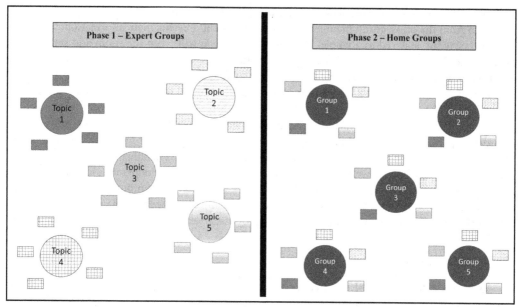

Figure 8-5. Jigsaw classroom.

Near the end of the fishbowl discussion, you will let the inside students know time is about to expire and provide each one with 30 seconds to give a final statement about a position or feeling on the content. The facilitator will summarize key points and make any observations or recommendations for the class. You can also allow time for verbal feedback and reflection, such as asking questions about what went well during the discussion, what helped or hurt the discussion, how they can improve discussion of the content, or if there is anything they would do differently.

Jigsaw Classroom

Another cooperative learning instructional method is the jigsaw classroom (also called group expert technique or home and expert groups). Interestingly, educators originally used this method of instruction to reduce the gap between students from various ethnic groups. Since the 1970s, educators have used this instructional method across a variety of educational settings, disciplines, and class sizes. Educational literature reports a jigsaw classroom is an effective and feasible way for students to engage in small group discussion and higher-level thinking. In this method of learning, each student is responsible for completing a portion that is essential for the group's understanding of the overall product. Therefore, we suggest you implement a jigsaw classroom when you have content that can be divided into equal parts among your students. It also works best with text-based learning material.

A jigsaw classroom can be broken into three phases. During phase one, you divide students into expert groups. These groups are called expert groups because the students become an expert on one specific topic. Your number of expert groups should match the same number of specific topics. Each student examines the assigned topic and works within their expert group to discuss the information, decide how to best teach others, and receive feedback and suggestions (Figure 8-5). This phase is important because less skilled students can learn and rehearse the course material with more proficient learners and vice versa.

Once students have completed their work in the expert group, you reorganize the class so that each new group (also called home group) has an expert for each topic (phase 2). Aronson and Patnoe (2011) suggest a group size between three and seven students with the ideal size being five to six students. Each student has a unique and vital contribution and teaches their home group about their topic. The students are interdependent because they cannot do well unless they pay attention to and learn from the other group members. After each student presents their information, the group should review the material as a whole. During this time, you will roam the room and serve as the facilitator and monitor roles and encourage your students to pay careful attention, ask clarifying questions, and encourage each other to present the topic effectively. Your expert group and home groups will work together in a 1-to-2 time ratio (e.g., 20 minutes in expert group and 40 minutes in home group).

Lastly (phase 3), you administer a quiz to hold the students accountable to the information. In order to perform well on the quiz, students must not only know their own topic but also know their other group members' topics. Although educational literature generally breaks down the jigsaw classroom into three phases, we suggest you add a fourth phase to this cooperative learning method. After your students have completed phase three (the quiz), provide a few minutes and/or strategies to summarize and debrief (e.g., the element of group processing described earlier in this chapter). Are you able to recognize or apply the five elements of cooperative learning in this instructional method?

Team-Based Learning

Team-based learning (TBL) is a cooperative learning instructional method used to develop group work and communication skills, improve knowledge retention, and maximize learner preparation, participation, and engagement. First discussed in 1982, educational literature provides a well-designed set of implementation principles with very little variation. Educators have demonstrated increased interest in this method of instruction, as evidenced by a growth from two publications in 2000 to approximately 80 publications in 2015; most (75%) of which occur in the United States. Although its roots are found in business education, health professional and medical education literature suggest TBL is an effective and feasible method appropriate for teaching the application of professional content. In addition, educators employing TBL often report a significant increase in energy and engagement during class. When using this method of instruction, your students will spend most of the class time engaged in group work. You can elect to implement this method within one or two classes or during the entire course.

You can break the implementation of TBL into four distinct phases (Figure 8-6). During the *pre-class preparation phase* (phase one), you will purposefully design and post the learning materials informed by your objectives (e.g., reading, additional resources, short videos). Your students complete these learning activities prior to class so they are familiar with key concepts and are prepared for class participation. Students are motivated to complete phase one because of the various activities that occur during phase two of TBL.

Prior to implementation of the *readiness assurance process* (phase two), you will prepare a short multiple-choice quiz (typically five to 20 questions) on the relevant concepts from the pre-class learning materials. As you write these questions, focus on key concepts as opposed to the picky details, but make sure the questions are challenging enough to stimulate good group discussion. During phase two, your students complete a number of activities during class. At the start of class, each student completes the quiz individually—called the *individual readiness assurance test (iRAT)*. Each student submits the iRAT for a grade.

Be aware of time during phase two! You should allow the same amount of time for the iRAT and tRAT (combined), feedback, and application portions of this phase.

Next, you will organize your students into groups that include five to seven members. Educational literature highly recommends you thoughtfully and strategically form these groups to ensure diversity of experiences, personalities, genders, and ethnicities. This action is important so that each group has adequate resources to complete learning activities and equal opportunities to develop cohesiveness by avoiding coalitions. As a group, the students collaborate to complete the exact same quiz an additional time—called the *team (or group) readiness assurance test (tRAT)*. As they are completing the tRAT, students discuss and defend

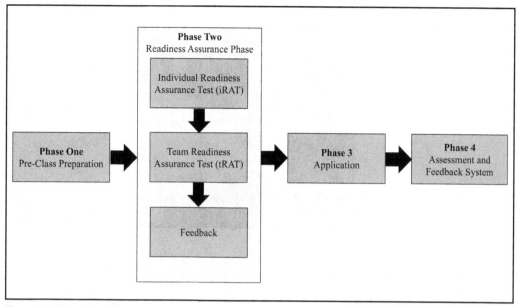

Figure 8-6. Team-based learning phases.

their knowledge and position in order to come to an agreement on the answer to each question (Figure 8-7). You can also encourage each group to explain and justify their answers to other groups. However, you should avoid providing the students with answers while they are taking the tRAT. Several scholars recommend having each group submit their quiz for an additional grade, so each student is motivated to contribute to the team and to learn the material prior to class.

Also in this phase, you will provide your students with feedback about the correct answers to the quiz. Some educational research discusses the use of an answer sheet or a scratch-off sheet (Immediate Feedback Assessment Technique) to provide the groups with real-time feedback about their answers. However, you will also likely want to provide verbal feedback during this time to clarify any concepts or misconceptions with which your students are experiencing challenges. Some educators prepare a brief presentation or discussion during this time. Your feedback on individual and group performance is vital to your students, so they adequately understand the concepts for the phase of application.

In phase three, the *application of course concepts phase*, you will carefully develop learning activities or assignments that require the group to put the course content they were previously tested on to work. Each group utilizes their critical-thinking skills to apply their newly learned knowledge to solve an authentic professional problem. As each group is working on this learning activity, you continue to roam the room to facilitate discussion as your students continue to polish their solutions. You can also implement a wrap-up discussion during this phase if you feel as though your students would benefit from revisiting challenging content. Educators find designing the assignments for this phase as the most challenging aspect of the implementation of TBL. However, literature proposes using the 4S structure for building an effective application-based group assignment (see Chapter 12). You will want to design an assignment that:

1. Possesses a problem that is **significant** to your students
2. Requires all the students to solve the **same** problem to promote learning within and between groups
3. Commands the students to make a **specific** decision using the course content
4. Requires each group to **simultaneously** report their decisions

Figure 8-7. Students engage in the team readiness assurance test.

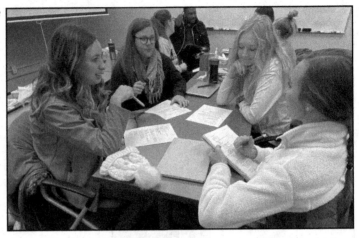

Lastly, in the final phase, you will create an *assessment and feedback system*. It is necessary for you to hold each student accountable to the group and for you to develop an effective way to assess group performance. Educational literature on the use of TBL recommends the use of various peer assessment mechanisms. However, similar to group work skills, you should not assume your students know how to use or have been exposed to peer evaluation. You might discuss or demonstrate or even offer your students a guide to giving appropriate and constructive feedback. If you lack time or interest in designing a peer assessment, several excellent instruments are available in literature (Table 8-5).

ADDITIONAL IMPLEMENTATION NOTES

- When possible, allow your students to select their topic for the cooperative learning activity.
- Let your students distribute or divide the cooperative learning activity according to their strengths and talents.
- Review your learning activity and consider your group size carefully; too small of a group will create a heavy workload, and too large of a group will reduce interactions and potentially foster too many ideas, which will be difficult to organize.
- Watch for excessive group work by reflecting on your entire course and communicating with your colleagues about their courses; when students are involved in numerous group projects, the workload becomes heavy and they lose motivation and interest.
- Remember, do not assume your students know how to perform well in groups, as poor functioning groups cause negative attitudes and increase the students' preference for working independently.
- Offer short meetings to check how each group is functioning and progressing toward goals.

TIPS AND TRICKS

- Devote an appropriate amount of time to carefully design and implement cooperative learning.
- Take the time to know your students better.
- Monitor learning closely.
- Incorporate cooperative learning instructional methods early in your course or program.

TABLE 8-5

Methods for the Assessment and Feedback System

AUTHOR/METHOD	DESCRIPTION
The Michaelsen Method	Students assign group members a score based on what they believe each member contributed to the overall group performance. For example, each student in a six-member group receives 50 points. Each student rates the group members with a minimum score of 7, an average of 10, or a maximum of 13.
The Fink Method	Each student receives 100 points and divides the points among each member.
Paul Koles	Each student completes a comprehensive instrument that is comprised of a quantitative section (e.g., rates on cooperative learning and interpersonal skills, self-directed learning) and qualitative section (asks questions about the most valuable contribution and most important area the individual could perform to effectively assist the group).

- Recognize your attitude and active participation are key factors in successful implementation for cooperative learning instructional methods. In a survey, 60% of educators did not implement cooperative learning instructional methods (despite evidence and theory) because they did not believe they were more efficient and reported lack of interest or organization (Thanh, 2011).

OPPORTUNITIES FOR FEEDBACK AND REFLECTION

Throughout this chapter, we have discussed the importance of individual and group feedback and reflection. We will further expand on previously mentioned examples and offer additional resources.

Self-Assessment

There are several self-assessment tools available in health professional education literature. However, in order for your students to engage in deeper thought about their performance in a group, we will offer questions your students can reflect on in a journal format. You can grade these prompts based on the quality and depth of their responses. Examples of prompts include:

- Describe your greatest contribution to your group.
- Describe an area in which you could improve your group performance. Discuss strategies you can implement to improve this area in future group work.
- Describe a challenge you encountered during group work and how you handled or would handle that challenge differently in the future.
- Provide examples of group work skills you demonstrated that your future colleagues would consider good practice.
- Explain skills you improved or obtained that your future clients would appreciate.
- Write a goal for your future individual performance in a group.

- Select one of the group work skills we discussed earlier in the semester. How did you demonstrate this group work skill during this project?
- Describe an instance when you provided a group member with constructive feedback, accountability, or resources. How will this benefit your future practice?

Peer Assessment

The literature consistently reports a need for educators to prepare their students for the peer evaluation process. You will need to provide clear and specific criteria and training on how to adequately use whichever method of peer assessment you select. A couple of strategies you can use are to provide your students with an exemplar of peer feedback, educate them on how to provide constructive recommendations, and allow them to practice using self and peer assessments. We also want to make you aware of a few additional challenges with peer feedback. These challenges include the potential for creating anxiety or a competitive and hostile learning environment, lacking confidence in other's judgments of work, disagreeing with or not understanding how to interpret contradicting feedback, or believing the educator should provide the feedback. When considering these potential challenges, decide if the peer feedback will be anonymous or nonanonymous. With anonymous peer feedback, students do not have the opportunity to exchange verbal information for clarification and may provide very irresponsible or harsh feedback. Lastly, in an integrative review of peer assessment in nursing education, scholars highly recommended to avoid grading peer evaluation and feedback for a grade, but instead grade on the quality of peer feedback the student provides on the assessment to assign a grade (e.g., you use the information to assign a grade, the students do not assign the overall grade).

One example of peer assessment in health professional educational literature is the TeamUP rubric. This assessment covers five domains of teamwork skills:

1. Project planning and management
2. Fostering a team climate
3. Facilitating the contributions of others
4. Managing conflict
5. Contributing to team project

Each domain includes a definition and description of the behavior. Group members do not "mark" or score each other, but give feedback using a color system (red, amber, yellow, and green). They can also write additional qualitative feedback in each domain to justify their color selection. The educator uses this information to assign each student a final score.

Group Processing

We recognize providing feedback on group performance is complex in terms of equality and student satisfaction. However, literature in nursing education outlines several recommendations for the assessment of group work. You will likely assign each student in the group the same grade based on the quality of the group's final product and achievement of learning outcomes. You will also reserve a small or even separate portion of each student's grade for the feedback found in the self and peer assessments. In addition, it is important for you to facilitate discussion within the group so students are not surprised by peer feedback and so each student can reflect on the group process and skills needed for successful outcomes. Therefore, one of the most important things you can do at the end of a cooperative learning activity is to provide regular time for group processing and reflection. Good group processing occurs when students reflect on which group member's actions were valuable or inadequate and when the students in the group make decisions about actions they should continue and/or change to achieve future learning goals. We have provided you with examples of questions:

- Discuss how well you communicated as a group. How could you improve this area for your future practice?
- How did the group learn to overcome any obstacles?
- What strategies helped the group achieve the learning goals? What strategies hindered the group's progress toward the learning goals?
- What would the group do differently if asked to solve the same problem an additional time?
- What skills helped the group's performance? What skills could be improved for future performances?
- How can the group better support and encourage its members?
- How will you use what you learned from working in this group in your future practice?
- When did your group realize they had decided on the best solution to the problem?

Take a moment and write down a few additional reflection questions you could include on self, peer, or group assessments.

APPLICATION TO OCCUPATIONAL THERAPY PRACTICE

Example 1: Implementation of Collaborative Learning in School System

In their research study, Wilson and Harris (2018) provide an excellent example of cooperative learning between teachers and occupational therapists in an elementary school setting. Using the Partnership for Change model, occupational therapists collaborated with teachers to develop universal design strategies to support students with special needs in their classrooms. In this situation, the two parties experienced the common goal of addressing students' priorities and achieving their learning outcomes. The teachers and educators cooperatively planned and implemented various learning strategies and group lessons. The teachers appreciated the ability to watch the occupational therapists model these new approaches, and they all received and provided feedback. Through collaborative learning, teachers and occupational therapists developed relationships and trust and provided support for all the students in the classroom.

Example 2: Implementation of Fishbowl Discussion in Your Department

Perhaps your department offers a monthly lunch and learn event, and it is your turn to design the educational experience. Your department has recently had challenges with discharge planning, so you select this topic for the event. Prior to the date, you create an "expert group" to provide information. You might include yourself, a social worker, or a caregiver as members of this group. You briefly meet to discuss the overall goal and organization of the event and decide what information each group member will research or provide. You meet one additional time to determine eight to 10 discussion questions and select a facilitator. On the day of the lunch and learn, you arrange the inner circle with a chair for each member of your group and two additional chairs. The rest of your department sits around the inner circle creating the fishbowl. You explain the fishbowl discussion process and the facilitator completes the 2-minute introduction. As the group discusses the answers to their questions, the individuals in the outer circle listen, take notes, or move to the inner circle to ask questions, clarify important points, or offer a different point of view or concern. Near the end of time, the facilitator provides a summary to the group and the outer circle offers feedback. Organizers of a recent medical conference implemented 10 fishbowl discussions to increase active participation of attendees. Following the conference, 169 attendees completed a survey about their experiences with the fishbowl discussion. A majority of these respondents (78.5%) recommended this method for future conferences and reported comfort in participating in the discussion.

Advantages

- Fosters group collaboration and social support
- Perceptions of ability to problem solve improve
- Engages in deep and meaningful learning
- Improves ability to become self-directed lifelong learners
- Increases student engagement and motivation
- Improves self-efficacy skills
- Fosters communication skills needed for future professional experiences (negotiation, conflict resolution, etc.)
- Enhances knowledge and skill performance
- Works well for any material and at any educational level
- Works for variety of practical skills
- Gives learners a sense of security with working with others similar to them
- Improves students' attitudes toward teamwork
- Has ability to be implemented with small and large courses
- Theory and evidence support these methods

Challenges

- Requires more effort and preparation from learners prior to class
- Requires training and commitment of the educators' time and effort
- Potential for competitiveness
- Requires educators to train students on group work skills and assessment and feedback systems

In the space below, list any additional advantages or challenges.

```



```

Brainstorm strategies for overcoming these challenges when implementing the use of cooperative learning instructional methods.

```



```

THREE THINGS YOU CAN DO TOMORROW TO IMPLEMENT COOPERATIVE LEARNING INSTRUCTIONAL METHODS WITH YOUR STUDENTS

1. Discuss with your colleagues about how you teach your students group work skills.
2. Review one form of self or peer assessment and think about how you can implement it in one of your courses.
3. Practice using the Examples of Essential Elements (see Table 8-4) when redesigning or developing a cooperative learning instructional method.

Cooperative Learning Instructional Methods Evidence Table

FISHBOWL

Author/Year	Study Objectives	Design and Participants	Intervention and Outcome Measures	Results
de Sam Lazaro & Riley (2019)	Researchers compared educational outcomes of a peer-led teaching approach using a fishbowl method to a traditional faculty-led teaching approach	Design: Post hoc analysis of 2 teaching methods Participants: 115 first-year graduate occupational therapy students Both groups of students enrolled in a 3-credit hour graduate course lasting 7 weeks	Intervention: Researchers divided students into 2 intervention groups based on the type of teaching method and course schedule The faculty-led teaching group employed instructional methods, such as assigned readings, traditional lectures, and large class discussions, to assist students in creating a "grid" assignment about theories in occupational therapy The peer-teaching group provided recorded lectures to be viewed before the start of class, and then included a fishbowl approach to discussion about a specific case study during each class session Outcome measures: Accuracy of responses on exams Researchers coded exam items at various levels of Bloom's Taxonomy of Cognitive Skills (knowledge, comprehension, application, analysis, synthesis, evaluation)	No statistically significant differences between the faculty-led group and peer-led teaching group in knowledge or comprehension of exam information No statistically significant differences between the 2 groups in application of exam information Peer-led teaching group performed better than the faculty-led teaching group in analyzing ($P = .036$), synthesizing ($P = .32$; $P = .009$) and evaluating ($P = .001$) exam information Overall, the 2 groups performed similarly on exam items requiring lower-level cognitive skills, such as knowledge, comprehension, and application of information Peer-led teaching groups performed better on exam items requiring higher-level skills, such as analysis, synthesis, and evaluation of information

(continued)

Cooperative Learning Instructional Methods Evidence Table (continued)

JIGSAW CLASSROOM

Author/Year	Study Objectives	Design and Participants	Intervention and Outcome Measures	Results
Nolan et al. (2018)	Researchers examined college students' academic performance after using jigsaw classroom instructional methods	Design: Cross-sectional posttest Participants: 126 students at the University of Scranton • Enrolled in a 200-level social psychology course • Enrolled between the fall semester of 2013 and fall semester of 2016	Intervention: Students completed 2 different jigsaw activities in the classroom The course instructor created groups of 3 students, designating each student as the "expert" on 1 of 3 topics within each group Each student learned necessary information about their assigned topic in preparation for each class session Students first met in large groups of students with the same topic, then split into their designated jigsaw groups to teach their peers about their assigned topic The instructor assessed students' knowledge about each topic using varying methods throughout the semester Outcome measures: Students' academic performance in the social psychology course, including: • Overall student performance • Topic preference on examinations • Student feedback	On short-answer test items, students frequently chose to write about the topic they were assigned to teach their peers (62.96% of students) when given the option Students scored higher on short-answer exam items related to the topic they taught to their jigsaw group as compared to the students who did not teach that specific topic Multiple-choice exam items showed no significant differences in academic performance between students who taught a specific topic and students who learned that topic from their peers The majority of students (80.65%) reported that the jigsaw method improved their understanding of their assigned topic as compared to the topics they learned from peers

(continued)

Cooperative Learning Instructional Methods Evidence Table (continued)

TEAM-BASED LEARNING

Author/Year	Study Objectives	Design and Participants	Intervention and Outcome Measures	Results
Burgess et al. (2014)	Researchers summarized available evidence on team-based learning (TBL) to inform curriculum and educators in medical education	Design: Systematic review Participants: Medical students Researchers included 20 articles in this review	Researchers searched the following databases: MedLine, PubMed, Web of Knowledge, Education Resources Information Center (ERIC) from 2002 to 2012 Inclusion criteria: • Medical students enrolled in undergraduate or graduate medical schools Exclusion criteria: • Excluded articles with individuals in residency training, continuing medical education, or continuing education • Students from other health care professions	Of the 20 articles, 14 discussed traditional TBL methodology while 6 described a modified approach The studies implemented problem-based learning in a wide range of topics; primarily in preclinical years Researchers implemented TBL for a wide range of sessions; the range of team size was 4 to 12 students per group Educators most commonly used random or alphabetical to assign teams Studies used individual and team tests in align with TBL recommendations; number of questions ranged from 10 to 13 In 11 studies, educators provided immediate feedback Literature suggests the 4S structure: • Significance: High-level-thinking problems of common real-world issues • Same: Teams worked on the same problems • Specific: Use of multiple-choice questions with 1 best answer • Simultaneous: Groups reveal responses at same time

(continued)

Cooperative Learning Instructional Methods Evidence Table (continued)

Author/Year	Study Objectives	Design and Participants	Intervention and Outcome Measures	Results
Chen et al. (2018)	Researchers aimed to understand the effectiveness of TBL in medical education	Design: Meta-analysis Participants: 1,545 pool participants Researchers included 13 studies in this review	Researchers included studies from inception to 2015 Researchers searched the following databases: CNKI, CBM, Chinese Wanfang, Classification of Instructional Programs (CIP), PubMed, Embase, Cochrane Library Inclusion criteria: • Investigated TBL in medicine disciplines • Used randomized/nonrandomized design • Compared TBL to traditional lecture-based learning • Discussed quantitative results	All studies used outcome measures of theoretical examination scores and surveys From the pooled data of the 13 studies, researchers reported TBL significantly increased exam scores when compared to lecture-based learning 4 studies reported learning attitudes and 5 studies reported learning skills; each pooled data in these areas demonstrated significance Randomization, level of education, or gender were factors that contributed to heterogeneity
Dearnley et al. (2018)	Researchers examined outcomes of students enrolled in nursing and midwifery educational programs when using TBL approaches	Design: Systematic review Selected 16 studies Participant inclusion criteria: student nurses, student midwives, nurses and midwives in undergraduate or postgraduate academic programs Participants could be in the pre/postregistration phase, but must be in the higher education setting	2 reviewers examined the titles and abstracts of each study and the eligibility of a study based on the specified inclusion/exclusion criteria Databases: CINAHL, MedLine, ERIC Search terms: team-based learning, nurse, nurses, nurse practitioner, midwife, midwives, midwifery Inclusion criteria: • International research papers • Published in English • Researched use of TBL as compared to the customary faculty-led lecture approach	3 studies showed improvements in levels of student engagement when using TBL methods 4 studies reported an increase in undergraduate nursing students' satisfaction after using TBL instructional methods 4 studies demonstrated improved academic attainment for students using TBL methods, although some improvements were limited to students who were initially lower performing as compared to their peers

(continued)

Cooperative Learning Instructional Methods Evidence Table (continued)

Author/Year	Study Objectives	Design and Participants	Intervention and Outcome Measures	Results
			• Outcomes must be related to progression, completion, attainment, retention, attrition, student satisfaction, or student dissatisfaction • Primary or secondary research Each study completed between 2011 and 2017	3 studies examined the correlation between TBL methods and increased practice development in nursing students, with 2 of these studies demonstrating significant improvements in practice examination scores for students using TBL methods 7 papers reported an improvement in the transformational aspects of learning, which included the students' experiences of personal or professional growth, when using a TBL instructional approach
Fatmi et al. (2013)	Researchers examined the effectiveness of TBL on learning outcomes in health professional education	Design: Systematic review Researchers included 14 studies in this review	Researchers searched the following databases: Physical Education Abstracts, Scopus, Web of Science, ERIC, OpenSIGLE, ProQuest Dissertations and Theses, MedLine, Embase, PubMed, CINAHL, Cochrane Library Inclusion criteria: • Medical students, residents, physicians, nursing students, pharmacy students, dental students, veterinary trainees, dietician trainees, clinical psychology trainees, other allied health professionals, interdisciplinary health professions • TBL in conjunction with lectures, workshops, small group learning, clinical teaching, or other teaching methods • Described TBL • Included a wide variety of outcomes • Included a wide variety of studies	Each study used knowledge outcome measures; 7 demonstrated statistically significant increase of TBL compared to control 4 studies did not report a significant difference; 3 did not report significant testing 1 study reported significance in learner reaction in favor of TBL

(continued)

Cooperative Learning Instructional Methods Evidence Table (continued)

Author/Year	Study Objectives	Design and Participants	Intervention and Outcome Measures	Results
Hong & Rajalingam (2018)	Researchers aimed to summarize current literature on TBL in medical education and create a questionnaire to gain further understanding	Design: Systematic review Researchers included 39 articles in this review	Researchers searched Web of Science database Researchers created a questionnaire to capture gaps in literature on implementation	Most articles reported educators used TBL in preclinical courses Mean class size was 152 with average group size 6.28 In most medical schools, educators use TBL less than 25% of curriculum as a complementary instructional method
Lang et al. (2019)	Researchers completed a meta-analysis to evaluate the effectiveness of TBL in pharmacy education in China	Design: Systematic review and meta-analysis Participants: 1,271 pharmacy students in China (pooled); 631 in experimental TBL group Researchers included 12 studies in this review	Researchers followed Preferred Reporting Items for Systematic Reviews and Meta-Analyses (PRISMA) guidelines and Cochrane Handbook Researchers searched the following databases: CNKI, Chinese VIP database, Chinese Wanfang, PubMed, Embase, Cochrane Library Inclusion criteria: • Students engaged in pharmacy education at a Chinese institution • Used TBL in pharmacy curriculum • Compared TBL to traditional lecture-based learning • Used outcome measures of theoretical scores, abilities • Randomized controlled studies	Students engaged in TBL received higher theoretical/knowledge scores on objective tests On the studies that explored students' enthusiasm for learning and self-study abilities, results favored TBL pedagogy Studies also demonstrated TBL improved students' thinking abilities 2 pooled studies suggest TBL improves students' communication
Reimschisel et al. (2017)	Researchers desired to summarize evidence on TBL in health professional education	Design: Systematic review Researchers included 118 articles in the systematic review	Researchers searched the following databases: PubMed, Web of Science, ERIC, Google Scholar Limited search to articles written in English	Almost half of studies investigated use of TBL with medical students (most common undergraduate medical students)

(continued)

Cooperative Learning Instructional Methods Evidence Table (continued)

Author/Year	Study Objectives	Design and Participants	Intervention and Outcome Measures	Results
				67 of the 118 articles compared TBL to another method of instruction; 42 of the 67 studies used a control group; most commonly compared to lecture Most common group size was 5 to 6 students Most common number of sessions was only 1, but a range of 1 to 90 Researchers most commonly use outcome measures related to attitudes and learning outcomes
Zachry et al. (2017)	Researchers compared graduate occupational therapy students' opinions of TBL instructional methods to more traditional lecture-based instructional methods in the classroom	Design: Posttest survey design Participants: First- and second-year occupational therapy graduate students Master of Occupational Therapy program at the University of Texas Health Science Center at Houston	Intervention: Instructors applied TBL methods to 2 occupational therapy courses that required application of course topics: • Leadership development • Occupational-centered practice in community mental health All students completed an assignment prior to class, individually completed an in-class assessment of knowledge, and then worked in assigned groups to complete the assessment together Instructors revealed the correct responses to the class and then later required students to apply the learned concepts to a different assignment Outcome measures: Survey to students at the close of each academic course	84% student response rate to survey (89 students) Students preferred more traditional lecture-based instructional methods in comparison to TBL ($P < .05$) Fewer students believed TBL methods increased their comprehension of course material (69%) as compared to a lecture-based approach (82%) Students reported that both instructional methods were beneficial in preparing for any course assessments of knowledge Most students (73%) reported that their learning experience was enhanced by the problem-solving aspect of a TBL approach

(continued)

Cooperative Learning Instructional Methods Evidence Table (continued)

Author/Year	Study Objectives	Design and Participants	Intervention and Outcome Measures	Results
			Survey included 5-point Likert scale rating students' perceptions of a TBL approach versus a traditional lecture-based approach; scale ranged from strongly disagree (-2) to strongly agree (2)	

COOPERATIVE LEARNING

Author/Year	Study Objectives	Design and Participants	Intervention and Outcome Measures	Results
Kalaian & Kasim (2017)	Researchers examined the outcomes of small group learning methods, as compared to traditional lecture-based teaching, in undergraduate health care students	Design: Meta-analysis Selected 19 studies for review 4,050 participants: Undergraduate college students; nursing and health science classrooms • 1,560 students in classrooms using small group learning methods • 2,490 students in classrooms using lecture-based methods	2 researchers coded descriptive statistics and features of interest from each study Databases: ERIC, ProQuest, CINAHL, JSTOR, PubMed Search terms: cooperative learning, collaborative learning, problem-based learning, small-group learning, peer learning, inquiry-based learning, peer-led team learning, team-based learning in combination with health or nursing Researchers also searched the *Journal of Nursing Education* and references of obtained articles Inclusion criteria: • Research compared academic outcomes of using a small-group learning method to using a traditional lecture-based learning method in undergraduate nursing or health science classrooms	Small group learning methods were shown to be effective in improving students' academic performance in 17 studies, as shown by positive effect sizes in each study When compared to lecture-based methods, small group learning was more effective in improving academic performance (weighted average effect size of 0.59) Effect sizes were larger in studies conducted in 2001 and later Efficacy of small group learning methods were dependent on the age of the college student participants, with first-year college students demonstrating the largest effect size Small group learning was more effective for groups consisting of 4 students or less Small group learning was more effective when students were able to self-select their groups rather than being assigned to a group

(continued)

Cooperative Learning Instructional Methods Evidence Table (continued)

Author/Year	Study Objectives	Design and Participants	Intervention and Outcome Measures	Results
			• Research did not use self-reported outcome measures • Research used a 2-group experimental research design, 2-group quasi-experimental (pre/post) research design, or 2-group comparative (post only) research design • Research included adequate descriptive statistics • Research published any time before December 2014 Random effects approach to meta-analysis and meta-regression methods	Exams created by an instructor, as well as courses being taught by a researcher rather than a traditional instructor, both increased the efficacy of small group learning methods Efficacy of small group learning methods was associated with the length of a class session (longer duration of instruction led to a relatively small increase in effect size)
Zhang & Cui (2018)	Researchers examined the implementation and efficacy of collaborative learning techniques in higher nursing education	Design: Systematic review Selected 29 studies for review Participants: Nursing students	Databases: CINAHL, PubMed, Google Scholar Search terms: Nursing, nursing education, collaborative learning, cooperative learning Inclusion criteria: • Researched use of collaborative learning/cooperative learning in university nursing education • Research report or learning practice report All studies published in English Each study completed from 1985 to present day	Majority of studies were descriptive research, with 1 study using randomized controlled design and 5 studies using quasi-experimental designs Most studies included collaboration-based learning techniques with other nursing students, but collaboration with other health care disciplines was growing in popularity The use of a jigsaw method was rarely used in the literature Collaborative learning methods were found to be effective for nursing students in both the classroom and clinical settings

(continued)

Cooperative Learning Instructional Methods Evidence Table (continued)

Author/Year	Study Objectives	Design and Participants	Intervention and Outcome Measures	Results
				An emerging area of interest is that of online collaboration methods, which have enabled international collaboration among nursing students
				Students demonstrated increased academic achievement when instructors used a collaborative approach to test taking
				Collaborative learning methods have culminated many positive impacts on student learning, including improvements in skill mastery, concept comprehension, professional behaviors, and the ability to communicate with others
				Nursing students reported collaborative learning methods positively contributed to the learning process

Adapted from American Occupational Therapy Association. (2002). AOTA's evidence-based literature review project: An overview (D. Lieberman & J. Scheer, Eds.). *American Journal of Occupational Therapy, 56*, 344–349. https://doi.org/10.5014/ajot.56.3.344

REFERENCES

American Occupational Therapy Association. (2002). AOTA's evidence-based literature review project: An overview (D. Lieberman & J. Scheer, Eds.). *The American Journal of Occupational Therapy, 56,* 344-349. https://doi.org/10.5014/ajot.56.3.344

Aronson, E., & Patnoe, S. (2011). *Cooperation in the classroom: The jigsaw method.* Pinter and Martin.

Burgess, A. W., McGregor, D. M., & Mellis, C. M. (2014). Applying established guidelines to team-based learning programs in medical schools: A systematic review. *Academic Medicine, 89*(4), 678-688. http://dx.doi.org/10.1097/ACM.0000000000000162

Chen, M., Ni, C., Hu, Y., Wang, M., Liu, L., Ji, X., Chu, H., Wu, W., Lu, C., Wang, S., Wang, S., Zhao, L., Li, Z., Zhu, H., Wang, J., Xia, Y., & Wang, X. (2018). Meta-analysis on the effectiveness of team-based learning on medical education in China. *BMC Medical Education, 18*(77), 1-11. https://doi.org/10.1186/s12909-018-1179-1

de Sam Lazaro, S. L., & Riley, B. R. (2019). Developing critical thinking in OT education: Effectiveness of a fishbowl approach. *Journal of Occupational Therapy Education, 3*(2), Article 1. https://dx.doi.org/10.26681/jote.2019.030201

Dearnley, C., Rhodes, C., Roberts, P., Williams, P., & Prenton, S. (2018). Team based learning in nursing and midwifery higher education: A systematic review of the evidence for change. *Nurse Education Today, 60,* 75-83. http://dx.doi.org/10.1016/j.nedt.2017.09.012

Fatmi, M., Hartling, L., Hillier, T., Campbell, S., & Oswald, A. E. (2013). The effectiveness of team-based learning on learning outcomes in health professions education: BEME Guide No. 30. *Medical Teacher, 35,* e-1608-e1624. http://dx.doi.org/10.3109/0142159X.2013.849802

Hong, J. M., & Rajalingam, P. (2018). Geographic trends in team-based learning (TBL) research and implementation in medical schools. *Health Professional Education,* 1-14. https://doi.org/10.1016/j.hpe.2019.11.005

Johnson, D. W., & Johnson, R. T. (1990). Social skills for successful group work. *Educational Leadership, 47*(4), 29-33.

Johnson, D. W., & Johnson, R. T. (1999). Making cooperative learning work. *Theory Into Practice, 38*(2), 67-73.

Johnson, D. W., & Johnson, R. T. (2005). New developments in social independent theory. *Genetic, Social, and General Psychology Monographs, 131*(4), 285-358.

Johnson, D. W., & Johnson, R. T. (2009). An educational psychology success story: Social interdependence theory and cooperative learning. *Educational Researcher, 38*(5), 365-379. http://dx.doi.org/10.3102/0013189X09339057

Kalaian, S. A., & Kasim, R. M. (2017). Effectiveness of various innovative learning methods in health science classrooms: A meta-analysis. *Advances in Health Science Education, 22,* 1151-1167. http://dx.doi.org/10.1007/s10459-017-9753-6

Lang, B., Zhang, L., Lin, Y., Han, L., Zhang, C., & Liu, Y. (2019). Team-based learning pedagogy enhances the quality of Chinese pharmacy education: a systematic review and meta-analysis. *BMC Medical Education, 19*(286), 1-12.

Nolan, J. M., Hanley, B. G., DiViertri, T. P., & Harvey, N. A. (2018). She who teaches learns: Performance benefits of a jigsaw activity in a college classroom. *Scholarship of Teaching and Learning in Psychology, 4*(2), 93-104. http://dx.doi.org/10.1037/stl0000110

Reimschisel, T., Herring, A. L., Huang, J., & Minor, T. J. (2017). A systematic review of the published literature on team-based learning in health professions education. *Medical Teacher, 39*(12), 1227-1237. http://doi.org/10.1080/0142159X.2017.1340636

Thanh, P. T. H. (2011). An investigation of perceptions of Vietnamese teachers and students toward cooperative learning (CL). *International Education Studies, 4*(1), 3-12.

Wilson, A. L., & Harris, S. R. (2018). Collaborative occupational therapy: Teachers' impressions of the partnering for change (P4C) model. *Physical & Occupational Therapy in Pediatrics, 38*(2), 130-142. http://dx.doi.org/10.1080/01942638.2017.1297988

Zachry, A. H., Nash, B. H., & Nolen, A. (2017). Traditional lectures and team-based learning in an occupational therapy program: Survey of student perceptions. *The Open Journal of Occupational Therapy, 5*(2), Article 6. http://dx.doi.org/10.15453/2168-6408.1313

Zhang, J., & Cui, Q. (2018). Collaborative learning in higher nursing education: A systematic review. *Journal of Professional Nursing, 34,* 378-388. http://dx.doi.org/10.1016/j.profnurs.2018.07.007

BIBLIOGRAPHY

Al Kawas, S., & Hamdy, H. (2017). Peer-assisted learning associated with team-based learning in dental education. *Health Professions Education, 3*, 38-43. http://dx.doi.org/10.1016/j.hpe.2016.08.003

Buhr, G. T., Heflin, M. T., White, H. K., & Pinheiro, S. O. (2014). Using the jigsaw cooperative learning method to teach medical students about long-term and postacute care. *Journal of the American Medical Directors Association, 15*, 429-434. http://dx.doi.org/10.1016/j.jamda.2014.01.015

Christen, A. (2009). Transforming the classroom for collaborative learning in the 21st century. *Techniques, 84*(1), 28-31.

Cooley, S. J., Burns, V. E., & Cumming, J. (2015). The role of outdoor adventure education in facilitating groupwork in higher education. *Higher Education, 69*, 567-582. http://dx.doi.org/10.1007/s10734-014-9791-4

Duers, L. E. (2017). The learner as co-creator: A new peer review and self-assessment feedback form created by student nurses. *Nurse Education Today, 58*, 47-52. http://dx.doi.org/10.1016/j.nedt.2017.08.002

Dutt, K. M. (1997). The fishbowl motivates students to participate. *College Teaching, 45*(4), 143. http://dx.doi.org/10.1080/87567559709596217

Gullo, C., Ha, T. C., & Cook, S. (2015). Twelve tips for facilitating team-based learning. *Medical Teacher, 37*(9), 819-824. https://doi.org/10.3109/0142159X.2014.1001729

Hastie, C., Fahy, K., & Parratt, J. (2014). The development of a rubric for peer assessment of individual teamwork skills in undergraduate midwifery students. *Women and Birth, 27*, 220-226. http://dx.doi.org/10.1016/j.wombi.2014.06.003

Hennessey, A., & Dionigi, R. A. (2013). Implementing cooperative learning in Australian primary schools: Generalist teachers' perspectives. *Issues in Educational Research, 23*(1), 52-68.

Jensen, G. M., & Mostrom, E. (2013). *Handbook of teaching and learning for physical therapists* (3rd ed.). Elsevier.

Johnson, D. W. (2003). Social interdependence: Interrelationships among theory, research, and practice. *American Psychologist, 58*(11), 934-945.

Michaelsen, L. K., Sweet, M., & Parmalee, D. X. (2008). *Team-based learning: Small-group learning's next big step*. Jossey-Bass Inc.

Mucke, J., Anders, H. J., Aringer, M., Chehab, G., Fischer-Betz, R., Hiepe, F. Lorez, H. M., Schwarting, A., Specker, C., Voll, E. R., & Schneider, M. (2019). Swimming against the stream: The fishbowl discussion method as an interactive tool for medical conferences: Experiences from the 11th European Lupus meeting. *Annals of the Rheumatic Diseases, 78*(5), 713-714.

Najdanovic-Visak, V. (2017). Team-based learning for first year engineering students. *Education for Chemical Engineers, 18*, 26-34. http://dx.doi.org/10.1016/j.ece.2016.09.001

Oldland, E., Currey, J., Considine, J., & Allen, J. (2017). Nurses' perceptions of the impact of team-based learning participation of learning style, team behaviours and clinical performance: An exploration or written reflections. *Nurse Education in Practice, 24*, 62-69. http://dx.doi.org/10.1016/j.nepr.2017.03.008

Riley, W., & Anderson, P. (2006). Randomized study on the impact of cooperative learning distance education in public health. *The Quarterly Review of Distance Education, 7*(2), 129-144.

Priles, M. A. (1993). The fishbowl discussion: A strategy for large honors classes. *The English Journal, 82*(6), 49-50. https://www.jstor.org/stable/820165

Saborit, J. A. P., Fernandez-Rio, J., Estrada, J. A. C., Mendez-Gimenez, A., & Alonso, D. M. (2016). Teachers' attitude and perception towards cooperative learning implementation: Influence of continuing training. *Teaching and Teacher Education, 59*, 438-445. http://dx.doi.org/10.1016/j.tate.2016.07.020

Smart, K. L., & Featheringham, R. (2006). Developing effective interpersonal communication and discussion skills. *Business Communication Quarterly, 69*(3), 276-282. http://dx.doi.org/10.1177/1080569906291231

Smith, M., & Rogers, J. (2014). Understanding nursing students' perspectives on the grading of group work assessments. *Nurse Education in Practice, 14*, 112-116. https://doi.org/10.1016/j.nepr.2013.07.012

Stewart, S. R., & Gonzalez, L. S. (2006). Instruction in professional issues using a cooperative learning, case study approach. *Communication Disorders Quarterly, 27*(3), 159-172.

Tolsgaard, M. G., Kulasegaram, K. M., & Ringsted, C. V. (2016). Collaborative learning of clinical skills in health professions education: The why, how, when and for whom. *Medical Education, 50*, 69-78. http://dx.doi.org/10.1111/medu.12814

Tornwall, J. (2018). Peer assessment practices in nurse education: An integrative review. *Nurse Education Today, 71*, 266-275. https://doi.org/10.1016/j.nedt.2018.09.017

Wong, F. M. F. (2018). A phenomenological research study: Perspectives of student learning through small group work between undergraduate nursing students and educators. *Nurse Education Today, 68*, 153-158. https://doi.org/10.1016/j.nedt.2018.06.013

Xu, J. H. (2016). Toolbox of teaching strategies in nurse education. *Chinese Nursing Research, 3*, 54-57. http://dx.doi.org/10.1016/j.cnre.2016.06.002

DISCUSSION-BASED INSTRUCTIONAL METHODS

Cynthia Clough, PhD, OT/L

BASIC TENETS

Discussion-based instructional methods have the potential to offer students transformational learning experiences by fostering rich exchange of ideas and perspectives that would not be available in a traditional lecture-dominated classroom. Through discussion, educators build classroom community where vulnerability, intentional listening, and empathetic understanding merge to create opportunities for all participants to experience transformation of values and perspectives. By explicitly including habits of intentional listening, questioning, critiquing, and exploration in classroom routines, they move discussions beyond basic conversation and dialogue. In this environment, students engage in challenging dialogue and respond to educators and peers without fear of judgment.

Classroom discussions promote sharing of perspectives and knowledge, which allows students to expand their creative problem-solving skills and generate new ideas for creating solutions. With the use of effective discussion groups, students feel empowered to use their voice both within and outside the classroom (Figure 9-1). This empowerment gives students real-time experience engaging in democratic debate, exploring complex social issues, sharing and hearing personal narratives, and developing civil inquiry with others who have similar and/or different perspectives. Discussion has the power to transform students in ways that make them recognizably different in their understanding and perspectives of their position in the world. In this chapter, we will discuss several ways you can implement discussion-based instructional methods in your courses.

Henderson, W. (Ed.). *Effective Teaching: Instructional Methods and Strategies for Occupational Therapy Education* (pp. 217-234).

Figure 9-1. Students engage in a classroom discussion.

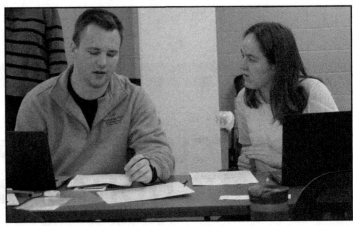

BACKGROUND

Society often views traditional college classrooms as being led by an educator who stands at the front of a lecture hall and delivers content to students. Students take notes, raise their hands to ask occasional questions, and respond to questions posed by the educator when confident their responses will be well-received. The traditional educator typically plans the delivery of content as a highly structured presentation. Freire (1979) referred to this model of education as the "banking" concept. In this model students "are the depositories and the educator is the depositor" (Freire, 1979, p. 72). Highly knowledgeable and expert-level educators deliver information to students who are expected to store that information for later recall.

This pervasive model of education does not promote inquiry, invention, or creativity. Rather, it promotes student dependency on educators for information and knowledge. They passively accept information without critical questioning and do not have opportunities to create or contribute to furthering knowledge development. In this type of environment, students often feel stifled and hesitant to speak up in class, question content, explore alternative perspectives, or share personal narratives relative to the topic. Furthermore, some students fear being wrong or ridiculed in front of their peers, making the classroom an intimidating experience. This type of fear may result in a code of silence enacted consciously or subconsciously by individual students and often by an entire class of students.

In response to concerns with traditional educational models, educators are increasingly using discussion-based instructional methods as a way to actively engage students in course content. Devised in the 1930s for students at a private boarding school, the *Harkness method* is among the earliest documented methods of deliberate engagement of students in discussion as a primary teaching method. Later in the 1970s, educators developed the jigsaw classroom (see Chapter 8) as a cooperative learning strategy that embedded discussions among students into classroom routines. William Fawcett Hill published *Learning Through Discussion* in 1977 and further challenged educators to reconstruct classrooms to include student engagement with content through discussion. *Learning Through Discussion* includes detailed steps for leading discussions, defining group roles for participants and leaders, and emphasizing active listening skills. Additionally, *Learning Through Discussion* facilitates the breakdown of reading assignments by having students address challenging vocabulary, identifying an author's main points, and applying content to other literature and personal experiences. Students engage in preparatory steps for discussions, so they arrive at class prepared to share rich personal connections to the reading and their interpretations and reflections of course materials.

Contemporary authors advanced these ideas by expanding on the use of discussion as a way of teaching. Brookfield and Preskill (2005, 2016) offer comprehensive guides to discussion-based instructional methods. They provide variations of discussion formats that can be applied to differing types of course content and adjusted based on class size, maturity of participants, experience of educators, and diversity of the classroom. Brookfield and Preskill (2005) posit that discussion is intricately tied to democracy and assert that educators need to practice and model nine distinct dispositions when using discussion in classrooms (see Appendix A): (1) hospitality, (2) participation, (3) mindfulness, (4) humility, (5) mutuality, (6) deliberation, (7) appreciation, (8) hope, and (9) autonomy. Through these dispositions, students and educators can engage in democratic discourse where every voice is valued, heard, respected, challenged, and explored.

THEORY

More than with any other instructional method, educators can create transformative learning opportunities when implementing well-planned classroom discussions. Students experience transformation when they feel "a deep, structural shift in basic premises of thought, feelings, and actions. It is a shift of consciousness that dramatically and permanently alters our way of being in the world" (Transformative Learning Center, n.d., para. 3). Transformational learning theory posits that through immersion in the experiences and perspectives of others, students experience a fundamental shift in their perspectives and are changed forever. Once transformed, students do not regress to a less informed position. Their perspectives may continue to undergo further transformation through exposure to new challenges and information, but they remain forever changed by the transformational process.

When educators model and teach the dispositions of discussion, they give students the tools to engage in transformative dialogue. These tools are intentional listening, critically reflecting, and "giving and taking" during discussion. In *intentional listening*, the educator ensures all students have equal opportunity to engage in dialogue and have their perspectives and experiences fully heard. When students strain to hear and understand, ask follow-up questions, and focus their energy and attention to what is expressed, they become open to expanding, establishing, and/or reflecting on their own previously held viewpoints. The students' ability to understand and establish new perspectives serves as the foundation for transformational learning.

Transformational learning theory suggests that *critical reflection* occurs throughout the educational process. An educator creates classroom conditions that encourage all students to deeply examine the roots of their perspectives, interpretations, and preconceived ideas while juxtaposing those against the experiences and perspectives of classroom peers. Through the careful selection of external sources, such as books, lectures, and literature that spark student interest, curiosity, and questioning, educators prime students to be transformed through classroom discussion. Students who engage in active listening to peers and openly share their experiences build a foundation upon which they can begin the process of inward self-reflection. Individual students and classroom groups negotiate meaning in ways that affirm and challenge existing frames of reference.

Educators transform learners through discussion when they engage in *give-and-take* experiences in speaking, listening, questioning, and witnessing. Through this give-and-take relationship, a "collective wisdom emerges that would have been impossible for any of the participants to achieve on their own" (Brookfield & Preskill, 2005, p. 4). In discussion-based instructional methods, educators enter dialogue with students as coinvestigators of problems, issues, literature, scholarship, and experience. They facilitate the means and methods of discussion through their selection of reading material, design of discussion groups, and guidance and modeling of intentional listening and reflective questioning.

IMPLEMENTATION

Take a moment in the box below to answer the following questions. How did an educator engage you in discussion that revealed unexpected perspectives that left you questioning the complexity of a topic in a way that you never imagined? How did an educator help you realize what seemed quite simple before was actually far more complex than you understood? How did the narratives, interpretations, knowledge, and perspectives of others offer you new ways to consider an issue, event, topic, and/or conceptual idea?

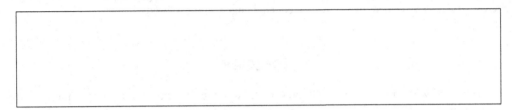

Effective educators create enlightening discussion moments, such as those you experienced in the box above. They spend time prior to class preparing to provide students with intriguing reading material, critical questions, complex problems, or case studies to contemplate and dissect with peers.

Before moving forward, we want to highlight that discussion in the classroom is not intended to replace all traditional methods of instruction. Educators will be most effective with discussion-based instructional methods when strategically blended with other instructional methods. Educators who are thoughtful in considering the nature of the content their students are examining will empower them to voice their perspectives, ask questions, and develop the classroom into a community. It is through discussion that educators can encourage students to engage in critical dialogue, informed questioning, and intentional listening—skills that will profoundly impact their ability to communicate in their professional practice.

Preparing for Discussion

In order to implement an effective discussion, educators begin with clearly defined learning objectives that address course content. Educators consider the nature of content to set the stage for the type of arrangements that will work best during the discussion. For example, if the purpose of discussion is to expand students' perspectives of social issues, then an educator might invite their individual experiences and personal interpretations of others' behaviors into a classroom dialogue. As the educator, your discussion preparation will need to account for individual challenges, personal narratives, and potentially contentious debate and deliberation among students about the meaning of social behaviors and personal experiences.

> Avoid assigning work that polices compliance with reading and other homework.

The educator's role is to set the stage for the topics, problems, issues, and concepts the students will explore during the class or course. Educators can foster a richer discussion and stay within the bounds of the learning objectives by creating a written assignment to hold the students accountable to outside readings. For example, you may pose a series of reflective questions that require students to interpret an author's intent. Remember, it is important that the educator does not assign questions that prompt students to simply skim the reading to quickly find and record answers to questions (e.g., low-level surface learning). Educators invite students to deeply engage with assigned content by asking them to compare, synthesize, and critique the literature (e.g., high-level deep learning). An example of this deeper learning includes asking students to compare the assigned reading to other course materials, associate the author's perspective to a perspective commonly expressed by people they know, or apply the author's message to personal experiences and/or case study scenarios. Educators assign preparatory learning activities for the primary purpose of creating opportunities for students to think critically about topics, connect personally with course content, and expand or challenge their previously held views.

One example of a preparatory worksheet is the *Talking Points* assignment (see Appendix B). Students complete the *Talking Points* worksheet as they are reading or shortly after they finish reading. At the top of the worksheet, students list the reference for the reading, any vocabulary words that were new to them (and their meaning), and a general statement of the author's message. They also learn about the author and gain a basic understanding of the author's experience and position regarding the course concepts. Students complete the two columns below the introductory information. In the left column, students cite three aha moments, take-away messages, or quotes that jumped out at them in the reading. They may include a direct quote or may paraphrase the author's point. We suggest you encourage students to include a page number in this column so they can direct peers to the quote or information during discussion. You and other students in the course gain a broader context for the text the students found interesting or meaningful.

In the right column, students write a personal connection that corresponds to each main point in the left column. They may include an experience they had, story they heard, previous view they held, their own internal contradictions with the material, or connections to other course work. The students bring the completed *Talking Points* worksheet to class in hard copy format. During small group discussion, each student shares their "talking points" and together they negotiate the meaning of the assigned reading. At the bottom of the worksheet, each student completes a handwritten summary of the discussion about what they learned, how they may think differently about the topic, or how their views changed or were challenged. This assignment typically enlightens students on what others found intriguing in the reading, how others relate to the topic on a personal level, and how the information connects to other scholarship.

Whether you use the *Talking Points* example offered in this chapter or another tool to prepare students for discussions, it is important to note that students often desire structure from educators to help focus their reading efforts. West (2018) found that students indicated a preference for preparatory work associated with reading assignments and were more likely to engage in classroom dialogue when they were held accountable for the reading material. West (2018) also relays that with the employment of preparatory assignments, "opening silence is now rare. I often hear students discussing the readings as they enter the classroom" (p. 152). We recommend that you use a tool that helps students connect with the material and requires them to think critically about the reading prior to the start of class.

Establishing Public Agreements

Educators have a responsibility to create an environment where students experience openness to sharing personal stories as well as their views and interpretations of course content (refer to Chapter 3). We recommend educators lead students in publicly establishing communication norms and expectations. These norms are referred to as *public agreements*. Public agreements are useful for various reasons:

- There is potential for some discussions to become contentious.
- Some students dominate conversations.
- Some students deliberately retreat from conversation.
- The power dynamics skew in favor of the more extroverted and confident students.

Some examples of public agreements include not interrupting a peer who is expressing a challenging position, not engaging in talk about peers' comments outside of the classroom setting, and showing respect for each student's right to hold differing positions on a topic. We recommend you encourage students to invoke established public agreements as a tool to address violations of civil discourse both inside and outside of the classroom. If necessary, you can have the class revisit and revise public agreements to ensure all students have opportunities to listen, share, and learn from the classroom community.

To initiate establishment of public agreements, it will be important for educators to explain the extent to which they will use discussion as a teaching and learning tool throughout the course. Beginning with turn-and-talk, you can offer a sentence completion prompt that students in close proximity to each other work on collaboratively. The following are examples of sentence prompts that educators can use to jumpstart discussion around public agreements:

- I learn best when . . .
- I shut down when . . .
- Speaking up is difficult when . . .
- From my instructor, I need . . .
- From my classmates, I need . . .

After small student groups respond to these prompts, the educator leads a large group discussion to find themes and commonalities that the entire class agrees are important. The large group discussion can be as simple as a verbal sharing by one student of each small group, having each group write their responses on a poster for a gallery walk, having one student summarize responses on a classroom white board, or having one student of each group write their responses in a shared document that is displayed in real time during class. In conjunction with the students, educators facilitate the discovery of major themes and commonalities among the responses and create statements of agreed participation behaviors that are displayed during each subsequent class period. The class should revisit their participation statements throughout the course and revise or add as they see fit. However, we recommend the number of public agreements be kept to 10 or fewer and not be delivered as "rules" but rather as agreements among all students of the class. By posting the agreements and reviewing before each discussion, educators create a classroom culture where students check each other's behavior, reframe questions, revise personal statements, and learn the basic dispositions of civil discourse.

Modeling Civil Discourse

To effectively facilitate fruitful discussion, educators need to model the behaviors they want their students to develop and create a climate that promotes community, democracy, and investment in learning. Of particular importance is for the educator to model appropriate ways to "call out" students when group agreements are broken and to demonstrate grace and professionalism in accepting feedback about their own missteps during discussion.

During discussions, educators implement effective strategies in the use of silence and plan time for reflection when students' sensibilities are at risk and intentional listening and productive discourse become endangered. When using silence as a deliberate strategy for reflection, educators and students can respond to each other by making statements, such as, "I need to think about that a minute" (Brookfield & Preskill, 2005, p. 46). When an individual shares a controversial or complex perspective, educators can ask their students to "sit with that" for a moment. We recommend providing students 1 to 5 minutes of silent reflection. In longer reflective silence periods, the educator has the opportunity to ask students to journal their thoughts, write down clarifying questions, relate a personal narrative to the discussion issue, and take note of additional information or context they need to better understand the discussed content. Educators who use silence will help their learners "learn that silence does not represent a vacuum in discussion" (Brookfield & Preskill, 2005, p. 46) but rather an opportunity to expand and explore new ideas.

In addition to learning to use silence as an active classroom discussion and reflection strategy, educators also need to be comfortable displaying and teaching active-listening skills. Students need to understand active listening goes beyond the well-known practice of parroting what others said to demonstrate the listening party heard and can repeat a message back. A student truly engaged

TABLE 9-1

Inner Chatter Thought Processes

1. Comparing ourselves to others
2. Second-guessing what others are saying
3. Rehearsing our responses to others
4. Judging and labeling people negatively
5. Adopting what others say
6. Focusing on advice giving
7. Placating others with insincere agreement and niceties

in deep active listening develops a bona fide understanding of the speaker's message regardless of whether the listener agrees or disagrees with the message. Active listeners show a sincere interest in developing understanding of viewpoints that challenge their own views and represent a departure from their longheld beliefs. They may not reach agreement and change their own positions through active listening, but they will better understand another person's position and personal experiences.

Another way to engage students in active listening is to help them recognize the need to "suspend one's inner chatter" while others are sharing experiences and perspectives (Palmer, 1998, p. 135). The *Learning Through Discussion* model suggests seven "inner chatter" thought processes that interfere with active listening skills (Table 9-1). Educators can remind students of these invasive thought processes prior to engaging in discussion by verbally stating a reminder at the start of a discussion, posting a list in the room, or having the seven types of inner chatter available as a tabletop handout.

We also recommend you give your students tools for responding to peers. Brookfield and Preskill (2005) pose seven types of questions that can be instrumental in deepening discussions and building understanding. We list the seven types of questions with examples in Table 9-2. Although Brookfield and Preskill (2005) suggest educators lead these types of questions, students can also ask each other these types of questions. Educators can also be deliberate about naming the type of questions they ask, so the students learn to frame questions in a nonoffensive manner and open questions by stating the type. For example, in response to a peer, a student can state, "I would like to ask for more evidence for your statement about the effectiveness of home programs. Where did you learn that?"

Another communicative behavior educators model and teach is the use of "I" statements in place of "you" statements. According to Kegan and Lahey (2001), "you statements provoke defensiveness; I statements characterize the speaker's experience and not the listener" (p. 100). For example, in a discussion with opposing and complex viewpoints, a student who responds to a peer with a statement such as, "You're not listening to what I'm saying, and you just don't get it," makes an accusatory statement that negatively characterizes the peer. The student hearing this statement is likely to become defensive and may try to repair in the face of public criticism. If the responding student's comment is reframed to characterize a personal experience with what has been expressed, it would sound more like the following statement, "I don't feel what I have expressed here is fully understood. When I heard the comment that I am playing the 'race' card, I felt frustrated and offended." This type of reframing is less likely to provoke the offending student into a defensive and self-protective response. Rather than being accusatory, the student speaking is offering personal feelings and experience with the dialogue. Using "I" statements to characterize one's feelings, interpretations, and experiences during a discussion maintains civility by being nonaccusatory and nonattributive toward peers.

TABLE 9-2

Seven Types of Questions for Discussion

TYPE OF QUESTION	EXAMPLES
1. Ask for more evidence	"I heard you say that parents of children with disabilities have higher rates of divorce than parents of typically developing children. I am curious about the source of that statement. Can you talk more about where you learned that?"
2. Ask for clarification	"I'm not sure I understood the point you made about use of family members as interpreters. I need clarification on why it is not a good practice to ask English-speaking family members to interpret for non-English speakers during an occupational therapy visit."
3. Ask open-ended questions	"That was a really interesting point. Can you tell me more about that experience? Can you share how you responded and what happened to the patient?"
4. Request a link to other content or previous discussions	"How do you think these research findings about opioid addiction in this population relates to the health disparities research we discussed last week? Do you see any connections?"
5. Ask for a hypothetical scenario to illustrate a point	"So, let's just say, for example, your patient does not receive funding for the power chair. What would be your next steps in helping meet her community mobility needs?"
6. Ask a cause and effect question	"What might be the consequences of implementing a falls prevention program in a senior living center? What do you anticipate will be the outcome?"
7. Ask for a summary or synthesis	"We have unpacked a lot of information today on health disparities. Take 5 minutes to synthesize what you learned about who is impacted by disparities, sources, or causes of disparities, and steps you can take to change health outcomes for those negatively impacted."

Take a moment to consider how you, as an educator, can model the use of "I" statements. Look at the first two "you" statements in the left column of Table 9-3. Note how the comments are changed to "I" statements in the right column; even positive comments have potential to convert to "I" statements. You can convey more clarity to students about the impact of their classroom contributions by using "I" statements. Try changing the last two statements yourself. Remember to think about how the behavior or situation impacts you, and center that impact and your feelings in the "I" statement.

Organizing Discussion Groups

When organizing discussion groups, educators have myriad options and should consider course content, class size, maturity of the students, extent to which the subject matter is provocative, and range of diversity of the students. Also keep in mind, student engagement in large group discussion is often enhanced by first creating small group discussions. Students in studies by both Ozment

TABLE 9-3

Converting "You" Statements to "I" Statements

"YOU" STATEMENT	"I" STATEMENT
"Please put your phone away during discussion. You are distracting the class and missing important information."	"I am finding it challenging to lead the class when it is unclear to me if everyone is receiving all of the information. I will be assured of your full attention if I know your phones are not in use during class."
"You did a nice job stating your point."	"I appreciate the depth and breadth of your responses. It was easy for me to follow your commentary, and I feel like I really understand your perspectives."
"You are cutting me off and interrupting class."	
"You must not have understood the authors' point in this reading assignment."	

(2018) and Benton (2016) appreciated small group discussions. Benton (2016) found students were able to offer views and interpretations several times on a given topic in small groups. Both authors found students benefitted from deepening relationships with peers and were able to find clarity of the content during small group discussions. We provide a few strategies we recommend for classroom discussion arrangements.

Peer-to-Peer

Evidence suggests the use of rigid classroom seating with students in traditional rows is the least effective arrangement for engagement; however, some educators face this type of classroom. In this situation, educators can structure peer-to-peer chats during class as a way to create active participation in the teaching and learning process. When using peer-to-peer discussions, students arrange in small groups with peers in close proximity. Typically, two to four students can comfortably engage in discussion when situated in fixed row seating (e.g., turn-and-talk or think-pair-share). Educators begin peer-to-peer chats by posing a question, problem, or issue for students to discuss. Students turn where they are seated and engage in discourse with their neighbors. In this arrangement, they are more likely to ask questions of each other than they are to ask the educator during the prompted "question" time. Peers may affirm with each other the presented information is confusing or they may offer their perspectives and interpretations for further clarification. If peers affirm confusion, students are more likely to collectively ask the educator for clarification during whole group questioning opportunities. Peer-to-peer chats often reduce intimidation for quieter and less confident students related to speaking and asking questions in front of an entire class. Following structured peer-to-peer chats, educators can ask students to "share out" with the class their significant questions, concerns, or perspectives related to the content. They can use this instructional method for building conceptual knowledge as well as for problem solving and developing rote and technical knowledge and skills.

Figure 9-2. Students engage in a discussion in a circle seating format.

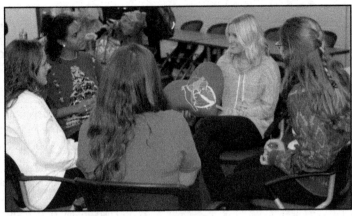

Circle and Cluster Seating

Circle and cluster seating arrangements work well when classrooms are flexible and chairs can be arranged in either large circles (20 to 24 students), medium circles (10 to 12 students), or small circles (four to six students). In these arrangements, students face one another so they are able to see who is speaking and observe the body language and active listening during the discussion. We recommend several strategies to assist in the management of student participation and speaking time. One strategy is to simply ask the students to use an object to pass or toss from one person to the next when contributing to the discussion (Figure 9-2). In addition, the educator can provide each student with a designated number of discussion chips (two to four per student). The educator sets an expectation that every student uses a minimum number of chips (at least one) for each discussion. These strategies assist the educator to even out participation among the more eager-to-speak students and those who are less inclined to speak up during class.

Another strategy for distributing discussion among students is the *three-person rule* (Brookfield & Preskill, 2016, p. 233). Educators use the public agreement process or simply create a discussion rule such that once a student asks a question or offers a perspective or idea, they wait for at least three other students to contribute before they make another contribution. You can ask students to take turns serving as the discussion moderator to help track responses using the three-person rule or you can expect individual students to track their own place in the response sequence.

One final effective strategy educators use to teach students to be active listeners is *timed talking*. In timed talks, the educator gives each student in the group a designated time frame (2 to 3 minutes) to share their perspectives, ideas, or talking points without interruption. They remind listeners to be mindful of body language and nonverbal messaging while another student is speaking. While a student is speaking, the listeners jot down questions that come to mind during the discussion. If a student finishes before the allotted time, listeners silently reflect for the remaining time. As noted previously, you should honor silent reflection and give students options to write notes, as this will serve as beneficial learning time versus a speaking gap that needs to be filled.

In circle and cluster discussions, students should continue to frame their questions using Brookfield and Preskill's (2005) seven question types (see Table 9-2). Educators allow question and reflection time once each student in the group has had a timed speaking turn. In this part of the discussion, educators create open question and response discussion or structure, so each student asks at least one question of a peer. If students are fully engaged and actively listening, they will likely have more questions than time permits. In that case, educators can use a follow-up assignment to deliver the remaining questions to each student, such as handwritten sticky notes, a journal passed among students, or a community white board where everyone can see the questions. Students can individually reflect upon the remaining questions between course meeting times and before optional in-class sharing out time. They can also respond to peer questions by turning in written responses as an assignment, posting responses on a discussion board, or adding their responses and reflections to a cumulative course journal.

Another discussion method educators can include to obtain a variety of perspectives in the learning process is *snowballing* (Brookfield & Preskill, 2016, p. 49). As a snowball rolls down a hill, it increases in size. In a discussion group, educators pose a question, idea, problem, or issue and ask students to silently reflect and write down their initial thoughts. Individual students turn to a peer and share reflections and find common ground or sources of disagreement. Each pair of students finds another pair with whom they continue to seek mutual understanding, points of disagreement, share confusion, and discuss other relevant reflections. The educator continues this process until all students are engaged in one large conversation or until the conversation snowballs to an effective group size. Brookfield and Preskill (2016) state they have found snowballing to be effective for groups as large as 65 with each student involved in the final discussion.

ADDITIONAL DISCUSSION-BASED INSTRUCTIONAL METHODS

High-Impact Quotes

Educators can select high-impact quotes for students to dissect and interpret as a way to help them build deeper understanding of conceptual knowledge. When left to read philosophical and theoretical work by themselves, students may find a quote to be obscure and difficult to interpret. However, when deconstructed as a small group, students are better able to derive meaning from a complex expression of ideas. For example, the following quote pertaining to the concept of identity as a social construct can be confusing and wordy for students on their own: "The structure by which that person identifies and becomes identified with a set of social narratives, ideas, myths, values and types of knowledge of varying reliability, usefulness, and verifiability" (Siebers, 2011, p. 15). When students break down this quote into manageable chunks and share their collective knowledge of socially constructed identities, they leave with a deeper understanding of the concept than if the educator had explained the quote or had left each student to their own interpretation. This type of discussion activity builds critical-thinking skills in the analysis of scholarly literature.

Multiple-Choice Debate

An additional method for active group discussion and lively debate is for educators to create multiple-choice format questions for students to respond to either individually or in small groups (four to six students). The educator begins by displaying the multiple-choice questions on a screen and posting the letters A, B, C, D, and E around the classroom. They ask students to stand next to the letter that represents their response to the question. With students lined up by the letter of their response, those in each group will discuss why they selected the response they did (Figure 9-3). In large classes, one student from a small group can represent the response of all the small group members. Other students can publicly defend the response question or comment from other groups. If a group gives a compelling argument for their response, students in other positions can change their response and move to the letter that matches their new response. They continue in discussion until all students agree on one **best** response or the educator decides to share the **best** answer. This type of activity not only helps students grasp content, but it also gives them opportunity to practice critical-thinking and problem-solving skills for test taking. It is important for you to remind students to adhere to previously written public agreements or classroom norms in their discourse so

Figure 9-3. Students engage in a multiple-choice debate.

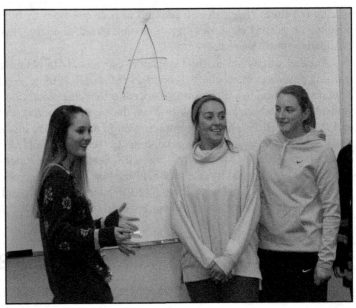

that positions can be clearly stated without interruption during these types of lively discussions. In addition, educators can structure the multiple-choice format for discussions using electronic polling apps or devices, such as clickers. Using this as an exam review offers a dynamic classroom experience in which students generally become quite animated.

ADDITIONAL IMPLEMENTATION NOTES

- Enhance discussions with practical case studies that require students to engage in cooperative group problem solving and shared critical thinking (see Chapter 12).

- Use discussion-based instructional methods for technical content, such as statistics, anatomy, kinesiology, and neurophysiology.

- Gain anonymous feedback at the end of a robust discussion by asking students to complete an "exit ticket"—this can identify themes that can be addressed during the next class.

Exit Ticket
Provide a notecard to students in which they share an aha moment, ask a clarifying question, identify concerns they have, or offer a closing remark about the class.

TIPS AND TRICKS

- Refrain from describing the classroom as a "safe space," as this implies a level of confidentiality you cannot promise individual students; state your own commitment to respecting the privacy of what is shared during discussions, but avoid making promises about the behavior of other students as they leave the classroom.

- Be aware of students' propensity to make eye contact as they share their responses with you as the educator. You may have to remove yourself from discussion circles, so students speak to each other rather than to you.

- Attempt to avoid the pitfall of responding to every student comment or statement. It is preferred to have students engage in discussion with each other without the power dynamic of an expert educator moderating their dialogue.

- Remain on the periphery of discussions and take silent notes without physically or verbally entering discussion groups as much as possible; step in as needed.
- Be prepared to offer your students opportunities to "touch base" with you in between discussions. They may feel the need to share their personal experiences with you after reflecting on the classroom discussion.
- Plan to provide one-to-one feedback to a student who, despite public agreements and "rules" for turn taking, does not demonstrate the dispositions of discussion that align with civility and respect for all students.

OPPORTUNITIES FOR FEEDBACK AND REFLECTION

It is important for educators to afford students opportunities to receive feedback from multiple sources. They need feedback about their contribution to and engagement in the discussion. Educators can create a quick peer feedback form that students share after a discussion. This can be in the form of a small notecard with prompts, such as:

- I really appreciated when you . . .
- From your contribution, I learned . . .
- One thing I can offer you for consideration when contributing to our classroom discourse is . . .

You may want to collect these feedback cards from students in subsequent classes so that you can provide them with tips and strategies for how they provide feedback to each other. Remember your ability to model and help students state comments that are productive and useful is important. Students may have a tendency to only provide positive comments or to be overly harsh with their criticism. In some discussion groups, you may elect to offer a point value for the feedback they provide each other to make sure they respect the process as a serious part of their learning.

It is most valuable to ask students to use feedback cards for the first few discussion groups or for some of the discussion topics that you anticipate being emotional or challenging. We recommend that you not expect every student to provide feedback to every peer. Receiving feedback from more than three to five peers may be overwhelming for students. Likewise, the more feedback cards an individual student is expected to complete, the less likely they are to offer thoughtful comments. It is reasonable for you to ask each student to provide feedback for three to five peers per class period. In addition, you can ask individual students to reflect on the cumulative feedback they receive and respond to that feedback. You facilitate a reflective practice that will assist in the development of dispositions of civil and democratic discourse when you ask students how they contribute to the classroom community.

Educators can also develop feedback cards to give to individual students following a class discussion. Focusing on a small number of students each class period will help you provide thoughtful and reflective individualized feedback. Consider listing three dispositions per feedback card. Give students feedback about discussion dispositions they employ well and those you would like them to focus on developing further.

APPLICATION TO OCCUPATIONAL THERAPY PRACTICE

Occupational therapy practitioners engage in discussions with their clients and families on a regular basis in all areas of practice. We can apply the concepts of public agreement, civil discourse, active listening, and discussion format in practical settings with individuals, families, groups, or populations. In addition, we can use the basic tenets of discussion when working with professional teams. In both formal and informal discussions, professional communication possesses the potential to become contentious and disordered if members are not able to engage with each other in a manner that promotes open sharing and intentional listening. We share two examples from professional practice to provide you with ideas about how to apply these discussion techniques to your practice setting.

Example 1: Team Meeting

In a school setting, occupational therapists work with a team to develop Individualized Education Plans (IEPs) for children with disabilities. In this process, team members potentially engage in an emotional experience fraught with varying opinions, perspectives, and ideas. Team members can be deliberate about modeling and using basic tenets of civil discourse to ensure the discussion around the strengths and needs of a child are positive and productive. Occupational therapists can model active listening during the most important and possibly most challenging aspects of highly contentious meetings. You can prepare yourself and your team members for an IEP meeting by reviewing the strategies for suspending inner chatter to ensure everyone is more available to fully hear every perspective. You can practice and perform responses by using "I" statements instead of "you" and other accusatory or defensive type of statements. Lastly, during meetings, you can ask specific questions for clarity and depth rather than challenging team members' positions and/or statements. These discussion practices have the power to increase the civility of discourse during challenging IEP meetings.

Example 2: Strategic Planning

A second example of employing discussion strategies in professional practice is the creation of public agreements among colleagues for participation in meetings that you and others agree have the potential to stir conflict and discomfort. For example, strategic planning meetings often include team members working through some variation of a strengths, weaknesses, opportunities, and threats analysis. Team members can establish public agreements prior to strategic planning meetings as a good preparatory activity to ensure civil discourse. Instead of the preparatory education-based exercise stated previously, you would want to ask colleagues to complete the following statements:

- I contribute most when . . .
- I shut down when . . .
- Speaking up is difficult when . . .
- From the team leader, I need . . .
- From my colleagues, I need . . .

Once the group establishes public agreements, you can employ turn-taking strategies for managing the flow of discussion. The three-person rule is one such strategy that could work well in a large group. If the group is managing a large or complex task, they can use the rotation option to divide and conquer the important issues. This strategy creates a more efficient and engaged team. Teams can also employ reflective silence, active listening strategies, use of questions as responses to colleagues, and employment of "I" statements during meetings to create civility, ensure democracy of voice, and be productive.

Advantages

- Students engage with course content in preparatory activities
- Most students feel compelled to prepare for class by completing reading assignments ahead of discussions
- Students can share their perspectives and hear the perspectives of others during discussions
- More students can actively learn
- Students gain experience in important professional soft skills, such as active listening
- Students experience transformation of learning
- Students co-construct knowledge with peers
- Educators emphasize personal experience and relationship to the course content in discussions

Challenges

- Students may not feel that discussion is a productive way to learn
- Educators may feel less opportunities to deliver specific content
- Some students may need more guidance than others with civility during discourse
- Some students may need emotional or psychosocial support during or after discussions
- Educators must closely monitor to ensure students uphold public agreements
- Educators need to gain skills in modeling discussion techniques

In the space below, list any additional advantages or challenges.

Brainstorm strategies for overcoming these challenges when implementing the use of discussion-based instructional methods.

THREE THINGS YOU CAN DO TOMORROW TO IMPLEMENT DISCUSSION-BASED INSTRUCTIONAL METHODS WITH YOUR STUDENTS

1. Look for natural breaks in the content where you can employ peer-to-peer chats.
2. Initiate use of the *Talking Points* worksheet for reading assignments.
3. Have *The Discussion Book: 50 Great Ways to Get People Talking* (2016) by Brookfield and Preskill available as a classroom resource.

REFERENCES

Benton, R, Jr. (2016). Put students in charge: A variation on the jigsaw discussion. *College Teaching, 64*(1), 40-45. http://dx.doi.org/10.1080/87567555.2015.1069725

Brookfield, S. D., & Preskill, S. (2005). *Discussion as a way of teaching: Tools and techniques for democratic classrooms* (2nd ed.). Jossey-Bass Inc.

Brookfield, S. D., & Preskill, S. (2016). *The discussion book: 50 great ways to get people talking.* Jossey-Bass Inc.

Freire, P. (1979). *Pedagogy of the oppressed. 50th anniversary edition* [2018]. Bloomsbury Academic.

Kegan, R., & Lahey, L. L. (2001). *How the way we talk can change the way we work: Seven languages for transformation.* Jossey-Bass Inc.

Ozment, E. W. (2018). Embracing vulnerability and risk in the classroom: The four-folder approach to discussion-based community learning. *Journal of the Scholarship of Teaching and Learning, 18*(2). 136-157. http://dx.doi.org/10.14434/josotl.v18i2.22448

Palmer, P. J. (1998). *The courage to teach: Exploring the inner landscape of a teacher's life.* Jossey-Bass Inc.

Siebers, T. (2011). *Disability theory.* University of Michigan.

Transformative Learning Center. (n.d.). Ontario Institute of Studies in Education of the University of Toronto (OISE/UT). https://legacy.oise.utoronto.ca/research/tlcentre/about.html

West, J. (2018). Raising the quality of discussion by scaffolding students' reading. *International Journal of Teaching and Learning in Higher Education, 30*(1), 146-160.

BIBLIOGRAPHY

Aronson, E., Blaney, N., Stephan, C., Sikes, J., & Snapp, M. (1978). *The jigsaw classroom.* SAGE Publications.

Kitchenham, A. (2008). The evolution of John Mezirow's transformative learning theory. *Journal of Transformative Education, 6*(2), 104-123. http://dx.doi.org/10.1177/1541344608322678

Merriam, S. B., & Bierema, L. L. (2014). *Adult learning: Linking theory and practice.* Jossey-Bass Inc.

Mezirow, J. (1997). Transformative learning: Theory to practice. *New Directions for Adult a Continuing Education, 74,* 5-12. John Wiley & Sons. http://dx.doi.org/10.1002/ace.7401

Rabow, J., Charness, M. A., Kipperman, J., & Radcliffe-Vasile, S. (2000). *William Fawcett Hill's learning through discussion* (3rd ed.). SAGE Publications.

Saputra, M. D., Joyoatmojo, S., Wardabum D. K., & Sangka, K. B. (2019). Developing critical-thinking skills through the collaboration of jigsaw model with problem-based learning model. *International Journal of Instruction, 12*(1), 1077-1094.

Smith, L. A., & Foley, M. (2009). Partners in a human enterprise: Harkness teaching in the history classroom. *The History Teacher, 42*(4), 477-496.

APPENDIX A

DISPOSITIONS OF DEMOCRATIC DISCUSSION

HOSPITALITY	Hospitality is demonstrated through mutual receptivity and respect among group members. Hospitality creates conditions for active participation, risk taking, and individual revelations of personal beliefs and perspectives.
PARTICIPATION	Participation is facilitated when conditions exist for all voices to be heard. This requires deliberate planning and strategizing of discussion arrangements. Group agreements regarding civility in discourse, turn-taking, and reflective responses to group members will set the stage for participation.
MINDFULNESS	Mindfulness is paying attention to and being aware of the whole conversation. Mindfulness requires intentional listening and questioning for understanding and clarity.
HUMILITY	Humility is being able to accept the limitations of one's own perspectives, experiences, and positions. Deep understanding of the value of others' positions and experiences as a point of learning about ourselves.
MUTUALITY	Mutuality is the genuine caring about the development of others' learning as one's own.
DELIBERATION	Deliberation is bringing evidence, data, and logic to the discussion from which to offer points and counterpoints for discussion. Entering discussion with willingness to be changed by the positions and information presented by others.
APPRECIATION	Appreciation is the expression of gratitude toward others. It is being appreciative toward the positions and experiences individuals are willing to share with the group.
HOPE	Hope is the deep sense that the effort toward problem solving, discussion, and building understanding is worth the effort and can make a difference.
AUTONOMY	Autonomy is the ability to stand for one's beliefs but also to be willing to have those beliefs challenged and evaluated by others.

Adapted from Brookfield, S. D., & Preskill, S. (2005). *Discussion as a way of teaching: Tools and techniques for democratic classrooms* (2nd ed.). Jossey-Bass Inc.

APPENDIX B

TALKING POINTS WORKSHEET

The purpose of this assignment is to increase your engagement with specific topics and to integrate concepts learned in the reading assignments with personal experiences and belief patterns. Sharing in class and discussing with peers will further enhance understanding of the reading and help each student ask and answer questions as well as clarify issues pertaining to the topic of the assigned reading.

Assignment Objective

Upon completion of this assignment you will have a deeper understanding of the assigned reading topic and be able to engage in personal and scholarly discussion of the information presented in the reading.

Instructions

Prior to in-class discussions, each student must complete the table below electronically and bring a printed copy to class. In the left column, summarize or quote material from the reading that is of particular interest to you. In the right column, state how you relate to the material (prior knowledge or beliefs). This column is meant to share how you process the reading and should be in short narrative forms with examples as needed to clarify your thoughts. Following class discussion, you will handwrite a summary at the bottom of the page stating how the discussion enhanced your understanding of the reading material. Turn in the assignment to the instructor before leaving class.

STUDENT NAME:	
TITLE OF READING ASSIGNMENT:	
BACKGROUND INFORMATION OF THE AUTHOR:	
OVERALL MESSAGE/INTENT OF AUTHOR:	
CHALLENGING VOCABULARY:	
List at least three take-away messages, aha moments, or new questions based on the reading. Include a passage, quote, and page number for each item to facilitate in-class discussion. Each article must have at least one take-away message or question.	*How does this relate to you, to your prior knowledge, your prior experiences, or your beliefs about the topic?*

10

INQUIRY-BASED INSTRUCTIONAL METHODS

Whitney Henderson, OTD, MOT, OTR/L

BASIC TENETS

As occupational therapy educators, we understand various challenges to practice, such as the lack of one simple solution or clear-cut answer and the need to frequently engage in professional dialogue. As future practitioners, our students must be able to communicate with policy makers, payers, managers and leaders, professional organizations, and other health care professionals. Our students will face challenges and conflicts in various environments and will need to articulate the value of our services at a societal and client level. Therefore, they require practice in addressing issues in a brief yet effective manner, articulating decisions based on evidence over personal opinions, developing well-reasoned and fluent arguments, and hearing the viewpoints of others with unprejudiced reasoning. When we use inquiry-based instructional methods in our courses, students gain experience with these important skills necessary for a successful professional practice.

Inquiry-based methods of instruction go beyond traditional discussion to promote personal and professional development at numerous levels. Scholars most widely cite the benefit of developing students' critical-thinking skills when implementing these instructional methods. However, health professional education literature provides several additional benefits relevant to the transition to professional practice, such as:

- Providing opportunities to complete a deeper analysis of topics
- Encouraging numerous points of view before arriving at a judgment or decision
- Thinking on their feet
- Taking responsibility for their own learning
- Appraising evidence and arguments
- Enhancing written and oral communication skills by determining what to say and how to say it
- Gaining confidence in their explanations and maintaining composure in front of others

Henderson, W. (Ed.). *Effective Teaching: Instructional Methods and Strategies for Occupational Therapy Education* (pp. 235-264).
© 2021 Taylor & Francis Group.

- Understanding the art of persuasion
- Developing teamwork skills
- Developing an appreciation for the complexity of practice
- Affording opportunities to apply information to changing or new situations

In this chapter, we will discuss the inquiry-based instructional methods of the Socratic method and debate.

Socratic Method

Additional Names in Literature:
Socratic instruction,
Socratic questioning,
Socratic techniques,
Socratic teaching,
Socratic disputation,
Socratic education,
Socratic practices,
Socratic framework

For centuries, educators have asked their students questions to facilitate learning. We use questions in various learning contexts for a variety of reasons, such as stimulating recall of previous knowledge, promoting comprehension of material, determining level of understanding, and building critical-thinking skills. The *Socratic method* is one instructional method educators can use to facilitate a deep discussion. Educational literature does not provide a generally accepted definition of this method. The most consistent definition of the Socratic method is when an educator poses a systematic series of pointed questions that challenge students' assumptions and beliefs, expose any contradictions, and generate new knowledge. Educators do not provide instruction or sway their students to a certain answer but instead test and examine the students' beliefs in order to create curiosity. There are a variety of terms used after the word Socratic to designate different aspects of this general approach. The most common terms are Socratic method, Socratic instruction, or Socratic questioning.

In the Socratic method, educators use open-ended questions to uncover the beliefs or knowledge students already possess or to identify current knowledge gaps. The students provide answers to questions that expose their perceptions and comprehension and their experiences with and attitudes about the content. Educators further ask questions to stimulate discourse, evoke doubt, or challenge assumptions and knowledge. These questions become increasingly difficult, but **do not surpass** the students' developmental level (e.g., the just-right challenge). When questions are posed properly, students are often inspired to expand on their own knowledge, take conversations to a deeper level, and have opportunities to consider others' viewpoints. They engage in an ongoing process of reflection, regulation, and refinement of their own thought processes. Educators employ this method to stimulate students' critical thinking and to build creative thought processes as they integrate and synthesize the course content.

You might be asking why the Socratic method is a good fit with occupational therapy education (example in Figure 10-1). As educators in occupational therapy, we must teach students to engage in lifelong inquiry of both existing and new knowledge of our profession. The Socratic method provides students with a framework to approach various questions in their professional practice. In this method of instruction, students develop the independent learning skills that are a cornerstone for being a successful health care professional. They begin to identify their own gaps in knowledge to further expand their knowledge. The clients, families, and communities we serve and the settings where we work are diverse and dynamic. When we implement the Socratic method, we encourage students to move beyond the textbook to further consider the impact of the various contexts. Students begin to recognize and evaluate issues from a broad range of perspectives, identify all relevant pieces of information, and notice consistencies across diverse events. Through this method, they assimilate information they already possess with new knowledge in order to problem solve and make the best decision in a particular situation.

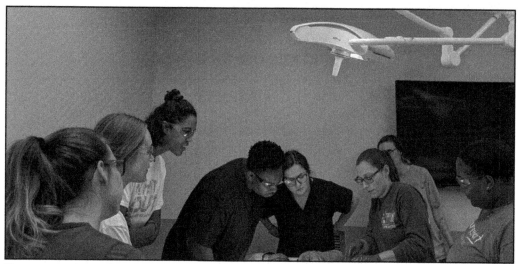

Figure 10-1. Educators implement the Socratic method with occupational therapy students during an applied anatomy lab.

Background of Socratic Method

What we know about this unique method of instruction dates more than 2,500 years ago. It is named after the creator, Socrates, who was a Greek philosopher and teacher in the 4th century B.C.E. Although considered the "father of Western philosophy," he did not record his beliefs about teaching and learning in written format. Much of what we have come to know about this method is credited to Plato, one of Socrates's proteges. Plato documented Socrates's beliefs about and reasons for this particular teaching practice. Since this time, the Socratic method has crossed temporal and geographical distances to influence our modern-day classrooms.

Socrates taught young Athenians to critically think by engaging them in thoughtful and deep discussion about relevant issues. He believed true knowledge resides within the student and the educator simply provides oversight, so they discover their own new realizations. Socrates was much more interested in developing his students' thought processes than conveying knowledge. Therefore, he asked them a series of important questions and required them to continuously test their answers against reason and fact in an honest debate. He would pose stimulating questions so his students could recognize their own misconceptions and further guide them to realize true knowledge via self-reflection.

Educators have implemented the Socratic method throughout history. Instructors in Germany, France, and Switzerland have referenced this method of instruction since the 16th century. However, scholars in the United States did not discuss the Socratic method in print until the mid-18th century. During this time frame, higher education employed traditional lecture and rote memorization. Because of increasing enrollment and mounting European literature, educators demonstrated interest in this instructional method. By the end of the Civil War, policy leaders and professors in education believed the Socratic method should be taught to future educators. Therefore, in the late 19th century, the Socratic method was widely mentioned in literature for K-12 education. By the early 20th century, departments and schools in higher education recognized the Socratic method as a highly relevant form of pedagogy, and it began appearing in various textbooks. In the literature, we recognize the most consistent use of this method in law and medical education. In medical programs, educators often use the Socratic method in the first 2 years of the program and on medical wards. However, there is a paucity of research with the use of this method in other health professional programs (see Inquiry-Based Instructional Method Evidence Table).

Table 10-1

Steps Students Use for a Debate

Students must:

- Define a problem
- Complete a comprehensive search for evidence and resources
- Appraise evidence to identify strengths and limitations
- Assess the credibility of various resources
- Develop a comprehensive understanding of the content
- Identify and challenge opposing assumptions with rebuttal evidence
- Recognize inconsistencies in resources and arguments
- Synthesize and prioritize pertinent and salient concepts
- Develop solutions to problems
- Examine, test, and refine their own beliefs
- Use effective communication, leadership, and teamwork skills

DEBATE

Educators have a long tradition with debate for a variety of topics in their classrooms. A *debate* is a structured process of discussion on a particular matter. Students actively take a position on an issue, provide opposing arguments and viewpoints grounded by theory and evidence, and attempt to convince others to agree. The observers of the debate actively listen, consider multiple viewpoints, ask questions, and can cast a vote at the end. When used as a method of instruction, we provide our students with immense opportunities to enhance relevant personal and professional skills and knowledge. In addition, our students usually demonstrate increased interest in and attention to course content when they participate in debate.

Take a moment and consider all the steps students must engage in to prepare for and perform well in a debate (Table 10-1). We can see the value of debate for fostering the complex and critical thinking required in educational and professional experiences.

Background

We can trace the use of debate as a teaching strategy to more than 4,000 years ago. Literature cites Protagoras in Athens as the "father of debate," but many Greek scholars and philosophers have perfected this form of rhetoric. Since 1823, Oxford University has established itself as a scholarly debating society due to a reputation for highly competitive debate teams. Many years later, McBurney (1952) published a chapter on the role of debate in a democratic society and suggested debate was an essential social tool to use when multiple solutions or no clear lines exist. Our political and legal systems and mainstream media have propagated the use of debates. Despite the long history, increased popularity, and use of the many beneficial steps and skills previously outlined, students on competitive university teams have traditionally been the only individuals regularly engaged in debate.

TABLE 10-2	
How Learning Internalizes Knowledge	
Stage 1	The student does not understand the educator and/or peers and requires explicit explanation and/or modeling.
Stage 2	The student has a limited understanding of the educator and/or peers, which encourages further discussion; requires regulation from the educator and/or peer.
Stage 3	The student has enough understanding to engage in coregulation of thoughts and understanding with the educator and/or peers.
Stage 4	The student internalizes information and self-regulates understanding and problem solving.

In literature, we note a rise in the use of debate as an instructional method. Educators in higher education settings use debate across numerous subjects, such as economics, engineering, psychology, sociology, history, math, and education. Similarly, health professional programs, such as dentistry, medicine, pharmacy, nursing, occupational therapy, and social work, are implementing this instructional method to teach their students complex and controversial topics in elective and professional development courses. However, our use of interprofessional debate remains scarce.

THEORY

One theory that can guide the use of inquiry-based instructional methods is Lev Vygotsky's dialectical constructivism, particularly the *zone of proximal development (ZPD)*. The ZPD is the difference between what the student can do independently and what the student can accomplish with support (e.g., the just-right challenge). In the ZPD, students work with educators or peers under guidance or in collaboration to successfully solve problems they could not solve on their own. Therefore, students **require** social interaction for cognitive change to occur in this zone. You can find this social interaction in the Socratic and debate methods of instruction.

Students bring a developmental history (e.g., experiences, values, beliefs, tools, skills) to the classroom (as discussed in Chapter 1). The educator provides the support structure for learning by facilitating reflection on experiences, assumptions, and beliefs. We see this structure by the way educators ask questions in the Socratic method and how the students must understand their own assumptions during the debate process. As the students interact with educators and peers, they share their histories. In these interactions, they are exposed to advanced systems of understanding, and learning becomes possible. The students experience cognitive changes and internalize interactions for future use and repeated application. As their internalization grows, they demonstrate the ability to use their knowledge and skills. Students internalize knowledge in four stages; three of these stages occur in the ZPD (Table 10-2).

In the ZPD, educators use instructional scaffolding to facilitate the performance needed for cognitive change. They provide students with selective assistance by asking them questions, directing their attention to a particular area, or offering them suggestions. Educators offer the most effective assistance when they tailor the assistance to the student. The educator gradually withdrawals the support as their students become more competent. As we discuss the implementation of the Socratic method later in this chapter, you will see how educators ask and scaffold their questions to achieve learning within the ZPD.

TABLE 10-3

Strategies for Creating a Psychologically Safe Environment

- Educate students that they can answer a question with "I don't know" without a consequence.
- Tell students there are several correct answers to a question, and if their answer does not match, it does not mean their answer was not right.

> Remember: Your behavior and demeanor greatly influence the student and environment.

- Communicate to students that they will not be punished for an incorrect answer.
- Allow students to ask questions or ask for assistance.
- Use "I" messages and avoid "you" messages, as these types of questions have the potential to create tension and halt conversation.
- "Might be…" or "I'm wondering…." statements demonstrate curiosity and show you do not have all the answers.
- Avoid interrupting a response.
- Maintain eye contact with the student that is providing the answer.
- Be mindful of your tone of verbal communication (e.g., avoid condescending or aggressive tones).
- Be mindful of your nonverbal communication, such as body language or facial expressions (e.g., avoid grimacing or crossed arms).
- Model openness.
- Correct or reprimand in a compassionate manner and provide clear explanations about shortcomings or misunderstandings.
- Reformat or abandon a question if you feel a sense of discomfort in the learning environment.

IMPLEMENTATION FOR SOCRATIC METHOD

Creating a Psychologically Safe Environment

Educational literature does not provide a manual or method for educators to systematically follow when implementing the Socratic method with their students. Despite this ambiguity, scholars frequently highlight the importance of fostering a psychologically safe learning environment. You are not employing the Socratic method by simply asking a series of questions. You must first cultivate a robust and synergistic environment to promote learning. Remember from Chapter 3, a student's emotional state affects their learning process. They need to feel safe to ask and answer thought-provoking questions and to share their thoughts and feelings within their community. **Safety equals learning**. Students feel safe when the educator creates a sense of trust, mutual respect, value, comfort, and support. In fact, when they feel psychologically safe, they often report feeling empowered to answer challenging questions. They also begin to appreciate the value of questions in guiding the expansion of their own knowledge. Please review Table 10-3 for a list of strategies for creating a psychologically safe environment.

Before moving forward, we want to make one important point. When fostering a psychologically safe environment, this does not mean you accept substandard performance. You should not ignore inadequate performance, overlook errors, or excuse a lack of effort. What makes the environment safe is your approach to identifying and correcting these issues, not your acceptance of these issues.

Take a moment to reflect on one of your memorable learning experiences as a student. Use the box below to write what the educator did that made you feel psychologically safe to explore the content. How can you include these additional strategies in your educational practices?

Asking Questions

In the Socratic method, you carefully construct a series of questions to create an exploratory conversation. You will not provide information directly to the students but instead use your thoughtfully designed questions to guide or lead them through the critical-thinking process. In order to use the Socratic method of instruction successfully, you will need to become skilled in asking the **right** questions to stimulate deep thinking to promote students' awareness and growth. In fact, educators asking the right questions is more important than students providing the right answers. Successful educators often consider their interactions with their students, understand where their students are developmentally, prepare a variety of questions, and anticipate their students' potential answers and spontaneous questions. When questions are poorly designed, students experience confusion and intimidation and reach limits in their ability to critically think.

> Be prepared for an "I don't know" answer during this phase.

In the Socratic questioning literature, you will notice two phases: the deconstructive phase and the constructive phase (Table 10-4). During the *deconstructive phase*, the educator asks demanding and difficult questions to challenge their students' beliefs. When the educator or peers challenge their beliefs, students become more prepared to think freely without feeling bound to their own ideas or assumptions. In this phase, the educator structures questions using two different mechanisms: the leading question and the evaluative components. The *leading question* is the most basic component and serves three purposes:

1. Focuses the students' attention to a specific area of content
2. Allows the educator to check their students' current level of knowledge
3. Affords the students opportunities to integrate a variety of resources

When asking leading questions, you do not want to request factual information but inquire in a way that **allows your learners to express their opinion**. After the leading question, you move to questions more *evaluative* in nature. You would want to word these questions in a way that **requires your students to evaluate, define, or abandon their point of view** (see Table 10-4). In this phase, remember there are no single correct answers, and the goal is not to determine the right answer as quickly as possible. Instead, the typical outcome of this phase is the students realizing how little they actually know or considered about the content.

TABLE 10-4

Phases of Socratic Method

PHASE	COMPONENT	EXAMPLE OF QUESTIONS
Deconstructive Phase	Leading	• In what ways does [topic] relate to our problem/discussion/issues? • How does [topic] relate to your future practice? • How does [topic] relate to what you saw in fieldwork? • What does [topic] mean to you? • What is [topic]? • How would you define the [topic]?
	Evaluative	• Is there another point of view we could approach [topic] with? • How does [XXX] relate or affect the [topic]? • What are potential conflicts with this [topic]? • Can you describe how you came to that belief? • What might change your mind?
Constructive Phase	Defense	• I am wondering how your definition fits with [different situation]? • How does this compare to [XXX]? • So [example of situation] means [related to student's definition]? • What evidence is there for [topic]? • Who might be in a position to know that information?
	Sequential Progression	• What changes could you make to your original definition? • What might be an alternative to [topic]? • If [XXX] and [XXX] are the case, what might also be true? • How can we find out? What other information do we need to formulate our response?
	Discontinuation	• What have you learned from this discussion? • If you were confronted with a similar problem next week, how would you approach it following this discussion? • Now that we have had this discussion, what do you think [topic] means?

Adapted from Overholser, J. C. (1991). The Socratic method as a technique in psychotherapy supervision. *Professional Psychology, Research, and Practice, 22*(1), 68-74; Oyler, D. R., & Romanelli, F. (2014). The fact of ignorance: Revisiting the Socratic method as a tool for teaching critical thinking. *American Journal of Pharmaceutical Education, 78*(7), Article 144; Toledo, C. A. (2015). Dog bite reflections—Socratic questioning revisited. *International Journal of Teaching and Learning in Higher Education, 27*(2), 275-279.

Following the deconstructive phase, the educator and students enter the *constructive phase*. During this phase, educators develop questions to encourage their students to arrive at new or altered understanding of the concept. Questions in this phase have three components: defense, sequential progression, and suspension or discontinuation. After the students have responded to your previous questions, you would advance to questions that **ask them to *defend* their answer**. When they defend their responses, they learn to clarify and articulate their rationale or approach to solving the problem. During *sequential progression*, you implement a shaping process to find the just-right challenge while students continue to refine their responses. When using these questions, students engage in higher order thinking and continue to advance their thoughts. Lastly, you would *discontinue questioning* once your students have had an opportunity to apply new information, re-examine their conclusion, or create a new idea about the content. In this final phase, it is beneficial if you provide reassurance about the progress your students have made in their learning and potentially step out of the Socratic role to provide further explanation from your point of view. At the end of this phase, your ultimate goals are to advance your students as far you can while engaging them in rich discussion with the content and improve their ability to evaluate and support their opinions with facts and evidence. Table 10-4 provides examples of questions for each phase.

> Some studies suggest educators predominately ask lower-order questions. Be aware—higher-order questions are key!

Using the previous examples, practice writing your own questions in Table 10-5.

Pimping Is Not the Socratic Method

When searching educational literature on the Socratic method, you will often discover the term *pimping*. Sometimes educators or clinical supervisors believe pimping is the same as the Socratic method. However, this belief is untrue as these two methods are distinctly different. Pimping is defined as a person in authority asking questions of their junior colleagues or students with the aim of reinforcing the power hierarchy. The primary difference between pimping and the Socratic method lies in the intent of the person asking questions and the perception of psychological safety of the student answering the questions. When educators abuse the Socratic method by demonstrating characteristics of pimping (Table 10-6), they **stifle their students' curiosity, critical thinking, and dignity**. In turn, students will not experience growth of important attributes of self-directed, lifelong learning. When the Socratic method is employed correctly, students are able to focus on constructing their schema for their professional knowledge, skills, and attitudes. Therefore, you will need to be aware of the blurred boundaries between these two methods.

IMPLEMENTATION FOR DEBATE

Before discussing the actual implementation of debate, we want to highlight an important notion. Although we discussed creating a psychologically safe environment in the use of the Socratic method, we believe this notion also applies to the instructional method of debate. Therefore, we encourage you to review this information with your students prior to the debate, so they each feel safe to express their arguments during this learning experience. In addition, your students will feel more comfortable with the debate process if they understand the intended learning outcomes, procedures, and assessment of performance. In one study, Hanna and colleagues (2014) provided students with a printed or electronic informational packet, which outlined how debates are positioned within the professional program, the intended learning outcomes, topics and team allocations, structure of the debate, methods of assessment and feedback, and the expectations for participation. In addition, these educators provided resources and dates of workshops to increase comfort in debate. Several other studies reported reviewing similar information via a discussion or presentation during a designated class. Lampkin and colleagues (2015) provided a 30-minute in-class overview,

TABLE 10-5

Writing Socratic Questions

PHASE	COMPONENT	EXAMPLE OF QUESTIONS
Deconstructive Phase	Leading	
	Evaluative	
Constructive Phase	Defense	
	Sequential Progression	
	Discontinuation	

which included similar information as the previously mentioned study. However, these researchers also offered a mock debate so their students could develop a clear grasp of the process. A majority of educators introduce this information near the beginning of the course because debate is typically a method that occurs throughout a semester.

Pre-Debate Decisions

When preparing, you will want to make a number of decisions prior to the debate. One decision is the type of assignments your students will complete in combination with debate participation. For example, educators in various studies require students to submit a written report (with references), a list of references that support their position, a presentation, or minutes from team meetings. In addition, you will want to consider if you will review reports or presentations prior to the debate to provide feedback and ensure the team adequately addresses the question. You could also elect to meet with each team as they develop their debate to provide guidance.

TABLE 10-6

Differences Between Pimping and Socratic Method

CHARACTERISTICS OF PIMPING	CHARACTERISTICS OF SOCRATIC METHOD
Educator poses questions to reinforce power hierarchy.	Educator serves as a guide or facilitator.
Educator appears politically motivated; encourages students to admire educator.	Educator centers questions around the students.
Educator asks extremely difficult or rapid questions.	Educator poses questions that are purposeful; considers the goal of the question.
Educator uses questions to evaluate students.	Educator asks questions that encourage students to apply the knowledge to a problem.
Educator asks questions to embarrass, belittle, or criticize students.	Educator does not rely on fear tactics to accomplish learning goals.
Educator intends to impose ignorance.	Educator intends to allow students to express knowledge and stimulate and integrate new knowledge; helps identify faulty reasoning or gaps in knowledge.
Educator poses threat to students' dignity and worthiness.	Educator fosters curiosity and critical thinking.

You will likely consider the number of students and the amount of course time you can devote when determining the size of each debate team. In health professional educational literature, we note a range from one student per team to 10 students per team. In large pharmacy courses (175 and 151 learners), educators divided students into groups of six to seven per team. Meanwhile, educators in physical therapy and nursing created three-to-five-person debate teams. A majority of literature suggests randomly assigning students to teams versus allowing students to select their teams. Once divided into a team, one study asked each group to assign roles (first speaker, second speaker, third speaker, report writer, minute taker, and team leader) to encourage all students to participate in the debate process. We recommend that you require each student to participate in a minimum of one portion of the debate process.

After creating debate teams, you are ready to assign each with a debate question and position. Evidence suggests debate is effective for controversial and ethical issues in practice, but we can also use for other important professional topics. For example, Griswold (1990) used debate to teach occupational therapy students about different delivery models in schools. The author gave the students a case study of a child in a school system and assigned one debate team a direct service model and one team an indirect service model. The students developed intervention according to the assigned model and debated how the delivery of occupational therapy services using their model would best meet the child's needs. You will want to pose questions in which students can only answer with an affirmative or negative point of view. As the students prepare for debate, they must consider both sides of the issue so they can rebut comments made by opponents, cover the full topic so they are not blindsided, and respond to weaknesses in their position.

Before moving forward, write down a few controversial or professional topics in occupational therapy that could be well-suited for a debate.

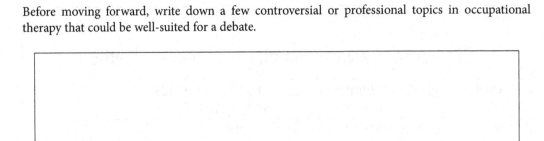

Interestingly, educators use multiple ways to assign debate topics. We will provide three examples for you to ponder in this step. One option is to just randomly assign each team with a question and position they will defend so they adequately prepare their argument in advance. Regardless of which side you assign, the students still gain a considerable amount of knowledge because they must learn about the strengths and weaknesses for each argument when preparing to respond to and present rebuttals. Second, you could ask each debate team to prepare an argument for both positions on the question. On the day of the actual debate, you would randomly assign (usually through drawing at random) which position the team will argue. One last option is to allow each group to select their question and position or to rank preference for a debate topic and position. We recognize that this strategy is the most learner-centered; however, we caution against its use to avoid bias and to promote an objective analysis of the topic.

Debate

You can structure your debates formally or informally; however, a formal debate structure provides your students with a useful guide for planning their arguments. Educational literature reports the most well-known debate structures are the Lincoln-Douglas style and the Oxford style. The primary difference between these two styles is that the Oxford style possesses a competitive feature in which the audience declares a winner through a majority vote. In the Lincoln-Douglas style of debate, there is no declared winner. Health care professional education literature suggests the Lincoln-Douglas style is most common because the students are active, and they easily understand the format. Therefore, we will use this format when outlining the steps to implementation (Table 10-7). However, we want you to be aware of other formats, so you can select which style best matches your needs. These formats include the British Parliamentary style, four-corner, impromptu, online, and think-pair-share debates.

In a majority of debate formats, the educator assigns one team an affirmative position and the other team a negative (opposing) position. Each team alternates turns speaking; whichever team is not speaking actively listens and does not interrupt. Regardless of the format, we typically see some form of three rounds in a debate—opening statements, rebuttals, and closing statements. You will want to assign each round a time limit and ensure that each team presents their information in the allotted time. In a majority of studies on the use of debate in health professional education, researchers allowed 20 to 35 minutes for each debate. On the day of the debate, you will want to arrange the room so the two debate teams are sitting across from each other and in front of the audience (Figure 10-2).

> Educators report that many of the students observing the debate wanted to be involved in the debate process.

We want to draw your attention to two additional questions to consider when implementing a debate. First, will you allow your students to use or take notes as they are debating? Second, will you let the audience actively participate by asking questions and providing comments? If you answer yes to the second question, just make sure to account for that time in your debate schedule. You will want to communicate the answers

TABLE 10-7

Steps of Lincoln-Douglas Debate

STEP	DESCRIPTION	APPROXIMATE TIME (MINUTES)
Affirmative Constructive	Opening argument: The student or group introduces the audience to their topic • Captures the audience's attention and interest • States the solution • States disagreements with valid reasoning and evidence • Concludes opening statement	6
Cross-Examination	The negative (opposing) construct asks questions of the affirmative construct	3
Negative (Opposing) Constructive	Opening argument: The student or group introduces the audience to their topic • Captures the audience's attention and interest • States position on topic • Supports observations with evidence and reasoning • Questions the affirmative construct with evidence • Concludes opening statement	7
Cross-Examination	The affirmative construct asks questions of the negative (opposing) construct	3
First Affirmative Rebuttal	The student or group responds to the negative (opposing) construct's observations by highlighting how it is not as strong or relevant as the affirmative construct to help rebuild the case for the side	4
Negative (Opposing) Rebuttal	The student or group: • Responds to the affirmative construct's observations • Makes final case that the negative construct is superior and that the affirmative construct has failed to adequately prove point • Summarizes and effectively concludes the debate	6
Second Affirmative Rebuttal	The student or group: • Responds to the negative (opposing) construct's observations • Makes final case that the affirmative construct is superior and that the negative (opposing) construct has failed to adequately prove point • Concludes the debate	3

Figure 10-2. Occupational therapy students participate in a debate.

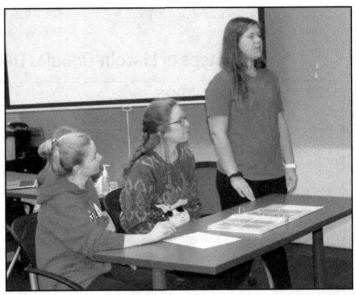

to these questions to your students prior to the debate. Lastly, if you elect to have the audience determine the winner of the debate, you will complete this step following closing statements. The audience selects a winner based on which team presented the best argument, not necessarily the position they support.

Role of Moderator

When implementing the instructional method of debate, you will likely serve the role of moderator. In this role, your primary responsibilities include setting and maintaining the rules of the debate and adhering to the allotted time set for each step. In addition, you will want to have knowledge of the content in case you need to step in and deliberately steer the dialogue in a certain direction, particularly if there is a certain issue the students need to contemplate. Lastly, you will need to possess awareness of your ability to hold opposing positions simultaneously in order to prevent biasing your students to one side.

Online Debate

In health professional literature, particularly pharmacy education, we notice an emerging trend in the use of debate in an online format. You could use this to supplement the face-to-face portion of your course or in a course taught entirely online. You would still want to provide a module outlining the details of debate and still need to make a number of decisions (e.g., group size, topic, debate format). In addition, you can use the discussion board feature found on most learning management systems or a website called www.createdebate.com. Vandall-Walker and colleagues (2012) provide a good example of a timeline for an online debate. On the first day, the students that are debating post their opening arguments while the other students in the course remain quiet. On day 3, the debaters post rebuttal arguments. The other students in the course contribute to the discussion in conjunction with the debaters until the sixth day. After the sixth day, the debaters summarize their argument and position on the debate and include any relevant feedback from the students in the course. The educator assesses the students using the same methods we discuss for in-class debate in the upcoming Opportunities for Feedback and Reflection section.

ADDITIONAL IMPLEMENTATION NOTES

- Pose questions with a purpose. You do not want your students involved in a guessing game of what you are thinking.
- Ask questions your students have enough knowledge to answer.
- Phrase your questions clearly and limit the number of action verbs per question.
- Sequence and balance questions; attempt to not ask too many questions.
- Avoid rapid fire questioning.
- Decide before class if you need lower-order questions to establish a foundation for higher-order thinking.
- Be strategic in your timing; allow silent pauses after posing questions so your students can consider the question, reflect on their knowledge, and formulate their responses.

  > Literature suggests pausing anywhere from 20 seconds to 1 to 2 minutes!

- Do not attempt to evaluate student performance.
- Students should feel a sense of closure at the end of the discussion or debate.

TIPS AND TRICKS

- Avoid asking questions that lead students to a specific answer and do not offer direct information.
- Read your students' facial expressions and body language to determine if a question needs to be rephrased.
- As you formulate questions before class, also develop additional questions in response to a variety of answers students might provide.
- Review your questions. Do you have a good mix of all cognitive domains? Are you meeting your learning outcomes?
- Do not attempt to fill silence by answering your own questions.
- Use the Socratic method in moderation with novice students.

OPPORTUNITIES FOR FEEDBACK AND REFLECTION

Educational literature provides several examples of ways to provide feedback and reflection following participation in debate. You can ask your students to complete a self-evaluation or a reflection paper, give a quiz before and after the debate to determine changes in knowledge or viewpoints, provide oral and written feedback via rubrics, or have the audience and group members contribute observational feedback via some sort of peer-evaluation method. Many studies on debate use a combination of methods. By incorporating peer feedback, you are also encouraging the audience of students to be active participants. Educators often use many of the following criteria when developing feedback methods for a debate: (1) preparation for debate, (2) knowledge of content, (3) professionalism, (4) argument reliability and validity, and (5) teamwork. Elliot and colleagues (2016) provide an example of the assessment criteria they used to provide feedback to their learners following a debate (Figure 10-3). In another study, Lampkin and colleagues (2015) wanted their students to openly engage in a debate without the fear of criticism from the educator. Therefore, they based

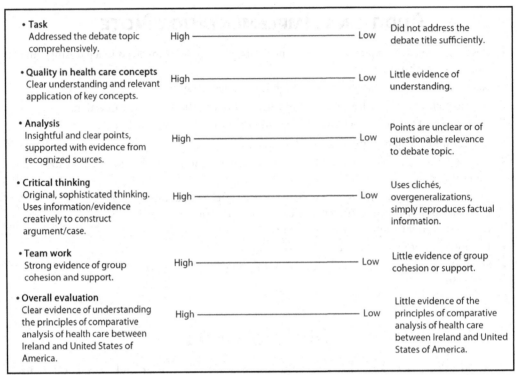

- **Task**
  Addressed the debate topic comprehensively.

  High ——————————— Low

  Did not address the debate title sufficiently.

- **Quality in health care concepts**
  Clear understanding and relevant application of key concepts.

  High ——————————— Low

  Little evidence of understanding.

- **Analysis**
  Insightful and clear points, supported with evidence from recognized sources.

  High ——————————— Low

  Points are unclear or of questionable relevance to debate topic.

- **Critical thinking**
  Original, sophisticated thinking. Uses information/evidence creatively to construct argument/case.

  High ——————————— Low

  Uses clichés, overgeneralizations, simply reproduces factual information.

- **Team work**
  Strong evidence of group cohesion and support.

  High ——————————— Low

  Little evidence of group cohesion or support.

- **Overall evaluation**
  Clear evidence of understanding the principles of comparative analysis of health care between Ireland and United States of America.

  High ——————————— Low

  Little evidence of the principles of comparative analysis of health care between Ireland and United States of America.

Figure 10-3. Example of assessment for debate. (Reproduced with permission from Elliott, N., Farnum, K., & Beauchesne, M. [2016]. Utilizing team debate to increase student abilities for mentoring and critical appraisal of global health care in doctor of nursing practice programs. *Journal of Professional Nursing, 32*[3], 224-234. https://doi.org/10.1016/j.profnurs.2015.10.009)

80% of the overall grade on the written report their students submitted prior to the debate with the remaining 20% devoted to preparedness and professionalism. We want to bring your attention to an interesting point as you design your course and assign grades. Many qualitative studies on the use of debate report students believed the workload was disproportionate to the grade due to the amount of time they spent meeting with a team and searching for evidence. For example, in a pharmacy education study, debate only contributed to 15% of the students' overall grade. Therefore, if you want your students to perceive that debate is valuable, you will want to give the feedback methods a comparative score.

Some scholars criticize debates because of the potential to dichotomize complex topics. However, we can address this concern through the facilitation of a discussion after the debate is over. In the Implementation section, you may have noticed a lack of time in the debate schedule devoted to discussion. While this is not a formal step in the debate process, we strongly encourage planning time for discussion and reflection. You can use this time to examine your students' professional reasoning and interpersonal skills and to ask your students to reflect on performance and feedback from you and their peers. We have provided a list of questions you can consider using during your post-debate discussion (Table 10-8). You can also ask your students to answer a few of these questions in a reflection paper. Interestingly, many educators report that students often continue to discuss after they leave class.

TABLE 10-8

Questions for Post-Debate Discussion or Reflection Paper

- How did the debate reinforce the material you have learned in this course or program?
- How did the debate change your view of the content?
- What challenge did you face as you prepared for or engaged in the debate?
- How did you feel about the topic prior to participation in the debate?
- What were the most valuable skills you gained from this debate that you can translate to your professional practice?
- What surprises or unexpected learning outcomes did you experience by engaging in this debate?
- Describe a power learning moment during the debate.
- Describe three things you learned by participating in the debate process.
- How can you use what you have learned in your future practice?

APPLICATION TO OCCUPATIONAL THERAPY PRACTICE

There are several examples of the use of the Socratic method with individuals participating in psychotherapy treatment. In psychotherapy treatment, therapists use Socratic questioning to guide a client's behavior and thought processes to facilitate achievement of their goals. Interestingly, Braun and colleagues (2015) found a positive relationship between a therapist that uses the Socratic method and improvement in symptoms of patients with depression. In this literature, you would detect similarities between this method and occupational therapy interventions related to coaching, cognitive-behavioral treatment, or guided discovery.

Example 1: Implementation of Socratic Method Principles During Group Intervention

Picture yourself facilitating a self-management group with individuals with chronic conditions. The group will be discussing healthy eating and exercise. You will use the Socratic method to understand and potentially change their beliefs about these topics. For example, your leading question could be, "What does eating healthy mean to you?" or "How would you define exercise?" After the group has provided their answers, you would create evaluative questions based on their responses. Examples of evaluative questions might include, "Describe why you believe exercise or eating healthy is important," "What is the appropriate amount of exercise?" or "How do you know the recommendations for healthy eating or exercise?" Next, you would move the group into the constructive phase by asking questions that require them to defend their answer. These questions might include, "Where else can exercise occur besides the gym?" "How can people who are unable to walk engage in exercise?" "Do you have to eat appropriate every meal to be considered a healthy eater?" or "How can healthy eating occur outside your home?" During sequential progression, you might ask questions, such as, "What changes could you make to your original beliefs or definition of healthy eating or exercise?" or "What might be an alternative solution to obtaining adequate exercise or healthy eating?" Lastly, you would discontinue the discussion by asking the group what they have learned from the discussion and how can they apply that new information to their life in the next week.

Example 2: Implementation of Socratic Method Principles During Intervention With Client With Depression

In this situation, you are working with a client experiencing depression impacting occupations, roles, and relationships. As the facilitator using the Socratic method, you could guide the client to widen their thinking about the situation or to think about the situation in another way. Examples of questions include:

- How do your feelings or thoughts impact your daily life?
- What do you believe or know about depression? How did you arrive at that belief?
- How could it be possible that individuals with these thoughts or feelings find ways to do [related to goals or roles]?
- What areas have you been successful in the past? What did that look like?
- What evidence do you have that your family believes [client's thought]?

Advantages

- When questions are well designed, the Socratic method can increase students' attention, curiosity, and critical thinking
- As students answer questions, the educator can gain insight into students' current perceptions and understanding of course content
- Educators can implement with students with a variety of abilities
- There is often no single correct answer to questions
- Can use with an individual or large groups of students
- Allows for horizontal learning (e.g., the students learn from each other)
- Provides an interactive method of learning
- Requires students are prepared for class
- Encourages students to think on their feet
- Can cover a large amount of complex content in a short period of time (debate)
- Learners gain proficiency in locating and appraising information from databases, professionals, and other resources (debate)

Challenges

- Ambiguous method of instruction, as there does not appear to be a generally accepted definition or description of the use of the Socratic method
- Demands a lot of time and effort to implement
- Requires tailoring to best meet the needs of each group of students
- Educators must create well-designed questions
- Students might consider questions straightforward and confrontational, creating anxiety, stress, fear, or pressure (pimping)
- Educators need to create a safe environment for sharing
- Students potentially report boredom while listening to other students
- Higher rate of improper execution (Socratic method)
- Potential to foster a competitive environment

In the space below, list any additional advantages or challenges.

Brainstorm strategies for overcoming these challenges when implementing the use of inquiry-based instructional methods.

THREE THINGS YOU CAN DO TOMORROW TO IMPLEMENT INQUIRY-BASED INSTRUCTIONAL METHODS WITH YOUR STUDENTS

1. Create a list of topics from the courses you teach in which your students could debate.
2. Review three different debate formats and decide which fits best with your students.
3. Use Table 10-5 to write questions for one topic you are teaching in the next 2 weeks.

Inquiry-Based Instructional Methods Evidence Table

SOCRATIC METHOD

Author/Year	Study Objectives	Design and Participants	Intervention and Outcome Measures	Results
Williams et al. (2018)	Researchers investigated faculty and student beliefs and experiences with pimping in pharmacy education	Design: Cross-sectional survey design Participants: 59 full- or part-time faculty with teaching responsibilities and 100 fourth-year pharmacy students at 2 universities Exclusion criteria: • Adjunct faculty, staff, or other faculty lines with sole focus on research	Intervention/outcome measures: Researchers developed 2 surveys; 1 for faculty with questions related to training and teaching experiences and 1 for students with questions related to experiences during pharmacy education Each survey contained 17 questions and a definition of pimping; researchers administered the survey electronically via Qualtrics	58% of respondents reported agreement with the reported definition of pimping with no significant differences between faculty and students Of the students, 60.6% reported faculty should use pimping sparingly and 22.3% reported faculty should avoid pimping; meanwhile, 45.8% of faculty suggested to use sparingly and 30.5% selected avoid use of pimping. The only significant difference was between faculty at the 2 pharmacy schools, as 1 group of faculty felt pimping should be used more sparingly when compared to faculty at the other institution Three fourths of faculty reported experience of pimping during their own training, but less than half reported use of the method during their educational practices. Similarly, almost 75% of students reported experience of pimping during pharmacy education. Students experienced pimping most frequently by nonfaculty pharmacists and most commonly when they were participating in rounds. Students reported they were stressed, challenged, and intimidated when experiencing pimping. A majority of students believed pimping improved ability to recall information, but less than half felt this method helped them apply and understand content

(continued)

Inquiry-Based Instructional Methods Evidence Table (continued)

Author/Year	Study Objectives	Design and Participants	Intervention and Outcome Measures	Results
Wood et al. (2016)	Researchers investigated emergency medicine residents' perception of "pimping" Researchers also evaluated if Socratic instruction enhanced emergency medicine residents' knowledge retention over traditional lecture–based learning	Design: Prospective, randomized controlled study Participants: 72 emergency medicine residents	Intervention: Researchers randomized groups of 3 to 4 emergency medicine residents to the instructional method, the Socratic method, or lecture–based learning to learn head trauma. Researchers trained 2 emergency medicine physicians to deliver the Socratic method. In the Socratic method group, residents answered a set of predefined questions. In the lecture–based learning group, residents engaged in traditional lecture format Outcome measures: After the intervention, each group completed a questionnaire related to their perceptions of pimping. Each group also completed a quiz 4 weeks after intervention	Of the 72 residents, 54% reported pimping is an effective method for teaching content most or all of the time. However, 82% of residents reported they would prefer use of the Socratic method at least some of the time Of the 72 residents, 57 completed the quiz 4 weeks after the intervention. Residents in the pimping group scored 66.2% and the nonpimping group scored 65.9% on the quiz. However, residents in the pimping group demonstrated higher average scores than the nonpimping group (59.6% versus 52.9%)
Zou et al. (2011)	Researchers implemented instructional methods to determine what type of teaching medical students in radiology preferred	Design: Posttest; survey design Participants: 65 third- and fourth-year medical students who attended a medical conference	Intervention: 90-minute radiology conference; the presenter implemented 2 instructional methods; 1 with radiological slides on a PowerPoint presentation similar to traditional lecture; the other required students to work in groups of 8 to 12 to interact and actively participate via a question and answer session Outcome measures: Survey	65 of 101 students who attended the conference completed the survey Most students (81%) reported preference for the interactive dialogue portion of the presentation; however, 65.7% reported preference for volunteering to answer questions versus being called on 70% of participants reported preference for viewing radiology films versus presenter reporting findings, and 72% of students reported pimping was an effective method of learning

(continued)

Inquiry-Based Instructional Methods Evidence Table (continued)

Author/Year	Study Objectives	Design and Participants	Intervention and Outcome Measures	Results
				The students felt the Socratic method made the presentation more interactive and forced preparation; however, reported cons of potential to be boring hearing other students answer and embarrassing if do not know the answer and are put on the spot

DEBATE

Author/Year	Study Objectives	Design and Participants	Intervention and Outcome Measures	Results
Choe et al. (2014)	Researchers compared action learning and cross-examination debate for bioethics education with nursing students	Design: Quasi-experimental; 2-group pre/posttest Participants: 93 undergraduate nursing students; 46 in the action learning method (ALM) class and 47 in the cross-examination debate (CED) class	Intervention: Students selected 1 of 2 nursing bioethics classes. Each class met 2 hours per week for 15 weeks ALM: Small groups of students (5 to 6) visited a clinical practice site, met with nurses, and listened to their experiences and cases of ethical issues. Each group selected 2 or 4 cases and determined solutions by researching/gathering information and participating in discussions CED: Students prepared for both sides of the debate. On date of debate, they randomly drew to determine which side of the argument they would defend. Students worked in groups of 4 Outcome measures: • Recognition of bioethical issues questionnaire; participants self-rated knowledge of bioethics and rated seriousness of bioethical issues	Each group of students demonstrated increased knowledge of bioethics. The ALM group demonstrated statistically significant more knowledge of bioethics after the course than the CED group Each group viewed bioethics education more positively after the class with no statistically significant differences between the 2 groups The ALM group reported a significantly greater need for bioethics education after the course than the CED group Researchers did not find significant difference about the perception of receiving sufficient bioethics education, but the ALM class did report higher scores Each student demonstrated an increase in ethical competence scores from pre to posttest with no significant differences between groups

(continued)

Inquiry-Based Instructional Methods Evidence Table (continued)

Author/Year	Study Objectives	Design and Participants	Intervention and Outcome Measures	Results
			• Bioethics education questionnaires (the experiences of bioethics education, need of bioethics education, and quality of bioethics education) • Ethical competence questionnaire	
Hanna et al. (2014)	Researchers evaluated a newly implemented debate method to teach pharmacy students about ethical issues	Design: Posttest design Participants: 151 second-year pharmacy students	Intervention: Students participated in debate workshops (2 workshops at 2.5 hours per workshop = total of 5 hours) and engaged in 5 hours of self-study. Each workshop included 2 debates Researchers divided students in groups of 8 to 10 students and assigned a side to 1 of 4 topics. When the group was not engaged in debate, they observed Outcome measures: • Team scores from peer and educator feedback; used the mean score with peer scores contributing to 40% and educator scores contributing 60% of the overall grade • Survey (8 questions)	The students scored an average of 25.9 out of 30; the range was from 23.2 to 28.7 Students scored highest on research skills and lowest on rebuttal skills On the survey, 77% of students reported agreed or strongly agreed debate changed opinion of an issue A majority of students (70%) reported agreed or strongly agreed that debate was a useful instructional method, with 49% suggesting educators use debate more frequently in pharmacy education Students indicated the most developed research skills and least developed rebuttal skills
Hartin et al. (2017)	Researchers aimed to develop evidence to support debate as an effective method for development of critical-thinking and communication skills with nursing students	Design: Posttest cross-sectional survey design	Intervention: Researcher included debates in tutorial sessions Outcome measures: Survey (11 focused questions on perception of debate)	First-year students positively supported the use of debate to improve grade, whereas third-year students did not support. Each group of students did not believe debate improved their research and writing skills, but the third-year students more strongly disagreed

(continued)

Inquiry-Based Instructional Methods Evidence Table (continued)

Author/Year	Study Objectives	Design and Participants	Intervention and Outcome Measures	Results
		Participants: 93 students enrolled in first- or third-year subject of a baccalaureate nursing degree, dual degree baccalaureate nursing/ midwifery, or Diploma of Health Sciences program		Students reported increased confidence and a fun, engaging, and nonthreatening environment
Lampkin et al. (2015)	Researchers implemented a debate series to assess students' perceptions of debates and the impact of debates on various skills (critical thinking, communication, public speaking, research methods, and teamwork)	Design: Quasi-experimental pre/posttest design. Participants: First-year professional pharmacy students	Intervention: 3-credit hour course; met 2 times per week for 50 and 110 minutes. Researchers used 5 debates related to various controversial self-care topics; students presented debates before lectures on the assigned topics. Students completed debates in groups of 6 or 7; the educators assigned debate topics and pro/con sides. Outcome measures: • Pre-debate and post-debate quizzes • Pre-course and post-course surveys	Students improved scores on each of the 5 quizzes from pre-debate to post-debate; range of 13% to 36% improvement. Anywhere from 9% to 31% of students changed opinion of topic following debates. Most students felt participation in debates assisted in learning material, but they did not feel observing the debates facilitated learning. 92% of students reported preparing for debates was at least slightly effective in improving skills. Students evaluated self as more competent in each of the 5 skills
Latif et al. (2018)	Researchers compared the effectiveness of role plays and debate on critical thinking and communication skills in problem-based learning (PBL) small group discussion	Design: Comparative cross-sectional survey design. Participants: 185 second-year undergraduate female medical students	Intervention: Researchers divided medical students into PBL groups of 1 to 13 members. Throughout the semester, they participated in PBL learning tasks. During the first semester of PBL, students participated in debate. In the following semester, students participated in 6 to 7 role plays and debates	Students reported role plays were more effective than debate in development of critical-thinking skills. Students positively rated debate and role play for improved communication and critical-thinking skills

(continued)

Inquiry-Based Instructional Methods Evidence Table (continued)

Author/Year	Study Objectives	Design and Participants	Intervention and Outcome Measures	Results
			Outcome measures: Questionnaire (8 questions)	70% of students reported role play better supported understanding real-life clinical scenarios Only 52% of students believed debates were relevant to real-life experiences; however, 76% of students believed debate opened their thinking over role plays Many students believed both methods changed their thinking/perspectives, eased potential communication, improved listening skills, and promoted teamwork
Mamtani et al. (2015)	Researchers evaluated the effectiveness of debate curriculum on patient safety and quality improvement competencies	Design: Cross-sectional, survey design (data collected over 2 years) Participants: 30 medical residents; unclear how many individuals on the committee completed survey	Intervention: 2 teams (senior-level resident and attending) participated in a debate of a mock clinical case for 30 minutes Outcome measures: • Survey (questions linked to specific milestones/competencies) to participants • Survey to clinical competency committee (questions related to ability to evaluate competencies)	71% of residents agreed or strongly agreed debates improved performance on topics by appraising literature and applying evidence-based medicine. In addition, 68% of residents agreed or strongly agreed they could describe concepts related to patient safety Approximately, one third of residents led a debate; each felt they could approach topic from an evidence-based perspective Committee reported it was easier to assess 3 competency areas from prior years
Moore et al. (2015)	Researchers saw if use of debate achieved course objective of critically evaluating clinical trials/guidelines to provide an opinion on controversies in pharmacy	Design: Posttest survey design Participants: 13 third-year pharmacy students	Intervention: Researchers divided the course into 6 topics and spent 2 weeks on each topic. During the first week, researchers implemented advanced patient cases. During the second week, students participated in debate of a controversial topic in groups of 4 to 5	A small majority of the students spent 5 to 10 hours preparing for each debate A majority of students (76.9%) preferred to present and observe debates that included PowerPoint presentations

(continued)

Inquiry-Based Instructional Methods Evidence Table (continued)

Author/Year	Study Objectives	Design and Participants	Intervention and Outcome Measures	Results
			Students debated 3 times during semester. When not debating, students observed debate. Outcomes measures: • Online survey asking questions about time spent preparing for event, preference for debate, role of debate in learning, etc. • Grading rubric (50% of course grade)	Students agreed or strongly agreed they met the course objective and that the debate facilitated this achievement Students also agreed or strongly agreed that debate improved their ability to apply information to patients, decide between certain medicines, present information, and think critically Students scored an average of 39.75 out of 40 on debate rubric
Peasah & Marshall (2017)	Researchers aimed to describe the process to incorporate debate, assess students' perceptions of debate, and evaluate debate performance	Design: Quasi-experimental pretest-posttest survey design Participants: First-year pharmacy students; 170 students in 2014 and 149 students in 2015	Intervention: Students attended class 2 hours per week. Researchers randomly assigned students into groups of 6 or 7. Students ranked topic and position preferences. Researchers assigned based on preferences. Researchers scheduled 1 debate per class, and it followed a lecture in 12 of the 16 classes. Students participated in debate for approximately 30 minutes Outcomes measures: • Online survey of opinion on topic and debate winner • Grades (team and individual performance) Researchers collected every day for 2 years (2 different classes)	In 2014, students did not grade peer performance. The educator gave an average grade of 99.65 out of 100. In 2015, the educator gave an average score of 68.8 out of 70. In 2015, students provided peer assessment and gave an average score of 28.26 out of 30 Researchers added survey questions to the 2015 cohort on the usefulness of debate for learning. 71% of students reported at least the debate would be useful at pretest and 83% reported usefulness at posttest Results demonstrated a statistically significant increase from pre to posttest on students indicating debates as useful or very useful Students performed better on midterm and final exams on the questions reflective of lecture content versus debate content

(continued)

Inquiry-Based Instructional Methods Evidence Table (continued)

Author/Year	Study Objectives	Design and Participants	Intervention and Outcome Measures	Results
Saito & Fujinami (2011)	Researchers aimed to evaluate the effect of a debate within a specialty track within periodontics education	Design: Cross-sectional pretest-posttest design Participants: 28 participants (full-time faculty, residents, and dentists completing a specialty course)	Intervention: Researchers divided participants into teams of 3 with 1 tutor. There were 5 judges and 13 audience members. Participants debated complex and controversial topics Outcome measures: • Judge Evaluation Sheet (17 items) • Pre and posttest (10 questions) • Feedback survey	Students on the affirmative teams demonstrated lower scores on time keeping, presentation performance, and response with evidence. In addition to these items, students on the negative team scored lower on rebuttal effectiveness and performance. When researchers compared mean scores to the affirmative and negative teams, there was a significant difference on quality of presentation and rebuttal performance 38% of the audience members demonstrated improvement in test scores after debate Of the participants, 88% of participants reported feeling stress related to debate
Strawbridge et al. (2014)	Researchers aimed to determine if debate was a useful strategy for pharmacy and physiotherapy students to learn together	Design: Quasi-experimental pretest-posttest design Participants: 76 pre-debate responses and 62 post-debate responses; 42 pharmacy students and 20 physiotherapy students The researchers used the pharmacy-only teams as a control group	Intervention: Researchers randomized students into 12 teams of 6 members. Of the 12 groups, 8 debate teams were interprofessional with physiotherapy and pharmacy students and the remaining 4 had only pharmacy students. Researchers randomly assigned the debate groups to a topic Outcome measures: • Survey (primary) • The Readiness for Interprofessional Learning Scale and the Attitudes to Health Professionals Questionnaire (secondary outcome measures for interprofessional education)	Students demonstrated a significant increase in opinion on 2 debate topics. Control group opinions did not change Students were significantly more likely to disagree with the idea that they do not like participating in debates following the course A vast majority of students (80%) felt the topics were challenging and that they developed critical-thinking skills (85%). More than 80% of students felt debate was an appropriate method to learn ethical topics Researchers reported no significant differences between the 2 groups or from pre to posttest in regard to interprofessional education attitudes

(continued)

Inquiry-Based Instructional Methods Evidence Table (continued)

Author/Year	Study Objectives	Design and Participants	Intervention and Outcome Measures	Results
Toor et al. (2017)	Researchers evaluated students' perceptions of a debate-style journal club to educate pharmacy students on critical analysis of literature	Design: Posttest survey design Participants: 17 fourth-year pharmacy students in ambulatory or acute care rotations	Intervention: Instead of a traditional journal club format, researchers assigned students a controversial topic or 2 similar drugs and asked to debate a side. Students participated in a debate for 15 minutes Outcome measures: Researchers created 8-question survey; 2 questions focused on attitude toward debate, 6 questions focused on agreement with statements related to skills	17 pharmacy students completed 6 questions, but only 12 students completed the comparison to traditional journal club format questions (the other students did not have a journal club experience to compare to) Students reported increased confidence in ability to locate, compare, and retain information from literature, and enjoyment and satisfaction with debate, but uncertainty with improvements in communication skills and drug information knowledge Of the students that completed the 2 questions related to comparison of the 2 methods, they reported uncertainty with the idea that debate improved knowledge retention and appraisal skills
Weeks & Laakso (2016)	Researchers formally evaluated student expectations and satisfaction with debate assignment	Design: Cross-sectional survey design Participants: 6 physiotherapy students enrolled in a clinical conference course completed first survey; 16 physiotherapy students completed the second survey	Intervention: Students participated in blended-learning capstone course. They completed debate that focused on professional, medical, legal, and ethical issues in physiotherapy practice. Students followed the modified British Parliamentary debate style in teams of 3 Outcome measures: • Individual grades • Online survey (1 was 2 weeks before debate to determine attitudes and perception of debate; 1 was a week after debate to further determine satisfaction and attitudes)	For pretest survey, all students felt engaging in dialogue on professional and ethical issues was important; 5 students reported anxiety or apprehension about engaging in a debate Of the 16 students, 11 enjoyed the debate; 50% of students reported increased confidence in professional dialogue skills

Adapted from American Occupational Therapy Association. (2002). AOTA's evidence-based literature review project: An overview (D. Lieberman & J. Scheer, Eds). *American Journal of Occupational Therapy, 56,* 344-349. https://doi.org/10.5014/ajot.56.3.344

REFERENCES

American Occupational Therapy Association. (2002). AOTA's evidence-based literature review project: An overview (D. Lieberman & J. Scheer, Eds.). *The American Journal of Occupational Therapy, 56,* 344-349. https://doi.org/10.5014/ajot.56.3.344

Braun, J. D., Strunk, D., Sasso, K. E., & Cooper, A. A. (2015). Therapist use of Socratic questioning predicts session-to-session symptom change in cognitive therapy for depression. *Behaviour Research and Therapy, 70,* 32-37. https://doi.org/10.1016/j.brat.2015.05.004

Choe, K., Park, S., & Yoo, S. Y. (2014). Effects of constructivist teaching methods on bioethics education for nursing students: A quasi-experimental study. *Nurse Education Today, 34,* 848-853. http://dx.doi.org/10.1016/j.nedt.2013.09.012

Elliott, N., Farnum, K., & Beauchesne, M. (2016). Utilizing team debate to increase student abilities for mentoring and critical appraisal of global health care in doctor of nursing practice programs. *Journal of Professional Nursing, 32(3),* 224-234. https://doi.org/10.1016/j.profnurs.2015.10.009

Griswold, L. A. S. (1990). Brief report—debate as a teaching strategy. *American Journal of Occupational Therapy, 54(4),* 427-428.

Hanna, L. A., Barry, J., Donnelly, R., Hughes, F., Jones, D., Laverty, G., Parsons, C., & Ryan, C. (2014). Instructional design and assessment: Using debate to teach pharmacy students about ethical issues. *American Journal of Pharmaceutical Education, 78(3),* Article 57.

Hartin, P., Birks, M., Bodak, M., Woods, C., & Hitchins, M. (2017). A debate about the merits of debate in nurse education. *Nurse Education in Practice, 26,* 118-120. http://dx.doi.org/10.1016/j.nepr.2017.08.005

Lampkin, S. J., Collins, C., Danison, R., & Lewis, M. (2015). Instructional design and assessment: Active learning through a debate series in a first-year pharmacy self-care course. *American Journal of Pharmaceutical Education, 79(2),* Article 25.

Latif, R., Mumtaz, S., Mumtaz, R., & Hussain, A. (2018). A comparison of debate and role play in enhancing critical thinking and communication skills of medical students during problem based learning. *Biochemistry and Molecular Biology Education, 46(4),* 336-342.

Mamtani, M., Scott, K. R., DeRoos, F. J., & Conlon, L. W. (2015). Assessing EM patient safety and quality improvement milestones using a novel debate format. *Western Journal of Emergency Medicine, 16(6),* 943-946. http://dx.doi.org/10.5811/westjem.2015.9.27269

McBurney, J. H. (1952). Chapter II: The role of discussion and debate in a democratic society. *The Bulletin of the National Association of Secondary School Principals, 36(187),* 22-26.

Moore, K. G., Clements, J., Sease, J., & Anderson, Z. (2015). The utility of clinical controversy debates in an ambulatory care elective. *Currents in Pharmacy Teaching and Learning, 7,* 239-248.

Overholser, J. C. (1991). The Socratic method as a technique in psychotherapy supervision. *Professional Psychology, Research, and Practice, 22(1),* 68-74.

Oyler, D. R., & Romanelli, F. (2014). The fact of ignorance: Revisiting the Socratic method as a tool for teaching critical thinking. *American Journal of Pharmaceutical Education, 78(7),* Article 144.

Peasah, S. K., & Marshall, L. L. (2017). The use of debates as an active learning tool in a college of pharmacy healthcare delivery course. *Currents in Pharmacy Teaching and Learning, 9,* 443-440. http://dx.doi.org/10.1016/j.cptl.2017.01.012

Saito, A., & Fujinami, K. (2011). Introduction of formal debate into a postgraduate specialty track education programme in periodontics in Japan. *European Journal of Dental Education, 15,* 58-62. http://dx.doi.org/10.1111/j.1600-0579.2010.00635.x

Strawbridge, J. D., Barrett, A. M., & Barlow, J. W. (2014). Interprofessional ethics and professionalism debates: Findings from a study involving physiotherapy and pharmacy students. *Journal of Interprofessional Care, 28(1),* 64-65. http://dx.doi.org/10.3109/13561820.2013.829423

Toledo, C. A. (2015). Dog bite reflections—Socratic questioning revisited. *International Journal of Teaching and Learning in Higher Education, 27(2),* 275-279.

Toor, R., Samai, K., & Wargo, R. (2017). Debate as an alternative method for medical literature evaluation. *Currents in Pharmacy Teaching and Learning, 9,* 427-432. http://dx.doi.org/10.1016/j.cptl.2017.01.009

Vandall-Walker, V., Park, C. L., & Munich, K. (2012). Outcomes of modified formal online debating in graduate nursing education. *International Journal of Nursing Education Scholarship, 9(1),* Article 15.

Weeks, B. K., & Laakso, L. (2016). Using debates as assessment in a physiotherapy capstone course: A case example. *Journal of University Teaching and Learning Practice, 13(3),* Article 8. http://ro.uow.edu.au/jutlp/vol13/iss3/8

Williams, E. A., Miesner, A. R., Beckett, E. A., & Grady, S. E. (2018). "Pimping" in pharmacy education: A survey and comparison of student and faculty views. *Journal of Pharmacy Practice, 31(3),* 353-360. http://dx.doi.org/10.1177/0897190017715393

Wood, S., Teran, F., Strayer, R., & Shah, K. (2016). Can active learning via the Socratic method improve knowledge retention amongst emergency medicine residents? *Western Journal of Emergency Medicine, 17(4.1).*

Zou, L., King, A., Soman, S., Lischuk, A., Schneider, B., Walor, D., Bramwit, M., & Amorosa, J. K. (2011). Medical students' preferences in radiology education: A comparison between the Socratic and didactic methods utilizing PowerPoint features in radiology education. *Academic Radiology, 18(2),* 253-256. http://dx.doi.org/10.1016/j.acra.2010.09.005

BIBLIOGRAPHY

Al-Darwish, S. (2012). The role of teacher questions and the Socratic method in EFL classrooms in Kuwait. *World Journal of Education, 2*(4), 76-84. http://dx.doi.org/10.5430/wje.v2n4p76

Boghossian, P. (2006). Socratic pedagogy, critical thinking, and inmate education. *The Journal of Correctional Education, 57*(1), 42-63.

Bruning, R. H., Schraw, G. J., & Norby, M. M. (2011). *Cognitive psychology and instruction* (5th ed.). Pearson.

Carey, T. A., & Mullan, R. J. (2004). What is Socratic questioning? *Psychotherapy: Theory, Research, Practice, Training, 41*(3), 217-226. http://dx.doi.org/10.1037/0033-3204.41.3.217

Carlson, E. R. (2017). Medical pimping versus the Socratic method of teaching. *Journal of Oral Maxillofacial Surgery, 75*, 3-5.

Charrois, T. L., & Appleton, M. (2013). Instructional design and assessment: Online debates to enhance critical thinking in pharmacotherapy. *American Journal of Pharmaceutical Education, 77*(8), Article 170.

Darby, M. (2007). Debate: A teaching-learning strategy for developing competence in communication and critical thinking. *Journal of Dental Hygiene, 81*(4), 1-10.

Doody, O., & Condon, M. (2012). Increasing student involvement and learning through using debate as an assessment. *Nurse Education in Practice, 12*, 232-237. https://doi.org/10.1016/j.nepr.2012.03.002

Dy-Boarman, E. A., Nisley, S. A., & Costello, T. J. (2018). It's no debate, debates are great. *Currents in Pharmacy Teaching and Learning, 10*, 10-13. https://dx.doi.org/10.1016/j.cptl.2017.09.016

Fani, T., & Ghaemi, F. (2011). Implications of Vygotsky's zone of proximal development (ZPD) in teacher education: ZPTD and self-scaffolding. *Procedia—Social and Behavioral Sciences, 29*, 1549-1554. https://dx.doi.org/10.1016/j.sbspro.2011.11.396

Haung, W. (2005). The Socratic method in medicine—the labor of delivering medical truths. *Family Medicine, 37*(8), 537-539.

Jha, S. (2013). Debates, dialectic, and rhetoric: An approach to teaching radiology residents health economics, policy, and advocacy. *Academic Radiology, 20*(6), 773-777. http://dx.doi.org/10.1016/j.acra.2012.12.017

Kennedy, R. (2007). In-class debates: Fertile ground for active learning and the cultivation of critical thinking and oral communication skills. *International Journal or Teaching and Learning in Higher Education, 19*(2), 183-190.

Launer, J. (2017). Socratic questions and frozen shoulders: Teaching without telling. *Postgraduate Medical Journal, 93*(1106), 783-784.

Magas, C., Dedhia, P., Barrett, M., Gauger, M., Gruppen, L., & Sandhu, G. (2017). Strategic questioning in surgical education. *The Clinical Teacher, 14*, 134-136.

Merida, D., Baratas, I., & Arrue, M. (2016). Guided University Debate (GUD): A new promising teaching and learning strategy for undergraduate nursing students. *Nurse Education Today, 45*, 69-71. https://doi.org/10.1016/j.nedt.2016.06.014

MIT OpenCourseWare. (2009). Lincoln/Douglas debate format [PDF document]. Retrieved from https://ocw.mit.edu/courses/comparative-media-studies-writing/21w-747-classical-rhetoric-and-modern-political-discourse-fall-2009/study-materials/MIT21W_747_01F09_study13.pdf

Sahamid, H. (2016). Developing critical thinking through Socratic questioning: An action research study. *International Journal of Education and Literacy Studies, 4*(3), 62-72.

Schneider, J. (2013). Remembrance of things past: A history of the Socratic method is the United States. *Curriculum Inquiry, 43*(5), 613-640. https://doi.org/10.1111/curi.12030

Stoddard, H. A., & O'Dell, D. V. (2016). Would Socrates have actually used the "Socratic method" for clinical teaching? *Journal of General Internal Medicine, 31*(9), 1092-1096. http://dx.doi.org/10.1007/s11606-016-3722-2

Tofade, T., Elsner, J., & Haines, S. T. (2013). Best practice strategies for effective use of questions as a teaching tool. *American Journal of Pharmaceutical Education, 77*(7), Article 155.

Whitman College. (2014). Lincoln-Douglas format and sample resolutions [PDF document]. https://www.whitman.edu/Documents/Academics/Debate/WNDI_LD_Starter_Kit_2014_v2.pdf

11

CONCEPT MAPPING

Whitney Henderson, OTD, MOT, OTR/L

BASIC TENETS

Concept mapping provides a powerful illustration of meaningful learning; students retrieve prior knowledge and connect new knowledge with these existing cognitive structures. By nature, individuals think in concepts and learn through written or spoken symbols. Students begin developing new knowledge by first understanding or observing the concepts they already possess. In other words, the knowledge the students have prior to implementation of a concept map provides the fuel for new learning. As students identify key concepts from new information, they connect this knowledge to prior knowledge by linking relevant ideas.

A concept map possesses several key components. A *concept* is defined as an event or object and is enclosed in a circle or box. The concept is designated by a *label*. In concept map literature, a label can also be called a *node*. Two or more concepts are connected by a *link* to demonstrate a relationship with a line or arrow. These connections create a *proposition* that represents a meaningful phrase. Another key feature of a concept map is the use of *cross-links*. Cross-links are relationships or links between concepts in different portions of the concept map. This feature allows students to understand relationships in different parts of their maps. A final concept map includes a framework of propositions that provides a schematic summary of what the student has learned (Figure 11-1).

In Figure 11-2, "adolescent obesity," "health," "occupations," "interventions," "individuals," "families," and "communities" are examples of concepts represented by labels (nodes), and "influences," "impacts," "of," and "with" are examples of links. The links that form the proposition, "adolescent obesity addressed by interventions with individuals," becomes a meaningful phrase. We can further expand the concept map by adding various interventions under individual, families, or communities. Those interventions can be cross-linked to occupations in the other portion of the map.

Henderson, W. (Ed.). *Effective Teaching: Instructional Methods and Strategies for Occupational Therapy Education* (pp. 265-286). © 2021 Taylor & Francis Group.

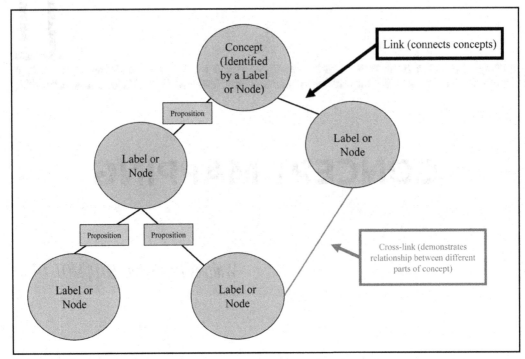

Figure 11-1. Components of a concept map.

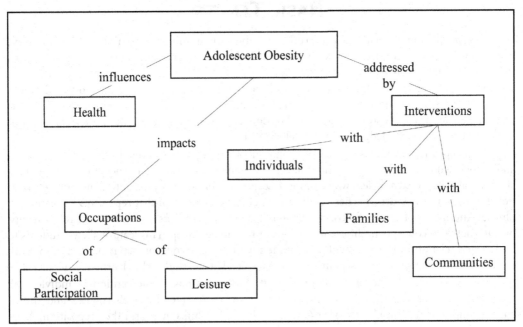

Figure 11-2. Example of a concept map.

BACKGROUND

Concept mapping is a schematic representation of a set of ideas that are linked in some way to form meaningful phrases. In the 1960s and 1970s, Professor Joseph Novak at Cornell University created concept mapping to understand students' knowledge before and after instruction on a topic. However, he quickly learned that a concept map could also foster meaningful learning (instead of traditional rote learning) and began to investigate the use of this instructional method with junior high students engaged in science coursework. By the early 1980s, this instructional method emerged in mathematics and science courses in higher education and became widely used across the world by the turn of the next decade. Novak (1990) reported concept maps can be used for **any** domain of knowledge. Currently, educators in higher education use concept mapping in a variety of ways: (1) as an instructional method in lectures, group discussions, and laboratory experiences; (2) to guide curricular development; or (3) to assess student learning. Educational literature also suggests that concept mapping can bridge the gap between theory and application of knowledge to practice when implemented in clinical education programs, such as occupational therapy.

THEORY

Novak (1998) developed concept mapping using David Ausubel's Assimilation Theory of Learning. He devoted considerable time and effort to understand Ausubel's work. Therefore, you will notice profound similarities between concept mapping and the Assimilation Theory of Learning. As stated in its name, the central idea of Ausubel's theory is *meaningful learning*. Meaningful learning requires three conditions:

> When students engage in meaningful learning, they use some of the same cells that already store information similar to the new knowledge.

1. The new material should be clear and presented in ways that relate to a relevant portion of the student's existing cognitive structure (e.g., what the student already knows).
2. The student must have relevant prior knowledge.
3. The student must choose to engage in meaningful learning (e.g., motivation).

Novak believed concept mapping was a powerful tool to engage students in meaningful learning because it provides a template or scaffold to help them organize and structure information. Novak and his colleagues wanted to find better ways to represent what the student knew and developed a method to operationalize the stages of meaningful learning. Ausubel (1963) outlined three stages students use concepts to engage in meaningful learning: (1) subsumption, (2) progressive differentiation, and (3) integrative reconciliation (Table 11-1). In these various stages, students actively engage with content as they organize and interpret information and further compare, contrast, and synthesize the information to produce a final product.

In addition, Ausubel made important contributions about differences between reception and discovery approaches to instruction. In *reception learning*, the educator presents all the content to the students in final form, and the students internalize the information, so that they can use the information at a later date. Students do not engage in independent discovery in this type of learning. In the current higher education landscape, educators would relate this type of learning to the instructional method of lecturing. Discovery learning is quite different than reception learning. In *discovery learning*, students independently identify concepts and discover the learning material for internalization. They must rearrange new information, integrate this information with existing cognitive structures, and reorganize the new combination to create some sort of end product (e.g., what students do when concept mapping). Ausubel (1963) reported that "…everyday problems of living are solved through discovery learning" (p. 17). In addition, concept mapping facilitates flexibility, decision making, and critical thinking, making this type of learning ideal for health professional education.

TABLE 11-1

Summary of Relationship Between Theory and Concept Mapping

STAGE	DEFINITION (According to Ausubel's Assimilation Theory of Meaningful Learning)	REPRESENTATION IN CONCEPT MAPPING
1. Subsumption	Provides base for linking new information to prior knowledge; when being linked, the new concept and stored information are slightly modified.	Student identifies concepts to answer the focus question or topic; begins to rank concepts and place lower-order concepts under higher-order concepts.
2. Progressive Differentiation	Continues to analyze and refine meanings of concepts; gives concepts more accuracy and specificity.	Student continues to create hierarchal structure of concept map; begins to ask questions about relationships between concepts.
3. Integrative Reconciliation	Recognizes new relationships in existing cognitive structure; synthesizes and integrates information together, forming a meaningful learning set.	Student links concepts together with lines and words to form meaning; looks for connections in various parts of map.

Adapted from Daley, B. J., & Torre, D. M. (2010). Concept maps in medical education: An analytical literature review. *Medical Education, 44,* 440-448; Novak, J. D. (1998). *Learning, creating, and using knowledge: Concept maps as facilitative tools in schools and corporations.* Routledge Taylor & Francis Group.

IMPLEMENTATION

Educators can use various approaches to introduce students to concept mapping. Similar to other ways of teaching, there is no best way for educators to introduce this instructional method. However, we use literature to provide a framework for implementation of concept mapping with your students.

Step 1: Propose a Focus Question

The educator begins by **proposing a focus question** that students will address in their concept map. A *focus question* is a specific question, problem, or issue that a concept map will help answer. Using the adolescent obesity example from before, we might ask students what types of occupational therapy interventions influence adolescent obesity? You can use your learning objectives to guide your focus question.

Step 2: Create List of Concepts

After identifying the focus question, the educator encourages students to **develop a list of concepts**, so the students become aware of the knowledge they already possess. For example, ask the students to:

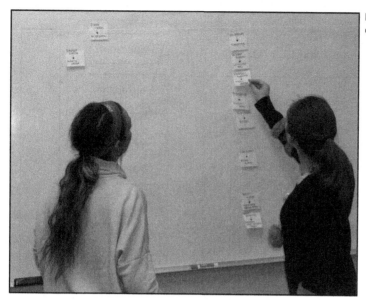

Figure 11-3. Students write concepts on sticky notes.

- Make a list of familiar words or objects related to the question or topic
- Select key words from a meaningful article or paragraph
- Describe what they think of when they think about an experience (i.e., observation or fieldwork experiences) related to the topic

Typically, a list of 15 to 25 concepts will be sufficient for students to construct their concept maps. Remember, the concepts are typically one to three words. The students can write each concept on a piece of paper, whiteboard, or computer. We like the use of sticky notes so students can continuously rearrange the concepts on a wall or whiteboard in later steps of concept mapping (Figure 11-3). The educator can also encourage students to use photos or pictures to represent concepts, which further taps into their creativity and motivation. For the question about types of adolescent obesity, students might write consultation, physical activity, nutrition, or education.

> How you ask the question or foster the development of the list of concepts fuels student motivation, an important factor for meaningful learning.

Write down three additional ways you could help the students create a list of concepts.

Step 3: Rank Concepts

After students create a list, they begin to **rank each concept**. The concepts that are broad are ranked higher than the concepts that are more specific. The students store the ranked concepts in the *parking lot* until they fit each one into their map (Figure 11-4). In the adolescent obesity example, the students have the concepts education, consultation, physical activity, nutrition, routines, technology, and telehealth ranked in their parking lot. The concepts remain in the parking lot until the students are ready to fit each into their map.

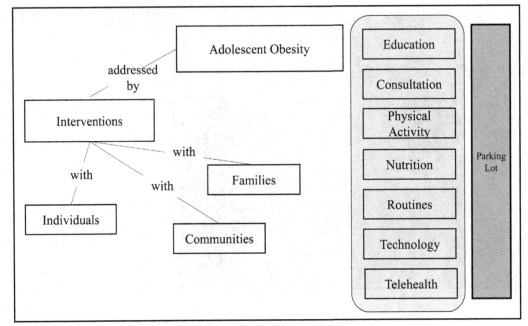

Figure 11-4. Example of a parking lot in concept mapping.

If working in small groups, students might disagree about the rank order of the concepts. The educator should view this conflict as a valuable social learning opportunity and facilitate discussion about the different meanings of a concept. Educators might also need to clarify concepts that are not clearly presented in learning activities in order for the students to negotiate a shared meaning of the concept. During this step, students can add or remove concepts during the ranking process if needed.

Step 4: Construct the Map

> If working in small groups, the educator must watch that everyone is participating!

Once a list of concepts is created, the students can begin to **construct their concept map**. A concept map is typically hierarchically structured with the general, most inclusive concepts at the top. Using their rank order, they place approximately one to three concepts at the top of their map. Students will then place two to four subconcepts under each of their broad concepts and continue placing subconcepts underneath, creating another level of hierarchy until completed. Novak (1998) suggests if there are more than four subconcepts per broader concept, they should consider creating an additional level in the hierarchy.

Step 5: Connect the Concepts

> Students report creating the propositional phrases as the most challenging part of constructing a map!

The students connect concepts with a line and a few linking words to form a proposition that demonstrates a meaningful relationship. When selecting linking words, the educator should instruct students to carefully consider and select these words. Oftentimes two or three words provide valid ways to link concepts; however, each word creates a slightly different meaning to the proposition. Students will want to select linking words that answer the focus question and clearly and accurately communicate the relationship. It may be beneficial to have the focus question in close proximity during this phase.

Step 6: Revise the Concept Map

Lastly, **concept maps must be revised**, as the first draft is certain to have a few imperfections. A majority of educational literature suggests students complete at least two to three revisions. The educator encourages students to continuously revise or redraw the structure of their concept map. During the revision process, students can continue to add, remove, or rearrange concepts and continue to look for clarity of relationships and links in different sections of the map (e.g., cross-links). In this final step, students need to ensure that other individuals can read and understand their concept maps.

ADDITIONAL IMPLEMENTATION NOTES

One exciting feature of this instructional method is that there is no one way to draw a concept map. While some students might struggle with this ambiguity, concept maps can help foster their creativity. As previously discussed, Novak and Gowin (1984) encourage the hierarchal structure of a concept map. However, in some educational literature, you will find the main concept in the center of the map with surrounding subconcepts. This type of map is called a *mind map* and is slightly different than a concept map. However, educators employ steps similar to those previously outlined to facilitate the development of a mind map.

In a traditional concept map, there are not typically arrows on the connecting lines because the hierarchical nature implies the direction of the relationship. If needed, students can add arrows to demonstrate the relationship between the two concepts is primarily in one direction or bidirectional. In addition, when creating a concept map, students have access to several online programs, such as CmapTools (https://cmap.ihmc.us/). They can create a concept map and download for discussion or assignment completion.

Educators can use concept maps in a variety of ways. For example, there are expert-generated versus learner-generated concept maps. In learner-generated concept maps, students fully develop the concept map. In expert-generated, the educator develops a portion and the students finish the concept map. Research supports the use of learner-generated over expert-generated because the students engage in more meaningful learning since they are the ones actually developing the concept map. Similarly, Montpetit-Tourangeau and colleagues (2017) asked two groups of students to interact with a concept map; one group finished the missing parts of an incomplete concept map, and one group simply studied a completed concept map. However, the educator should use caution when using these varied forms because the students might not be fully engaging in meaningful learning.

TIPS AND TRICKS

- Inform students of the purpose and benefits of concept mapping; emphasize it is a learning activity not an "add-on" assignment. Many students initially resist the idea of concept mapping as a learning tool. It could be beneficial for educators to provide a video or discuss evidence supporting use of concept mapping to increase student buy-in.
- Devote class time to show students how to construct a concept map.
- Give clear instructions.
- If first learning to construct a map, pick a domain of knowledge that is very familiar to the students.
- Clearly define how the concept map relates to the learning objective(s).

- Provide an authentic context so students have to solve real-world problems (this assists to provide the motivation for meaningful learning).
- Allow time for students to briefly discuss concept maps.
- Use concept maps even after completion (e.g., apply to another scenario later in the course).
- Consider timing of when this instructional method is introduced (e.g., allow time for students to become familiar with concept mapping, when academic load is lower).

OPPORTUNITIES FOR FEEDBACK AND REFLECTION

In this section, we will provide educators with several strategies they can use to promote student reflection and feedback following the completion of a concept map. First, the educator can facilitate discussion. King and Shell (2002) provide several examples of rich discussion questions, such as:

- What additional information do you need in your concept map (e.g., What is missing?)?
- Explain how [concept A] relates to [concept B].
- How does [concept A] influence [concept B]?
- Where are your gaps in knowledge or what do you need to learn more about?
- How can you use the concept map to guide your occupational therapy practice?

The educator can ask additional questions to assist students to identify the gaps in their knowledge, such as:

> You can also teach students to ask themselves or each other these questions!

- Is this the only [subconcept] that influences [concept]?
- Have you thought about this [subconcept]?

Similarly, the educator can ask "what if" questions. We will return to our example about adolescent obesity. Perhaps in their concept maps, the students identified social factors that influence adolescent obesity. The educator asks, "If you were to create a YouTube video about healthy eating behaviors and physical activity, what impact would this intervention have on adolescent obesity?" The students could review their concept map to determine how the subconcept of media influences other areas in their concept map, so they can truly understand the impact of their intervention.

One last strategy the educator can implement is to simply ask the student(s) to explain their concept map (Figure 11-5). They can either explain their map to the educator or discuss and compare their concept map with a peer in the class. In their study with social workers and mental health nurses, Bressington and colleagues (2011) reported that participants found concept maps useful for reflecting on what they learned, and that reflecting increased their confidence and ability to challenge their own practice. Similarly, in another study, a group of students that created concept maps and discussed in teams with feedback from peers and the instructor experienced more improvements in problem solving than students that created concept maps without feedback.

What other questions can you ask or ideas can you use to facilitate discussion and reflection of a concept map?

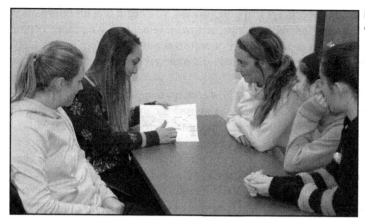

Figure 11-5. Student explains a concept map.

APPLICATION TO OCCUPATIONAL THERAPY PRACTICE

Similar to educators' use of students' prior knowledge, occupational therapy practitioners should attempt to understand their clients' prior knowledge and what information they are acquiring during the teaching-learning process. In occupational therapy practice, concept mapping can serve as a valuable tool to **link newly acquired knowledge to previous knowledge** when implementing education, or be used to reveal and discuss emotional factors that influence one's cognitive thought processes. We will outline two examples of how occupational therapy practitioners can use concept mapping with the clients and families they serve in their everyday practice.

Example 1: Implementation During Client Education

Perhaps you are working with a client or a group of clients to provide education on pain management strategies. Therefore, the central concept is pain. You ask your client(s) to freely write words that the concept of pain evokes. You implement the steps previously outlined, and the client ranks the various words and begins to create links and propositions between the words (i.e., concepts). Next, you implement patient education regarding strategies for reducing and managing pain. You might even modify your patient education materials (if time) depending on what the client(s) already knows and places on the map. You then ask the client(s) to complete the concept map an additional time without reviewing the first one. As you review the second concept map, you gain information about what the client learned (i.e., which concepts became more accurate or specific, which concepts remained stable, or what changes occurred in relationships between concepts).

Example 2: Facilitate Discussion and Understanding of Emotional Responses

Occupational therapy practitioners working in inpatient or community-based mental health practice settings can use concept mapping to understand their clients' experiences. For example, you can ask a focus question, such as:

- "What words or sentences describe a good day?"
- "What important changes do you notice in your life when you are feeling well?"
- "What words or sentences describe good care?"

As you guide the client through the concept mapping process, you begin to gain information about health care use, social supports and relationships, self-management of symptoms, coping strategies, feelings, and expectations. You can ask further questions about the concept map to identify areas of needs and strengths and define treatment goals and intervention strategies. In turn, the client engages in reflection.

Wilson and Mandich (2018) provide an example of how concept mapping can be used in occupational therapy practice. In their feasibility study, they examined the use of concept mapping in combination with the Cognitive Orientation to Daily Occupational Performance approach with 10 adolescents with autism. The participants completed a training session on how to use software to develop their concept maps with Cognitive Orientation to Daily Occupational Performance. They broke down a task (goal) and developed a plan via concept mapping before executing and checking their plan. After checking their plan, the participants made changes to their concept maps. Several of the participants provided qualitative feedback about the value of concept mapping.

Advantages

- Used for any topic and in a variety of learning contexts
- Completed individually, in small groups, or as a class
- Implemented with all developmental levels (studies with children as young as first grade)
- Used multiple ways (instructional method, outcome measure, outline for a paper)
- Involves high-level and low-level cognitive process (students must remember basic facts but also evaluate and compare concepts)
- Allows educator to understand what their students already know
- Allows educator and students to discuss and debate meanings
- Facilitates reflection of the learning process
- Students can improve concept mapping abilities with practice
- Fun and interactive
- Can display maps for further discussion and reflection
- Allows students to reduce comprehensive information
- Literature provides quantitative methods for scoring concept maps
- Ability to use as an outcome measure to demonstrate change in learning

Challenges

- Educators require resources to be good facilitators of concept mapping
- Potential for student resistance and engagement (particularly if they have been engaged in rote learning)
- Initially, educator must thoughtfully design activities and provide guidance and training to teach novice concept mappers the technique
- Requires practice to develop quality concept maps
- Requires time to complete task and for mastery
- Educator must determine what competencies the concept map will develop or address
- Difficult to determine what are the main characteristics of an excellent concept map (i.e., size, quality)

In the space below, list any additional advantages or challenges.

Brainstorm strategies for overcoming these challenges when implementing the use of a concept map.

THREE THINGS YOU CAN DO TOMORROW TO IMPLEMENT CONCEPT MAPPING WITH YOUR STUDENTS

1. Search for a video about concept mapping to help introduce the idea to your students.
2. Think of one topic in your course that students could create a concept map for.
3. Create an account with an online concept mapping program.

Concept Mapping Evidence Table

Author/Year	Study Objectives	Design and Participants	Intervention and Outcome Measures	Results
Bixler et al. (2015)	Researchers aimed to determine if small group concept mapping improved the critical thinking of medical students	Design: Nonexperimental pilot study; pre/posttest single group design Participants: 27 senior medical students in a neonatal elective course	Intervention: Researchers provided a 1-hour introduction to concept mapping. They divided students into groups of 4 to 6 members. The students constructed 4 maps in class during a 4-week course. They also completed readings prior to class Outcome measures: • California Critical Thinking Disposition Inventory (CCTDI) • California Critical Thinking Skills Test (CCTST) • Knowledge via test (multiple choice) • Survey	Students increased scores from pre to posttest, an average of 35% on knowledge test Students demonstrated no significant differences on the CCTST score from pre to posttest. Students scored high on pretest Student scores strong on CCTDI, particularly in areas of inquisitiveness and confidence in reasoning 63% of students felt concept mapping was easy to use, but only 42% reported this method provided a deeper understanding of a topic A majority (57.9%) reported concept mapping required too much time and 68.4% reported preferences for didactic lectures versus concept mapping
Daley & Torre (2010)	Researchers review literature on the use of concept maps as an instructional method for medical students Researchers discussed implications for the teaching and learning in medical education and provided direction for future research on use of concept mapping in medical education	Design: An analytical literature review Participants: Health professional students	Literature search between 1989 and 2009 Searched: Academic Search, Education Resources Information Center (ERIC), EBSCOhost, PsycINFO, PsycArticles, PubMed, MedLine, CINAHL, Embase Inclusion of 35 articles 2 researchers reviewed each paper and grouped papers into 4 themes	Of the 35 articles, 16 occurred in medical education, 13 in nursing education, 2 in veterinary education, and 1 in dentistry education In medical education, the 4 functions of concepts maps include: • Promotes meaningful learning • Provides additional resource for learning • Allows educator to provide feedback to students • Assesses learning and performance

(continued)

Concept Mapping Evidence Table (continued)

Author/Year	Study Objectives	Design and Participants	Intervention and Outcome Measures	Results
				Majority of articles suggest concept mapping facilitates meaningful learning, critical thinking, and problem solving
				Concept maps can be a useful resource, but more research is needed
				Growing body of evidence that concept maps can be used to provide students feedback and as an assessment strategy in medical education
				Found no studies that a concept map had a detrimental effect in medical education
Grice (2016)	The researcher investigated the use of concept mapping in 2 courses on students' perception and attitudes	Design: Posttest survey design Participants: 37 first-year occupational therapy students in biomechanics course and 32 second-year students in a hand orthopedic unit of a biomechanics process course	Intervention: First-year students created a concept map on anatomical areas of elbow, forearm, wrist, hand, hip, and knee Second-year students created a concept map on 5 different injuries or pathologies; the researcher provided students with a list of 10 to select from The researcher provided an example of a map and resources for map completion Outcome measures: • Rubric • Survey	Approximately 97% of students completed the survey Students reported the aspects of a concept that had the greatest impact on learning was the way it assisted to organize and access information and assisted to comprehend the material Students believed concept maps required them to dig deeply into course material and required them to think more about the information

(continued)

Concept Mapping Evidence Table (continued)

Author/Year	Study Objectives	Design and Participants	Intervention and Outcome Measures	Results
Hsu et al. (2016)	Researchers aimed to demonstrate differences in competency, cognitive load, and learning satisfaction with nursing students enrolled in a neurological care course	Design: 2-group pre and posttest experimental study Participants: 213 sophomore nursing students in the medical or surgical portion of the curriculum 2 of the 4 groups randomly assigned to experimental or control group	Interventions: Each group of students completed 12 hours of education separately (4 hours were laboratory experiences) Control group: Objective-based training Experimental group: Use of concept map for outcome-based training Outcome measures: • Survey • Competency Inventory of Nursing Students • Cognitive Load Scale of Neurological Nursing • Learning Satisfaction Scale of Neurological Nursing • Concept Map Scoring Scale	Each group of students demonstrated increased nursing competency scores from pre to posttest. Researchers found no significant differences between the 2 groups at posttest. The experimental group demonstrated lower mean cognitive load scores and higher mean learning satisfaction scores than the control group
Jaafarpour et al. (2016)	Researchers assessed the impact of concept mapping in academic achievement with nursing students	Design: Quasi-experimental, crossover design Participants: 64 nursing students (freshmen); students divided into 2 groups of 32 students	Intervention: Group A constructed a content map of the course content for each class. Group B completed multiple-choice quizzes about the content of each class. Each group engaged in 8 weeks of lecture on fundamentals of nursing After 8 weeks, the students participated in the other method Outcome measures: • Cumulative test (at week 8 and week 16) • Concept map scores • Questionnaire (student perception; 2 times)	In each phase, the group that completed the concept map scored higher on cumulative tests than the quiz group As the course progressed, students received higher scores on concept maps The highest score on the questionnaire related to the students' belief that the concept map was a time-consuming activity, and the lowest score related to the students' belief that sharing concept maps helped address misunderstandings

(continued)

Concept Mapping Evidence Table (continued)

Author/Year	Study Objectives	Design and Participants	Intervention and Outcome Measures	Results
Montpetit-Tourangeau et al. (2017)	Researchers compared effectiveness of concept map study versus concept map completion on meaningful learning of physical therapy intervention Researchers compared concept map study and concept map completion between novice and advanced learners Researchers compared cognitive load of a concept map study versus concept map completion and compared cognitive load of a posttest used to assess learning between the 2 groups	Design: Randomized controlled trial (RCT; 2x2 factorial design) Randomly assigned to concept map completion or concept map study Participants: 61 second-year physical therapy students in Canada	Students attended 3-hour course on concept mapping Concept map study: Study a completed concept map Concept map completion: Students completed the missing parts of an incomplete map 3 phases: • Pretest at start and 5 months later (ability to problem solve 4 clinical cases entailing a movement disorder) • 130 minutes of guided learning (80-minute online session with examples and activities related to concept mapping and 50-minute posttest) • 4-week self study (online access to learning materials and 50-minute delayed posttest) Outcome measures: • Pre and posttests • Rating Scale Mental Effort	Students in the concept map completion group demonstrated higher scores than the participants in the concept map study group on near and far transfer Students in the concept map study condition demonstrated higher conceptual knowledge at immediate posttest; however, on delayed posttest, there was not a difference between the 2 groups on conceptual knowledge Results demonstrated a significant effect on prior ability (novice versus advanced) and learning condition (concept map study or concept map completion) on conceptual knowledge but not near or far transfer
Mukherjee et al. (2018)	Researchers investigated the effectiveness of concept mapping on test scores and utility of concept mapping with pharmacy students	Design: Cross-sectional pre/posttest Participants: 47 third-year pharmacy students	Intervention: Researchers provided students handout on concept mapping. The students practiced in groups. Students completed concept map on pain management topic	64% of students reported they are visual learners on survey Students demonstrated improvements on 8 of the 10 questions from pre to posttest. Students improved from 62% on pretest to 70% on posttest (neither statistically significant)

(continued)

Concept Mapping Evidence Table (continued)

Author/Year	Study Objectives	Design and Participants	Intervention and Outcome Measures	Results
			Outcome measures: • Test (10 multiple-choice questions; pre/posttest) • Survey (posttest)	Majority of students (92%) reported concept mapping was effective method for improving learning. 55% reported learning most when they discussed and created maps. 38% of students reported the greatest challenge in organizing concept map
Pudelko et al. (2012)	Researchers explored literature to determine benefits of concept mapping on student learning in health professional education Researchers analyzed the methods used in concept mapping research Researchers focused on articles that researchers used concept mapping as a teaching and learning strategy	Design: Critical analysis Participants: Health professional students	Literature search between 2000 and 2011 Searched: MedLine, EBSCOhost, Academic Search Inclusion of 65 articles 2 coders reviewed each paper in 4 phases	24 of the 65 articles were theoretical; 41 of 65 studies were empirical studies • 31 of the 41 studies were pre-experimental • Other 10 articles between quasi-experimental and experimental 62% of the articles published in nursing education; 14% in medical education Majority of articles approached concept mapping using Novak's or Buzan's theory 40% of papers used concept mapping to develop care plans Educators reported using concept mapping to promote meaningful learning or critical thinking In majority of articles, educators combined concept mapping with other instructional methods Majority of students appreciated concept mapping; some articles reported students would not use in future because too difficult and time-consuming

(continued)

Concept Mapping Evidence Table (continued)

Author/Year	Study Objectives	Design and Participants	Intervention and Outcome Measures	Results
				3 studies reported improvements in problem solving for students engaged in concept mapping versus traditional teaching
Radwan et al. (2018)	Researchers explored relationship between concept mapping scores and clinical reasoning skills with medical students	Design: Cross-sectional analytical Participants: 55 sixth-year medical students (pediatric content)	Intervention: Researchers provided a workshop to inform students on the concept mapping process. Students completed concept maps during the first session. Researchers scored the concept maps. During the second session, students completed the script concordance test (SCT) on pediatrics Outcome measures: • Concept map scores • SCT	Students scored an average of 37.2% on the SCT There was a statistically significant correlation between mean concept map scores and total scores on SCT
Sargolzaie et al. (2019)	Researchers evaluated the effect of concept mapping on medical students' knowledge of rabies prophylaxis	Design: Cross-sectional, pre/posttest survey design; 2 groups Participants: 80 medical interns; 40 students per group	Intervention: Researchers trained group 1 with concept maps Researchers trained group 2 with readings An educator provided lecture to each group Outcome measures: Questionnaire (researcher developed to assess knowledge)	There was no statistical difference between the 2 groups on pretest scores Posttest scores of both groups significantly increased, but the mean scores of the 2 groups were significantly higher in the concept map group
Si et al. (2019)	Researchers investigated how the argumentation of a concept map during problem-based learning (PBL) impacts medical students' clinical reasoning skills	Design: Cross-sectional; pre/posttest design; 2 groups Participants: 95 first- and second-year medical students	Intervention: Researchers randomly assigned students to PBL groups of 7 to 8 members Students constructed concept maps related to the case according to Toulmin's structure of arguments and presented to the group. Researchers followed with brief lecture	Second-year students demonstrated significantly higher posttest scores on the Quality of Individual Arguments (no difference between 2 posttests) First-year students demonstrated significantly higher posttest scores on the Quality of Individual Arguments and significantly higher scores on posttest 2 versus posttest 1

(continued)

Concept Mapping Evidence Table (continued)

Author/Year	Study Objectives	Design and Participants	Intervention and Outcome Measures	Results
			Outcome measures: (3 times—before, after first PBL session, after second PBL session) • Individual problem-solving test • Assessment of the quality of arguments • Assessment of clinical problem-solving performance • Concept map presentation rubric	Second-year and first-year students demonstrated significantly higher scores on posttest 1 from pretest on problem-solving performance and significantly higher scores on posttest 2 versus posttest 1 Second-year students demonstrated significantly higher mean scores than first-year students at posttest 1 and posttest 2
Torre et al. (2017)	Researchers evaluated medical students' perceptions of the value of group concept mapping and examined how group concept mapping constructed and organized knowledge	Design: Posttest survey design Participants: 39 fourth-year medical students	Intervention: Researchers assigned students into 3 or 4 members per group to complete a concept map during their 1-month medicine rotation. An educator provided an introduction to concept mapping and computerized program at the start of the rotation The students completed the concept map on a clinical scenario. They constructed the concept map, sent to the group, made edits, and sent to educator. Each group determined how they collectively developed the map. Students presented maps at the end of their rotation Outcome measures: • Questionnaire • Evaluation of concept map	95% of medical students completed the questionnaire More than half of students made changes to the concept map that another student constructed 89% of students found value in feedback from the group 81% of students felt the concept map was useful for helping them understand important relationships and concepts with 72% suggesting maps facilitated learning integration of basic and professional concepts Students reported challenges in learning concept mapping software and inability to make changes while working with other members of the group Students made maps with a range of 41 to 192 concepts with a median of 67.5 concepts

(continued)

Concept Mapping Evidence Table (continued)

Author/Year	Study Objectives	Design and Participants	Intervention and Outcome Measures	Results
Tseng et al. (2011)	Researchers measured short- and long-term changes in registered nursing students' competencies after applying a PBL concept mapping during a course	Design: Quasi-experimental design (nonequivalent experimental and control groups); longitudinal Participants: 120 registered nursing students; 51 in experimental group and 69 in control group	Experimental group: Researchers divided the 51 students into 4 PBL groups Students enrolled in 3-credit-hour course, which included introduction to PBL and application of concept mapping (spent 42 hours in PBL and concept mapping) Control group did not take course Outcome measures: • Demographic inventory • Critical thinking scale (CTS) • Self-Directed Learning Readiness Scale • Students' performance in PBL tutorial sessions questionnaire Researchers collected data 3 times; before course, immediately following course, and 6 months after course	Students in the control group reported higher scores on the CTS, Self-Directed Learning Readiness Scale, and PBL tutorial sessions questionnaire than the experimental group at pretest However, the scores of the experimental group were significantly higher at immediate posttest and 6-month posttest than the control group. Students in the experiential group demonstrated significant growth at posttest data points suggesting long-term effect on competencies related to critical thinking and self-directed learning
Vadlapatla et al. (2014)	Researchers evaluated pharmacy students' perceptions of a new concept mapping assignment	Design: Posttest survey Participants: 46 first-year pharmacy students	Intervention: Researchers created concept map assignment to assist students to understand connection between dosages Each student designed 2 concept maps; 1 was an individual, and 1 was a group. Students could use any format for concept map (online tool, hand-drawn, etc.) Outcome measures: • Survey (9 questions) • Concept map grade	Researchers gave an average grade of 3.9 out of 4 More than 90% of students agreed or strongly agreed concept maps enhanced ability to learn conceptual topics, reinforced content, and challenged intellect

(continued)

Concept Mapping Evidence Table (continued)

Author/Year	Study Objectives	Design and Participants	Intervention and Outcome Measures	Results
Yue et al. (2017)	Researchers investigated effectiveness of concept mapping on development of critical thinking in nursing education	Design: Systematic review and meta-analysis Participants: Total sample size; 1,204 participants (nursing students or nursing clinicians in continuing education)	Literature search between 1998 and 2016 Searched: PubMed, Web of Science, Embase, CENTRAL, CINAHL, CNKI Inclusion criteria: • RCT or non-RCT with comparison study • Participants included nursing students or nurses in continuing education • Intervention was concept mapping • Outcome measure included critical thinking • Reported sample size, mean difference and confidence interval of critical thinking scores 2 researchers independently reviewed each article 13 studies included for qualitative analysis and 11 studies included for meta-analysis Outcome measures: • CCTDI • CCTST • CTS	Researchers used CCTDI in 7 studies; results of meta-analysis indicated concept mapping had significant effect on critical thinking, particularly affective dispositions (open-mindedness, truth-seeking, analyticity, systematicity, self-confidence, inquisitiveness, and maturity) Researchers used the CCTST in 3 studies; the overall score of critical thinking was higher in the intervention group versus the control group Researchers used the CTS in 2 studies; the overall score of critical thinking was higher in the intervention group versus the control group

Adapted from American Occupational Therapy Association. (2002). AOTA's evidence-based literature review project: An overview (D. Lieberman & J. Scheer, Eds.). American Journal of Occupational Therapy, 56, 344-349. https://doi.org/10.5014/ajot.56.3.344

REFERENCES

American Occupational Therapy Association. (2002). AOTA's evidence-based literature review project: An overview (D. Lieberman & J. Scheer, Eds.). *The American Journal of Occupational Therapy, 56,* 344-349. https://doi.org/10.5014/ajot.56.3.344

Ausubel, D. P. (1963). *The psychology of meaningful verbal learning.* Grune & Stratton.

Bixler, M. G., Brown, A., Way, D., Ledford, C., & Mahan, J. D. (2015). Collaborative concept mapping and critical thinking in fourth-year medical students. *Clinical Pediatrics, 54*(9), 883-839. http://dx.doi.org/10.1177/0009922815590223

Bressington, D. T., Wells, H., & Graham, M. (2011). A concept mapping exploration of social workers' and mental health nurses' understanding of the role of the approved mental health professional. *Nurse Education Today, 31,* 564-570.

Daley, B. J., & Torre, D. M. (2010). Concept maps in medical education: An analytical literature review. *Medical Education, 44,* 440-448.

Grice, K. (2016). Concept mapping as a learning tool in occupational therapy education. *Occupational Therapy in Health Care, 30*(3), 309-318. http://dx.doi.org/10.3109/07380577.2015.1130886

Hsu, L. L., Pan, H. C., & Hsieh, S. I. (2016). Randomized comparison between objective-based lectures and outcome-based concept mapping for teaching neurological care to nursing students. *Nurse Education Today, 37,* 83-90. http://dx.doi.org/10.1016/j.nedt.2015.11.032

Jaafarpour, M., Aazami, S., & Mozafari, M. (2016). Does concept mapping enhance learning outcome of nursing students? *Nurse Education Today, 36,* 129-132. http://dx.doi.org/10.1016/j.nedt.2015.08.029

King, M., & Shell, R. (2002). Critical thinking strategies: Teaching and evaluating critical thinking with concept maps. *Nurse Educator, 27*(5), 214-216.

Montpetit-Tourangeau, K., Omer Dyer, J., Hudon, A., Windsor, M., Charlin, B., Mamede, S., & van Gog, T. (2017). Fostering clinical reasoning in physiotherapy: Comparing the effects of concept map study and concept map completion after example study in novice and advanced learners. *BMC Medical Education, 17*(238), 1-23. http://dx.doi.org/10.1186/s12909-017-1076-z

Mukherjee, S. M., Cabrera, A., & Silva, M. A. (2018). Evaluation of group concept mapping during advanced pharmacy practice experiences. *Currents in Pharmacy Teaching and Learning, 10,* 1616-1623. https://doi.org/10.1016/j.cptl.2018.09.009

Novak, J. D., & Gowin, D. B. (1984). *Learning how to learn.* Cambridge University Press.

Novak, J. D. (1990). Concept maps and vee diagrams: Two metacognitive tools to facilitate meaningful learning. *Instructional Science, 19,* 29-52.

Novak, J. D. (1998). *Learning, creating, and using knowledge: Concept maps as facilitative tools in schools and corporations.* Routledge Taylor & Francis Group.

Pudelko, B., Young, M., Vincent-Lamarre, P., & Charlin, B. (2012). Mapping as a learning strategy in health professions education: A critical analysis. *Medical Education, 46,* 1215-1225.

Radwan, A., Nasser, A. A., Araby, S. E., & Talaat, W. (2018). Correlation between assessment of concept maps construction and the clinical reasoning ability of final year medical students at the faculty of medicine, Suex Canal University, Egypt. *Education in Medicine Journal, 10*(4),43-51. http://dx.doi.org/10.21315/eimj2018.10.4.5

Sargolzaie, N., Sargazi, S., & Lotfi, G. (2019). Concept mapping as a tool to improve medical students' learning about rabies surveillance. *Journal of Education and Health Promotion, 8*(132). http://dx.doi.org/10.4103/jehp.jehp_132_18

Si, J., Kong, H. H., & Lee, S. H. (2019). Developing clinical reasoning through argumentation with concept map method in medical problem-solving. *The Interdisciplinary Journal of Problem-Based Learning, 13*(1), 1-16. http://dx.doi.org/10.7771/1541-5015.1776

Torre, D., Daley, B. J., Picho, K., & Durning, S. J. (2017). Group concept mapping: an approach to explore group knowledge organization and collaborative learning in senior medical students. *Medical Teacher, 39*(10), 1051-1056.

Tseng, H. C., Chou, F. H., Wang, H. H., Ko, H. K., Jian, S. Y., & Weng, W. C. (2011). The effectiveness of problem-based learning and concept mapping among Taiwanese registered nursing students. *Nurse Education Today, 31,* e41-e46. http://dx.doi.org/10.1016/j.nedt.2010.11.020

Vadlapatla, R., Kaur, S., & Zhao, Y. (2014). Evaluation of student perceptions of concept mapping activity in a didactic pharmaceutics course. *Currents in Pharmacy Teaching and Learning, 6,* 543-549. http://dx.doi.org/10.1016/j.cptl.2014.04.014

Wilson, J., & Mandich, A. (2018). Concept mapping and the CO-OP approach with adolescents with Autism Spectrum Disorder: Exploring participant experiences. *Open Journal of Occupational Therapy, 6*(4), Article 3. http://dx.doi.org/10.15453/2168-6408.1455

Yue, M., Zhang, M., Zhang, C., & Jin, C. (2017). The effectiveness of concept mapping on development of critical thinking in nursing education: A systematic review and meta-analysis. *Nursing Education Today, 52,* 87-94. http://dx.doi.org/10.1016/j.nedt.2017.02.018

Bibliography

Aguiar, J. G., & Correia, P. R. M. (2017). From representing to modelling knowledge: Proposing a two-step training for excellence in concept mapping. *Knowledge Management & E-Learning, 9*(3), 366-379.

Chiu, C. H., & Lin, C. L. (2012). Sequential pattern analysis: Method and application in exploring how students develop concept maps. *The Turkish Online Journal of Educational Technology, 11*(1), 145-153.

Daley, B. J., Morgan, S., & Black, S. B. (2016). Concept maps in nursing education: A historical literature review and research directions. *Journal of Nursing Education, 55*(11), 631-639. http://dx.doi.org/10.3928/01484834-20161011-05

Daley, B. J., Shaw., C. R., Balistrieri, T., Glasenapp, K., & Piacentine, L. (1999). Concept maps: A strategy to teach and evaluate critical thinking. *Journal of Nursing Education, 38*, 42-47.

Daugherty, J. L., & Dixon, R. A. (2012). Mapping concepts for learning and assessment. *Technology and Engineering Teacher, 71*(8), 10-14.

Franca, S., d'Ivernois, J. F., Marchand, C., Haenni, C., Ybarra, J., & Golay, A. (2004). Evaluation of nutritional education using concept mapping. *Patient Education and Counseling, 52*(2), 183-192.

Hung, C. H., & Lin, C. Y. (2015). Using concept mapping to evaluate knowledge structure in problem-based learning. *BMC Medical Education, 15*(1), 212. http://dx.doi.org/10.1186/s12909-015-0496-x

Kinchin, I. M. (2014). Concept mapping as a learning tool in higher education: A critical analysis of recent reviews. *The Journal of Continuing Higher Education, 62*, 39-49. http://dx.doi.org/10.1080/07377363.2014.872011

Klem, S., van Broeckhuysen-Kloth, S., van Vliet, S., Oosterhuis, L., & Geenen, R. (2018). Personalized treatment outcomes in patients with somatoform disorder: A concept mapping study. *Journal of Psychomatic Research, 109*, 19-24. https://doi.org/10.1016/j.jpsychores.2018.03.009

Laight, D. W. (2004). Attitudes to concept maps as a teaching/learning activity in undergraduate health professional education: Influence of preferred learning style. *Medical Teacher, 26*(3), 229-233.

Langlois, M. A. (2004). Using concept mapping to promote coordinated school health programs. *Journal of School Health, 74*(3), 105-107.

Liese, B. S., & Esterline, K. M. (2015). Concept mapping: A supervision strategy for introducing case conceptualization skills to novice therapists. *Psychotherapy, 52*(2), 190-194.

Mok, C. K. F., Whitehill, T. L., & Dodd, B. J. (2014). Concept map analysis in the assessment of speech-language pathology students' learning in problem-based learning curriculum: A longitudienal study. *Clinical Linguistics & Phonestics, 28*(1-2), 83-101. http://dx.doi.org/10.3109/02699206.2013.807880

Novak, J. D., & Canas, A. J. (2008). The theory underlying concept maps and how to construct and use them [PDF document]. Technical Report IHMC Cmap Tools, Florida Institute for Human and Machine Cognition. Retrieved from https://cmap.ihmc.us/docs/theory-of-concept-maps.php

Torre, D. M., Durning, S. J., & Daley, B. J. (2013). Twelve tips for teaching with concept maps in medical education. *Medical Teacher, 35*, 201-208. http://doi.org/10.3109/0142159X.2013.759644

Wilberforce, M., Batten, E., Challis, D., Davies, L., Kelly, M. P., & Roberts, C. (2018). The patient experience in community mental health services for older people: A concept mapping approach to support the development of a new quality measure. *BMC Health Services Research, 18*(1), 461. https://doi.org/10.1186/s12913-018-3231-6

Yeo, C. M. (2014). Concept mapping: A strategy to improve critical thinking. *Singapore Nursing Journal, 41*(3), 2-7.

CASE-BASED INSTRUCTIONAL METHODS

Meredith Gronski, OTD, OTR/L, CLA

BASIC TENETS

Case-based learning (CBL) and *problem-based learning (PBL)* are learner-centered instructional methods that place a problem or scenario at the center of the activity to stimulate acquisition of new knowledge, skills, or attitudes. These instructional methods contextualize learning in authentic scenarios and emphasize problem-solving to support an independent and lifelong learning mindset. CBL and PBL share a common goal of discovery through small group

Additional Names in Literature: project-based learning, integrated learning, patient-centered learning, pathway models

problem solving of a practical case or scenario. However, in PBL, educators employ an *open-inquiry approach* because they serve as facilitators that play a minimal role in the learning process. They allow students to struggle to define the problem, explore related topics, and resolve the presented problem how the small group deems suitable. In CBL, educators provide a slightly more structured *guided-inquiry approach* by sharing the responsibility with the students for creating closure on key learning objectives for each session. The educator guides the students back to the learning objective(s) if they begin to stray. Although CBL and PBL use a structured small group format, these instructional methods differ from cooperative learning (Chapter 8) because of the unique use of a facilitator to develop new understanding through collaboration and problem resolution of contextual case scenarios.

Henderson, W. (Ed.). *Effective Teaching: Instructional Methods and Strategies for Occupational Therapy Education* (pp. 287-316). © 2021 Taylor & Francis Group.

BACKGROUND

In the 1950s, graduate medical education materialized case-based approaches in response to the growing sense that intense didactic lecturing of foundational science courses was ineffective for student learning. Educators found this type of instruction exhausting and were unable to tap into medical students' internal motivation to learn and apply new knowledge and skills. Medical school faculty at McMaster University began a philosophical reconstruction of their entire curriculum when they found their students were able to recite fragmented biomedical knowledge from rote memorization but unable to solve clinical problems during residency training. Therefore, they created a more learner-centered approach that afforded opportunities to incorporate interprofessional learning. In 1969, McMaster University initiated PBL, and later in 1980, Howard Barrow authored the first tutor guidelines grounded on a strong educational and cognitive psychology conceptual framework.

In the mid-1980s, the panel on the General Professional Education of the Physician and College Preparation for Medicine, sponsored by the Association of American Medical Colleges, produced a report making recommendations for changes in medical education to: (1) promote independent problem solving, (2) reduce lecture hours and scheduled class time, and (3) evaluate the ability to learn independently. These recommendations strongly supported the implementation of PBL in medical education and proliferated across other health professional education programs. Medical educators have widely used PBL for more than 60 years and support this instructional method as a means to generate health care professionals better prepared to be problem solvers and lifelong learners. The objectives of this approach include:

- Acquisition of a rich body of deeply understood knowledge
- Development of effective clinical problem-solving skills, self-directed learning, and high-quality interpersonal skills
- Growth of an insatiable curiosity and desire to continually learn

Occupational Therapy Education

Similar to the objectives of PBL, occupational therapy education focuses on obtaining a deep understanding of knowledge, developing high-quality skills, and fostering an internal drive to learn. In the mid-1990s, we note the emergence of PBL in health professional education. Royeen (1995) documents one of the first uses of PBL in occupational therapy education. The author outlines the program's approach to implementing PBL in an effort to transform occupational therapy education to enhance a focus on professional reasoning and clinical reflection. As occupational therapy education grew to focus on professional reasoning skills, educators documented the various types of reasoning students and practitioners use in CBL and PBL instructional methods:

- *Scientific reasoning* is the rational and logical thought process in which a practitioner engages in order to generate a hypothesis about performance limitations and seeks ways to test the clinical hypothesis through assessment practices.
- *Interactive reasoning* is the process of understanding the perspective and experience of another person, such as when a practitioner takes an occupational narrative or completes the occupational profile.
- *Conditional reasoning* is the ability to imagine a variety of opportunities or outcomes for a given clinical scenario. This is the process by which practitioners can envision outcomes in the future for their clients based on their choices of intervention approaches.
- *Pragmatic reasoning* is a practitioner's ability to consider contextual factors (such as reimbursement and client access to transportation) and how they impact daily life and the therapeutic process.

TABLE 12-1				
The Autonomy Continuum for Motivation				
MOTIVATION SOURCE	External rewards or punishments (e.g., quiz grade)	Self-imposed thoughts (e.g., pride, guilt)	Value, importance, enjoyment of a behavior or activity	Activity or behavior is perceived as part of one's self or identity
LOCUS OF CAUSALITY	External locus of control	Somewhat external locus of control	Somewhat internal locus of control	Internal locus of control
Controlled	⟵―――――――――――――――――――――――⟶			Autonomous

Adapted from Niemiec, C. P., & Ryan, R. M. (2009). Autonomy, competence, and relatedness in the classroom: Applying self-determination theory to educational practice. *Theory and Research in Education, 7*(2), 133-144.

Similar to medical education, occupational therapy education has advanced beyond the use of passive didactic lecturing to more integrated active learning strategies, such as CBL and PBL (see Case-Based Learning Instructional Methods Evidence Table).

THEORY

Case-based instructional methods (CBL and PBL) heavily rely on and aim to develop student motivation and autonomy. In *self-determination theory (SDT)*, authors assume that inherent in human nature is the drive to be curious about one's environment and a desire to gain and internalize knowledge and skills. This innate drive to learn is supported or limited by competency, relatedness, and autonomy. An individual's *competency* refers to their self-efficacy or confidence that they can learn and achieve the learning objectives. *Relatedness* refers to an individual's sense of connectedness to the material they are presented to learn. *Autonomy* refers to the individual's sense of control over their own mode and rate of learning.

SDT presents several assumptions about motivation and the mechanisms that drive the innate tendency to seek knowledge and learning. In *intrinsic motivation* (autonomous), individuals behave and perform based on what they find enjoyable, sustainable, or significant in absence of an external reward of incentive. It is important to note that in order to sustain intrinsic motivation, students must feel satisfied in both their level of competence and level of autonomy. In *extrinsic motivation* (controlled), individuals require rewards, punishments, or pressures to drive learning behaviors. An example includes educators using graded assessments (e.g., tests, quizzes, papers), which may create a sense of expectation or stress in students that promotes cramming, examining concepts on a shallow level, or rotely memorizing content. This continuum from internal to external motivation aligns with a student's locus of control or sense of autonomy (Table 12-1).

Through the use of CBL and PBL, educators foster internal motivation and autonomous learning through supported open and guided inquiry approaches integral to these instructional methods. These learner-centered instructional methods inherently promote an internal locus of control and self-regulation of learning by considering views of other individuals, offering opportunity for choice, and expecting students will take greater responsibility for skill and knowledge acquisition.

SDT also suggests an element of relatedness drives a student's motivation to learn. Students inherently want to feel connected to and experience a sense of belonging in their learning environments. In CBL and PBL instructional methods, educators facilitate this element by collaborating with students to establish group structure and function on a foundation of mutual respect from the onset. When students experience the three elements of competency, relatedness, and autonomy, they will expend more academic effort and be more willing to engage in learning activities, which result in high-quality outcomes.

IMPLEMENTATION

Essential Elements of a Good Case Study

Occupational therapy educators use cases to facilitate the application of core knowledge and progression of professional reasoning skills. As students transition to graduate education, they are often focused on memorization and recitation of core concepts and may struggle with grasping the nuances of client scenarios embedded in more complex and authentic contexts. Educators offer a variety of case formats to support diverse learning needs and opportunities. They can also vary the amount and type of details in cases. In some scenarios, educators write cases with limited details, which may be useful to allow students to think critically about potential pathways and outcomes. In other learning scenarios, they create a case with extensive details about personal and contextual factors, including assessment results, which may be useful in directing students to a particular outcome.

Educators should first consider the learning objectives and type of professional reasoning they desire to target in order to determine which specific details of a case should be included or left out. For example, if the learning objective is for the students to develop a plan of assessment strategies and intervention approaches for the client's identified priorities and needs, the educator should provide a case with background information and some hints about long-term limitations if the areas of concern are left unresolved. Alternatively, if the learning objective is for students to grow empathy and an emotional connection during the discussion of an ethical dilemma, the educator should provide a case that illustrates the client's lived experience, emotional perception, and specific dialogue with meaningful family members and health care providers.

In which of your own learning activities would you want to include more details in a case to facilitate learning? When would you want to include fewer details?

Paper Cases

Educators typically present written cases in narrative format to target each type of professional reasoning depending on the content of the case. They can reveal the entire case in full during the initial presentation or in smaller portions (e.g., one page at a time) to mimic how practitioners authentically encounter information in practice. In the latter structure, educators give students one or two prompts or questions to consider after each portion of the case to incrementally develop knowledge (Figure 12-1).

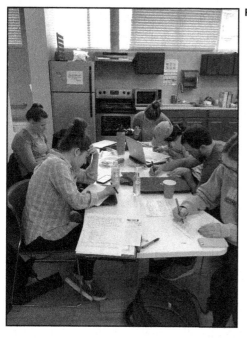

Figure 12-1. Students review a paper case during PBL.

Video Cases

In a video case, educators provide students with visual and auditory information about the client and scenario. Traditionally, they create or use a video to portray a client performing an assessment, completing an occupation-based task, or describing perspectives, values, or experiences. When educators employ the use of a video, they foster additional types of professional reasoning, such as interactive and conditional, because the students really begin to consider the client's perspectives, strengths, and challenges. In many situations, educators can portray cases with more complexities with video cases than are possible in a written paper case.

Simulated Cases

In a simulated case, the educator trains an actor to perform as a client by providing a description of the social-emotional background, scripted responses, and simulated movement and behavioral manifestations. In this method, the educator moves beyond the role of writing a case. Although this type of case often requires additional time and expense to train actors, educators are often able to maximize student development of professional reasoning through a "serve and return" method of engaging in real-time therapeutic communication and problem solving. Because the case is simulated, educators can institute "time outs" for reflection and feedback to reduce students' fears of doing something wrong. For more information on creating simulated cases, please refer to Chapter 7.

Live Cases

Educators seek individuals living in the community with a certain condition, context, or performance to serve as a client in a case. Ideally, these individuals are aware of occupational therapy services. In live cases, students have the unmatched opportunity to hear, feel, see, and comprehend the true lived experience of the individual. When real clients share their lived experiences of illness, disability, context, adaptation, and recovery, students obtain access to the highest level of professional reasoning. Educators may also translate live cases to paper or video for longevity or present a hybrid format of the different case types.

TABLE 12-2

Tips for Good Case Construction

- Tells a story
- Possesses a current temporal, technological, and culture context (within 5 years)
- Includes a subjective perspective (quotations or an emotional standpoint)
- Creates ability to relate, connect, or empathize with the central figure
- Holds potential to provoke conflict or an ethical dilemma
- Provides variety in pedagogical utility (multiple learning pathways)
- Includes several client and contextual factors with obvious occupational performance concerns
- Situates in a discernable service delivery setting
- Is not too long

Regardless of format, educators should structure cases so there are multiple learning pathways and practical problems to solve. They should write cases to tell an intriguing story within a contemporary context. We provide additional tips for constructing a good case scenario in Table 12-2.

Essential Elements of Problem-Based Learning

Educators employ the central element of PBL when they present a practical problem to students with no to minimal foundational or prior knowledge about the elements they need to solve the case. The students gain knowledge and professional reasoning skills through the process of struggling, identifying learning needs, delegating tasks, and collaborating to provide solutions. Students discover new knowledge and develop new skills during the presentation of the contextual case rather than theoretically learning about skills and interventions and subsequently applying to the case. This notion is called *situated learning* in which students more effectively engage in learning activities when rooted in a meaningful and authentic context that is relatable to everyday practice. This type of learning supports the core concepts of competency, relatedness, and motivation highlighted in self-determination theory. It is important for educators to understand the assumptions about this form of constructivist learning, which serves as the basis for PBL.

- Individuals construct their own knowledge and socially co-construct from interactions with the environment; knowledge cannot simply be transmitted.
- There are many perspectives related to every situation.
- The culture and context in which individuals exist distributes meaning and reasoning and provides the tools for learning.
- Individuals obtain knowledge embedded in relevant contexts.

Educators execute these assumptions in PBL by organizing students into groups of five to eight with one instructor or practitioner serving as a facilitator—often called the *tutor*. The tutor supports the problem-solving process, models positive group dynamics, and ensures student accountability. In some instances, the tutor may probe students to deepen their inquiry and understanding of a topic or skill. However, they are **not** knowledge disseminators or content experts. In addition, they should not guide or dictate learning objectives but rather allow students to be wholly and

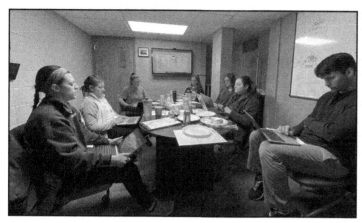

Figure 12-2. Students discuss case to establish learning objectives.

collaboratively responsible for the generation of their own learning (Figure 12-2). During the student-directed learning process, they complete learning activities that they design for themselves in order to resolve the problem scenario as it is presented (Table 12-3). When applied to occupational therapy curriculum, PBL groups may identify a need to learn through role play, service learning, field trips, or assessment practice.

During each class session, the tutor typically provides a time for each student to report to or teach the group about the assigned learning objective. As learning evolves, students share their hypotheses, revisit the problem, and reject some ideas and advance others as they obtain new information or insights. At the end of each session and periodically throughout the course, the tutor asks students to summarize, reflect, and integrate their learning. For each problem presented, the tutor needs to hold a minimum of two tutorial sessions, where the students work collaboratively as a group under the facilitation of the tutor, and one independent learning session, where students work more independently toward common objectives in preparation to report back to the group. Depending on the complexity of the problem, there can be anywhere from two to six class sessions devoted to working through a case.

Essential Elements of Case-Based Learning

Educators follow a more structured *guided inquiry method* to achieve knowledge and professional reasoning objectives but utilize the situated and student-led learning strategies found in PBL. A key component of this instructional method is educators must design a case in which students must arrive with some level of fundamental knowledge they can utilize and apply to achieve the learning objectives. In CBL, educators require students to pull from previously or concurrently learned material or skills in order to solve a practical case scenario. Similar to PBL, a skilled tutor facilitates a collaborative learning process with students arranged in small teams. They provide students background information about a client and include a practice scenario or problem to solve. In CBL, the students still typically lead the small group sessions, but the tutor provides a more structured guideline of what must be accomplished during each session and targets learning objectives to achieve by the end of the case. For example, the tutor may devote the first session to initially analyzing the case, brainstorming, and setting intervention priorities. In subsequent sessions, they may have students target specific strategies, such as writing an evaluation report or role playing a treatment session. In this situation, the educator expends a significant amount of time and effort preparing items, such as outlining the learning objectives and creating the flow of each session across multiple cases for a semester.

TABLE 12-3

Steps of a Problem-Based Learning Case

STEP	STUDENT IS	TUTOR IS
1. Clarify unknown terms, concepts, or diagnoses in the case.	Making a list of learning needs or looking up information/resources in real time.	Facilitating breadth of knowledge to ensure students have complete information before defining problem; may be asking students if they know specific information about a concept before allowing the process to continue.
2. Define the problem.	Creating a list of what they need to accomplish or learn and delegating tasks to each other.	Ensuring students stay within course objectives and scope of occupational therapy; may be checking for understanding of practice setting limitations.
3. Analyze the problem and brainstorm as many different factors or possible explanations for the case.	Selecting possible frames of reference or suggesting potential evaluation plans; reporting out evidence for each possible evaluation or intervention approach.	Supporting depth of analysis; using probing questions if students are missing key factors.
4. Analyze possible explanations and hypotheses and begin to generate a rational explanation for the underlying concern. Reject some explanations and hypotheses if needed.	Selecting possible frames of reference or suggesting potential evaluation plans; reporting out evidence for each possible evaluation or intervention approach.	Analyzing and critiquing quality of resources used by students; using probing questions if students are missing key resources or concepts.
5. Formulate a self-directed learning objective and assign each group member to spearhead one.	Identifying and implementing opportunities to advance knowledge and skills; may be suggesting role play, video model therapeutic interaction, in-context site visits, or content expert consultations.	Assisting students to determine what is realistic in course time frame and space; supporting accountability for depth of skill practice and ensuring engagement by all students in the group.
6. Fill in gaps for their assigned learning objective through an independent study.	Working independently with resources to analyze hypotheses; developing evaluation and/or treatment plans for case.	Ensuring accountability and effective use of time.

(continued)

TABLE 12-3 (CONTINUED)

Steps of a Problem-Based Learning Case

STEP	STUDENT IS	TUTOR IS
7. Report findings to the group and integrate new knowledge with existing hypotheses to generate a comprehensive explanation or solution to the problem (debrief).	Reflecting and reporting out to group on how learning activity outcomes were supported (or not) by evidence, experiences, and expertise.	Supporting student reflection and analysis of their learning outcomes; suggesting further consultation with a content expert (as needed).
8. Assess own learning and performance and the learning and performance of peers through a formal evaluation tool.	Completing student evaluation tool and practicing the skill of seeking and giving feedback through this written and face-to-face reflection session.	Completing student evaluation tool and modelling feedback strategies; asking for feedback regarding their own group facilitation skills.

Adapted from Schmidt, H. G., & Moust, J. H. C. (2000). Factors affecting small-group tutorial learning: A review of research. In D. H. Evensen & C. E. Hmelo (Eds.), *Problem-based learning: A research perspective on learning interactions* (pp. 19-51). Lawrence Erlbaum Associates Publishers.

During CBL, students apply prior knowledge and professional reasoning skills to new contexts and cases, solve problems, and obtain new knowledge to adapt prior knowledge to effectively approach future cases and professional practice. We highlight similarities and differences between these two instructional methods in Table 12-4. It is important to clarify that without the guided inquiry of the tutor facilitating the learning objective of each group, the process is not a CBL approach. This differs from simply reviewing relevant information in class and asking students to apply it to a case in small groups (case study learning activity).

Specific Case-Based Learning and Problem-Based Learning Facilitation Strategies

In both CBL and PBL, it is critical that the inquiry process is student-led and facilitator supported. Educators must promote a learning climate of open communication and trust so the group dynamics can develop and students can brainstorm and take risks without the fear of failure or negative outcomes (see Chapter 9). In a supported environment, students can test ideas and work through assumptions without anxiety of what grade they will receive. They also gain confidence and increased communication.

> Students can benefit from a tutor outside core faculty to gain different perspectives and to feel less like they are constantly evaluated.

One way educators can facilitate a supportive group structure and context is to utilize well-trained adjunct instructors or clinicians as tutors to assist in group facilitation. The role of the tutor is of utmost importance to the success of the CBL or PBL process. They must actively engage all students in the inquiry and problem-solving process. Tutors may support learning by assigning or encouraging students to take on assigned roles (Table 12-5) or more directly asking specific group members to share their perspective or explain how they came to a particular viewpoint or hypothesis.

TABLE 12-4

Differences and Similarities Between Elements of Problem-Based Learning and Case-Based Learning

INITIAL TOPIC	Student	Unknown **PBL**	General Topic Shared **CBL**	Full Case Provided
	Faculty	Unknown	General Topic Shared	Full Case Provided **PBL** **CBL**
PREPARATION	Student	None **PBL**	Some **PBL**	Significant **CBL**
	Faculty	None	Some	Significant **CBL**
CONTROL	Student	No Direction	Some Guidance **CBL**	Direct Discussion **PBL**
	Faculty	No Direction **PBL**	Some Guidance **CBL**	Direct Discussion
DATA SEEKING (during/after case)	Student	None Sought	Some Sought **CBL**	Significant **PBL**
	Faculty	None Sought **CBL**	Some Sought **PBL**	Significant

Reproduced with permission from Srinivasan, M., Wilkes, M., Stevenson, F., Nguyen, T., & Slavin, S. (2007). Comparing problem-based learning with case-based learning: Effects of a major curricular shift at two institutions. *Academic Medicine, 82*(1), 74-82.

TABLE 12-5

Potential Student Roles in
Case- or Problem-Based Learning Groups

SCRIBE	Takes notes on the discussion, creates to-do lists for the group
TIMEKEEPER	Ensures all objectives are covered in allotted session time; gives 5- or 10-minute warnings
RESEARCHER	Looks up information in real time to keep the discussion moving when the group has a question or needs more information
ARBITRATOR/ MONITOR	Ensures that all comments are productive and respectful
DEVIL'S ADVOCATE	Asks clarifying questions to ensure the application of knowledge is in-depth and accurate

The tutor should not feel the expectation to know everything about the case or how the case should be solved. Instead, the tutor calls on students (at the appropriate time) to seek out information and evidence from reliable sources when the group gets stuck. Some specific tips for effective CBL and PBL facilitation include:

- Have the group set ground rules during the initial session
- Discuss or assign different group roles for each case or session
- Foster open communication and acceptance to build trust among group members
- Do not dominate the session as the tutor
- Reflect on and monitor your facilitation strategies
- Probe students for deeper understanding; ask why (see Chapter 10)
- Foster healthy debate between group members
- Ask open-ended questions
- Provide specific feedback to students
- Ensure the students know the role of the facilitator

What questions can educators ask to facilitate discussion and guide the CBL and PBL when students get stuck?

Training for Tutors

As educators develop the structure of a PBL or CBL course, it is critical that all tutors apply the learning principles and strategies equally. Each tutor will bring their unique experiences and personality to their group; however, the application of facilitation strategies, expectation of rigor, and accountability must be consistent. It is helpful for the course coordinator to hold an orientation or training session so that the tutors are familiar with the context of the course within the rest of the curriculum and to provide the full view of expectations and assignments within the course.

The course coordinator can provide tutors with foundational readings from this chapter and ask they review in addition to other literature prior to beginning the semester. If the tutors are expected to give any formal feedback to students (e.g., documentation, written feedback on assignments) as a part of the cases, the coordinator will need to train them to utilize a rubric, which may be helpful for consistent feedback and expectations across all students.

Finally, it is important to allow time for the tutors to review the cases and any background case notes for the class prior to the beginning of the course. They should have access to resources the students will likely utilize and be knowledgeable about what additional resources (assessment tools, videos, adaptive equipment) are available for students to access during the CBL or PBL process.

OPPORTUNITIES FOR FEEDBACK AND REFLECTION

As with many other instructional methods in this book, it is essential educators and students provide feedback and engage in reflection on the group learning process to further develop their professional reasoning skills. Educators must devote time to the core component of group reflection at the end of each PBL or CBL session. When providing in-the-moment feedback during a session, educators teach students to use approaches that start with positive aspects, pause for processing, and follow with areas that need improvement. It is also helpful for tutors to model a follow up to feedback with an action planning statement to help students envision how they will utilize constructive feedback.

It is also valuable for the tutor to have each student in the small group set one or two development goals for the length of the course. Students can write goals related to how they contribute during sessions, how they will engage in different group roles, how well they prepare for sessions, or how well they professionally communicate with peers. Educational literature also encourages tutors to engage students in some sort of midterm and final evaluation. In addition, forms of peer, tutor, or self-evaluation can offer multiple levels of feedback and reflection. In these forms of evaluation, students traditionally rate areas related to level of engagement in the learning process, amount of preparation for sessions, professionalism and dependability, quality of information sources, ability to give and receive feedback, and group participation dynamics. You can refer to Chapter 8 to further review peer, self, and group feedback and reflection strategies.

APPLICATION TO OCCUPATIONAL THERAPY PRACTICE

Example 1: Application of Problem-Based Learning Process in Adolescent Transition Planning Groups

Middle school students who receive special education services begin to participate in their own individualized education planning process. In this situation, occupational therapy services often focus on supporting these students to set their own goals after graduation from high school, practice daily living skills, and negotiate personal and professional relationships. Occupational therapy practitioners may use the PBL process when working with a small group of adolescents in middle or high school to facilitate knowledge and skills to support their post-secondary success. This group may be collaborative with the school counselor, social worker, or speech language pathologist. The tutor can use a real-life problem scenario that prompts the students to develop hypotheses and strategies for successful navigation. Examples of case scenarios could potentially include:

- Being late for work and missing the city bus
- Only having enough money to pay two out of three expenses
- Getting two invitations to concurrent social events
- Being invited for a job interview at the same time as a previously scheduled doctor's appointment
- Planning and using a weekly schedule or agenda

The PBL tutor can apply the steps of the PBL process (see Table 12-3) to assist the group of teenagers to gather any additional information needed, define the problem, set objectives, and analyze the potential solutions. The group will benefit from the reflective process at the end to determine if their solutions would be effective and on their own effectiveness as a group.

Example 2: Application of Case-Based Learning Process in Clinical Team Meetings

Occupational therapists across a variety of settings often participate in a weekly or monthly meeting time to discuss challenging cases or program outcomes. Oftentimes, health professionals lose focus and diverge productive solution-oriented discussion during these meetings. Health professionals can select one member of the group to lead the meeting and implement the use of a CBL method with structured guided inquiry agenda. In order for this method to be successful, health professionals would need to adequately prepare for meetings and participate in training because time is often limited and multidisciplinary in nature.

Advantages

- Develops intrinsic and extrinsic motivation
- Encourages self-reflection and critical evaluation of one's own skills and contributions
- Fosters problem-solving and critical-thinking skills
- Requires teamwork and effective collaboration
- Typically results in high student satisfaction
- Covers a wide range of clinical knowledge and skills
- Provides real-time flexibility to meet individual learning needs
- Specific content expertise not required for staffing

Challenges

- Requires significant time and resources to create
- Students are dependent on each other; if one student does a poor job researching objective, it impacts the entire group
- Requires good group dynamics
- Potentially requires significant time for evaluation and feedback

In the space below, list any additional advantages or challenges.

```



```

Brainstorm strategies for overcoming these challenges when implementing the use of PBL or CBL instructional methods.

```



```

THREE THINGS YOU CAN DO TOMORROW TO IMPLEMENT CASE-BASED LEARNING AND PROBLEM-BASED LEARNING INSTRUCTIONAL METHODS WITH YOUR STUDENTS

1. Start including clinician lab assistants to case study group work to facilitate inquiry and learning.
2. When using case studies for learning, be intentional about how much structure you provide (or do not provide).
3. Start brainstorming how to convert class time to several consecutive PBL or CBL sessions.

Case-Based Learning Instructional Methods Evidence Table

Author/Year	Study Objectives	Design and Participants	Intervention and Outcome Measures	Results
Azer & Azer (2015)	Researchers reviewed available evidence on group interaction in problem-based learning (PBL)	Design: Systematic review Participants: Health professions (majority of studies from medicine) Researchers included 42 studies in this review	Included articles between 1999 and 2013 Researchers searched the following databases: PubMed, Embase, PsycINFO, HighWire; also searched discipline-specific journals Inclusion criteria: • Qualitative or descriptive studies on group interaction during PBL • Assessed different factors that would affect the tutor-student relationship or peer-to-peer relationship • Explored impact of group interaction on learning Exclusion criteria: • Studies that did not include designs outlined above • Papers that lacked abstracts • Not written in English • Studies that assessed PBL tutorials or long-term impact • Training tutor programs • Papers that introduced PBL • Study did not match criteria for PBL	Studies used a variety of methods and outcomes for assessing group interaction during PBL Of the studies, 43% used video recording to assess the group interaction; others mention the use of focus groups, or interviews Numerous factors impact group interaction (e.g., tutor's background, student training, peer feedback) Only 5 studies examined the impact of group interactions on learning Researchers reported no conclusive evidence in regard to the impact of group interaction on student learning during PBL
Bassir et al. (2014)	Researchers completed a review to compare effectiveness of PBL to traditional methods in dental education	Design: Systematic review	Researchers searched the following databases: MedLine, Education Resources Information Center (ERIC), PsycINFO, CINAHL, Web of Science; also searched 2 dental education journals	Researchers classified each study as weak quality Of the 17 studies, 13 compared PBL to another method

(continued)

Case-Based Learning Instructional Methods Evidence Table (continued)

Author/Year	Study Objectives	Design and Participants	Intervention and Outcome Measures	Results
		Participants: Predoctoral and postdoctoral dental students Researchers included 17 articles in the review	Inclusion criteria: • Study completed with predoctoral and postdoctoral dental students • Used PBL as a course or curriculum • Described intervention as PBL • Studies included a control group of traditional methods • Included a quantitative outcome measure of the effectiveness of PBL Exclusion criteria: • Not written or available in English • Did not compare PBL to traditional methods • Did not clearly describe methodology or outcomes • Lacked statistical analysis	Researchers reported limited number of well-designed studies However, data in available studies suggest PBL does not negatively influence factual knowledge acquisition, but improves ability to apply knowledge to clinical situations, and enhances students' perception of preparedness
Galvao et al. (2014)	Researchers assessed effectiveness of PBL in the education of pharmacy students	Design: Systematic review and meta-analysis Participants: Undergraduate and graduate pharmacy students Researchers included 5 studies in this review	2 researchers reviewed articles Researchers searched the following databases: MedLine, Embase, Scopus, CINAHL, Web of Science, ERIC, Academic Search Premier, Wilson Education Full Test, ProQuest, Latin American and Caribbean Health Sciences Literature, SciELO; hand searched pharmacy education journals and pharmacy websites Researchers included articles that implemented a controlled study that compared PBL to traditional methods in pharmacy education. They desired outcomes of student learning	3 of 5 studies used randomization Following the meta-analysis of the 5 studies, the results on final and midterm outcome measures significantly favored those students that participated in PBL Researchers reported no differences on subjective assessments between PBL and traditional teaching methods

(continued)

Case-Based Learning Instructional Methods Evidence Table (continued)

Author/Year	Study Objectives	Design and Participants	Intervention and Outcome Measures	Results
Jay (2014)	Researchers determined occupational therapy students' perceptions of PBL	Design: Retrospective analysis Participants: First, second-, third-, and fourth-year occupational therapy students	Intervention: Students participated in PBL curriculum Outcome measures: Questionnaire (after participation in PBL curriculum; end of year); 22 closed-ended questions	Of the 22 questions, 4 explored students' attitudes toward group work in PBL curriculum; first-, second-, and fourth-year students reported strong affiliation to work in groups; third-year students reported more varied responses In regards to attitudes with working toward tutors, first- and second-year students reported positive attitude with tutor; fourth-year students reported more varied responses; third-year students demonstrated a more neutral attitude Only 2 questions addressed learning objectives; more than half of first-year and fourth-year students reported positive perception of learning objectives; second- and third-year student had neutral responses In terms of questions related to self-directed learning, a majority of students fell between neutral and strongly agree that PBL facilitated this skill Students reported agreement that they liked structure of PBL and they learned more from this format than from other traditional courses
Jin & Bridges (2014)	Researchers aimed to determine the effects of educational technologies in PBL in health science education	Design: Systematic review Participants: Dentistry, medicine, and speech and hearing science students	Researchers searched the following databases: ProQuest, Scopus, EBSCOhost Searched for articles from 1996 to 2004	Of the 28 studies, 20 explored the application of a variety of software and digital learning objects Majority of studies used questionnaire for outcome measurements

(continued)

Case-Based Learning Instructional Methods Evidence Table (continued)

Author/Year	Study Objectives	Design and Participants	Intervention and Outcome Measures	Results
		Researchers included 28 articles for analysis	Inclusion criteria: • Dentistry, medicine, and speech and hearing science students • PBL was a key pedagogy in the curriculum • Included learning software, digital learning objectives, plasma screens, or learning management systems • Studied effects of technologies on student learning and educator engagement during PBL	Primary reason for inclusion of technology was to serve as an aid or supplement or a replacement for traditional formats The educational technologies appeared to fit with PBL method Students and educators reported positive outcomes for learning Students and educators also reported several challenges (e.g., infrastructure, technological support)
Kong et al. (2014)	Researchers aimed to compare effectiveness of PBL and traditional lectures on nursing students' critical thinking skills	Design: Systematic review and meta-analysis Participants: 985 nursing students'; 439 in PBL, 546 in control Researchers included 9 studies in this review	Researchers searched the following databases: PubMed, Embase, CINAHL, CENTRAL, ProQuest, CNKI Inclusion criteria: • Randomized controlled trial (RCT) • Included nursing students • Implemented PBL as an experimental group • Used traditional lecture method as control group • Assessed critical thinking as an outcome measure • Reported sample size, mean differences, and 95% confidence interval	Most studies demonstrated low risk of bias 7 of 9 studies reported overall critical thinking scores; 2 of these studies demonstrated no significant differences between PBL and traditional lecture, while others demonstrated statistically significant differences; pooled effect size favored PBL 6 studies implemented PBL for a semester and demonstrated no significant difference between the 2 groups; a study for use of PBL over 2 semesters demonstrated significant difference in favor of PBL

(continued)

Case-Based Learning Instructional Methods Evidence Table (continued)

Author/Year	Study Objectives	Design and Participants	Intervention and Outcome Measures	Results
			Exclusion criteria: • Non-RCT • Included other participants other than nursing students • Used other interventions besides PBL • Did not assess critical thinking • Reported incomplete data (or lacked complete data)	
Li et al. (2019)	Researchers compared effectiveness of PBL to traditional teaching methods of nursing students and nurses' professional communication	Design: Systematic review Participants: Nursing students or nurses; 1,065 nursing students from different levels of education; 40 nurses at hospitals; 49 medical staff Researchers included 12 articles in this review	Researchers searched the following databases: MedLine, PubMed, Embase, PsycINFO, Cochrane Library, CNKI, Wanfang Data, VIP Database Inclusion criteria: • Used a RCT or quasi-experimental design • Included participants of nursing students or nurses • Implemented use of PBL • Assessed communication as an outcome measure • Reported sample size and process • Published in English or Chinese from years 1990 to 2018 Exclusion criteria: • Described other studies than ones described above in inclusion criteria • Included other participants than listed above	In these studies, the length of PBL intervention ranged from 4 hours to 1 year Of the 12 studies, 9 were pre/posttest design; sample size ranged from 12 to 240 Studies included a wide array of outcomes to measure communication Of the 12 studies, 11 demonstrated PBL developed nurses' or nursing students' communication skills; only 1 reported no significant differences between PBL and traditional learning methods

(continued)

Case-Based Learning Instructional Methods Evidence Table (continued)

Author/Year	Study Objectives	Design and Participants	Intervention and Outcome Measures	Results
Liu et al. (2019)	Researchers desired to examine the theoretical scores (exams and questionnaires) following PBL with students in pharmacology education	Design: Meta-analysis Participants: Students engaged in pharmacology education; pooled sample size was 4,406 students; 2,137 in experimental PBL group; 2,269 in control lecture-based learning group Researchers included 34 articles in this review	Researchers searched the following databases: EBSCO, PubMed, Web of Science, ProQuest Dissertations and Theses, ERIC, Embase, Cochrane Database, CNKI, VIP Database, Wanfang Data, CBM Searched for articles between 1965 and 2017 Inclusion criteria: • Included quantitative outcome measures on student learning • Used experimental and comparative study designs • Examined effectiveness of PBL (experimental group) to lecture-based learning (control group) • Dependent variable included theoretical scores • Investigated PBL within pharmacology education	Sample sizes ranged from 10 to 189 students Of the 34 articles, 19 were with medicine students, 9 with pharmacy, and 6 with nursing PBL intervention ranged between 3 months to 1 semester All studies examined theoretical knowledge scores Of the 34 studies, 26 demonstrated statistically significant differences between PBL and traditional lecture-based learning on theoretical scores; the others demonstrated no difference Pool effect size demonstrated significant differences in scores favoring PBL No significant bias noted with sensitivity analysis In the studies that used a questionnaire, a majority of students reported enthusiasm for PBL
Ma & Lu (2019)	Researchers used a meta-analysis to determine effectiveness of PBL in pediatric medical education in comparison to traditional methods	Design: Meta-analysis Participants: 1,003 medical students; 509 in PBL; 494 in lecture-based learning Researchers included 12 studies in this review	Researchers implemented Preferred Reporting Items for Systematic Reviews and Meta-Analyses (PRISMA) guidelines Researchers searched the following databases: CNKI, Wanfang Data, China Science Citation Database, CBM, PubMed, Embase, CENTRAL	All studies reported knowledge score data; PBL significantly increased scores compared to traditional lecture 5 studies reported on skill scores; PBL significantly increased skill scores compared to traditional lecture

(continued)

Case-Based Learning Instructional Methods Evidence Table (continued)

Author/Year	Study Objectives	Design and Participants	Intervention and Outcome Measures	Results
			Inclusion criteria: • Included participants of pediatric medical students in China • Used PBL in experimental group and traditional lecture-based learning in control group • Used a controlled trial in pediatric medical education • Included outcome measures of knowledge scores, skill scores, or case analysis scores	4 studies reported case analysis scores; PBL significantly increased scores on case analysis compared to traditional lecture

Merisier et al. (2018)	Researchers explored the influence of questioning during PBL in nursing education	Design: A scoping review
		
		Participants: Nursing students
		
		Researchers included 22 articles in this review; 19 were empirical studies
			Researchers reviewed the following databases: CINAHL, Embase, ERIC, MedLine, PubMed
			
			Included studies published between 1973 and 2017
			
			Inclusion criteria:
			• Empirical studies published in French or English
			• Included clinical reasoning and questioning
			
			Exclusion criteria
			• Published outside of date range
			• Non-English or Non-French
			• Addressed the 2 concepts of clinical reasoning and questioning, but did not provide a link between
				Researchers identified 5 themes after review of the articles
				• Critical thinking
				  ○ Studies primarily reviewed impact of questioning during PBL on critical thinking versus clinical reasoning
				• Nature of questions asked
				  ○ Many studies classified questions according to Bloom's taxonomy; many were low cognitive level questions
				• Effect of high-level questions on critical thinking
				  ○ Not many high-level questions asked with inconclusive results among all studies

(continued)

Case-Based Learning Instructional Methods Evidence Table (continued)

Author/Year	Study Objectives	Design and Participants	Intervention and Outcome Measures	Results

				• Beyond nature of questions asked
				  ◦ Noted use of 2 patterns; strategic questioning, which includes low-level questions followed in progression by high-level questions; nonstrategic used random questions with no specific goal
				• Questioning and PBL
				  ◦ Few studies actually found on this topic

Nkosi & Thupayagale-Tshweneagae (2013)	Researchers desired to review literature of impact on PBL on critical thinking and learning with nursing students	Design: Systematic review Participants: Nursing students Researchers included 17 studies	Researchers searched the following databases: Africa-Wide Information, EBSCOhost, PubMed, Science Direct, Google Scholar Searched articles published from 2005 to 2012 Inclusion criteria: • Studies in any country included • Student nurses • Addressed PBL either qualitatively or quantitatively • Published in English Exclusion criteria: • Included participants from other fields of study • Included other interventions besides PBL	Researchers reported several themes: • Students in Thailand and Taiwan reported unhappiness with PBL due to the heavy workload it requires • Students reported if the information is clear, they experienced increased self-esteem and confidence; they experienced opposite if information was vague • Educators reported lack of resources as a challenge to implementing PBL Researchers reported articles demonstrated no clear evidence that PBL promoted critical thinking; some evidence supported the use of PBL for development of research skills Studies reported students performed well on exams and could interpret concepts independently

(continued)

Case-Based Learning Instructional Methods Evidence Table (continued)

Author/Year	Study Objectives	Design and Participants	Intervention and Outcome Measures	Results
O'Donoghue et al. (2011)	Researchers conducted a systematic review to obtain a comprehensive summary of research and to identify further research needs	Design: Systematic review Participants: Various therapy professions Researchers included 6 papers	5 research team members use Cochrane Effective Practice and Organisation of Care and PRISMA Researchers searched the following databases: ERIC, Academic Search Premier, PsycINFO, Embase, PubMed, CINAHL, Scopus, Web of Science Inclusion criteria: • Professional entry-level therapy students • Intervention of problem-based learning based on Barrow's characteristics • RCTs, controlled trials, interrupted time series, controlled before and after studies, qualitative data • Included outcome measures on accumulation of knowledge, performance, approach to learning, or student satisfaction	3 of 6 studies were in physical therapy education; 1 in occupational therapy, dietetics, and podiatry 3 of 6 studies investigated an entire PBL curriculum, while the other 3 studies reviewed 1, 2, or multiple PBL modules Only 1 study used a randomized design 3 of 6 studies were high quality and the remaining 3 were low quality 3 studies examined students' knowledge; 1 suggesting higher knowledge in PBL with the other 2 demonstrating no significant differences between PBL and the control group 2 studies include clinical performance with no differences between PBL and the control group 4 studies reviewed PBL impact on approach to learning; in 1 study, the PBL group performed significantly better than the control group on tests of deeper understanding and cognitive skills; 2 showed no significant differences and 1 demonstrated a negative effect

(continued)

Case-Based Learning Instructional Methods Evidence Table (continued)

Author/Year	Study Objectives	Design and Participants	Intervention and Outcome Measures	Results
Qin et al. (2016)	Researchers desired to complete a meta-analysis to compare effects of PBL and traditional lecture-based learning on the improvement of the environment of medical education	Design: Systematic review and meta-analysis Participants: 673 medical students (pooled from studies) Researchers included 6 studies in this review	2 reviewers assessed each article with the Cochrane Collaboration tool Researchers searched the following databases: ERIC, PubMed, Google Scholar, CNKI, Wanfang Data Inclusion criteria: • Study compared PBL to traditional lecture-based learning • Used quantitative outcome measure that focused on medical education environment • Written in any language • Used PBL as the experimental intervention approach • Used lecture-based learning as the only instructional method in the control group • RCT • Reported sample size, mean differences, and standard deviations between the 2 groups • Used the Dundee Ready Educational Environment as an outcome measure Exclusion criteria: • No control group • Lecture not only method in control group • Non-RCT • Did not evaluate environment; used other tools to evaluate outcome • Incomplete data • Duplication	Most studies considered low risk of bias Studies demonstrated moderate heterogeneity; pooled effect size demonstrated significant difference on the medical education environment scores in support of PBL Of the subscores of the Dundee Ready Educational Environment, several areas supported PBL (e.g., perception of teachers, perception of learning, perception of atmosphere)

(continued)

Case-Based Learning Instructional Methods Evidence Table (continued)

Author/Year	Study Objectives	Design and Participants	Intervention and Outcome Measures	Results
Sayyah et al. (2017)	Researchers desired to complete a systematic review and meta-analysis to compare PBL to conventional educational methods in undergraduate medical courses in Iran	Design: Systematic review and meta-analysis Participants: Health professional students from disciplines of nursing, medicine, dentistry, and others Researchers included 23 studies in this review	Researchers searched the following databases: PubMed, Scopus, Embase; also reviewed additional external resources Inclusion criteria: • Example application of PBL instructional method as a stand-alone method or combination with lecture model in Iranian medical schools • RCT and non-RCT Reviewed studies that examined a continuous outcome, such as examination scores	Researchers used pooled effect size, which demonstrated favor of PBL when compared to traditional lecture-based learning 12 of the 23 studies demonstrated high methodological quality Further analysis support the use of PBL in isolation versus mixing with other instructional methods
Shin & Kim (2013)	Researchers synthesized effect of PBL in nursing education to answer the following questions: • What is the magnitude of the effect of PBL on nursing education? • What levels of evidence and evaluation have most influence on effect size?	Design: Meta-analysis Participants: Nursing students Researchers included 22 studies in this review	Researchers searched the following databases: EBSCO, MedLine, Web of Science, ProQuest Dissertations and Theses, ERIC, PsycINFO Selected articles from 1972 to 2012 Inclusion criteria: • Used quantitative outcome measures that assessed student learning or student reasoning processes • Included enough data to calculate effect size • Employed experimental, quasi-experimental, or descriptive and comparative design that examined effectiveness of PBL • Studied nursing students • Written in English	Effect sizes were positive for PBL when students demonstrated improved performance Researchers found a medium-to-large effect size on the impact of PBL in nursing education Researchers reported PBL had positive effects on satisfaction with training, skill courses, and clinical education with nursing students

(continued)

Case-Based Learning Instructional Methods Evidence Table (continued)

Author/Year	Study Objectives	Design and Participants	Intervention and Outcome Measures	Results
	• What research method variables have most influence on effect size? • What studying/learning contexts have most influence on effect size?			
Tsigarides et al. (2017)	Researchers completed a systematic review to determine if medical education with PBL influences students' career paths; they compared PBL versus traditional lecture-based learning on career selection	Design: Systematic review Participants: Medical students Researchers included 11 studies	2 researchers used the STROBE and CONSORT checklists to assess studies Researchers searched the following databases: MedLine, PubMed Central, Cochrane, ERIC Inclusion criteria: • Written in English • No date limitations Exclusion criteria: • Studies focused on academic performance, national test results or student demographics • Studies that did not discuss PBL Each study compared outcomes of the participants in PBL based curriculums versus non-PBL curriculums	Of the 11 studies, 7 were retrospective cohort In 7 of the 11 students, there were no significant differences in career choice between PBL and non-PBL curriculums In 1 study in Canada, they found significantly lower number of graduates from PBL curriculum employed in primary care (only study suggesting this association)

(continued)

Case-Based Learning Instructional Methods Evidence Table (continued)

Author/Year	Study Objectives	Design and Participants	Intervention and Outcome Measures	Results
Zarea Gavgani et al. (2015)	Researchers reviewed evidence to determine differences between digital case scenarios and paper-based scenarios on clinical reasoning during PBL	Design: Systematic review and meta-analysis Participants: 222 students from health and medical sciences Researchers included 5 studies in this review	2 researchers reviewed each article following PRISMA guidelines and appraised article with CASP guidelines Researchers searched the following databases: MedLine, Scopus, CINAHL, Web of Science, Google Scholar Studied articles from 2003 to 2013 Inclusion criteria: • RCT that included digital case scenarios versus paper-based scenarios during PBL medical education • Included multimedia scenario, video case, or online-guided scenarios • Published in English Exclusion criteria: • Nonrandomized control design • Nondigital scenario was not included	Researchers reported no significant differences on clinical reasoning skills between digital and paper-based scenarios; the effect of both methods were similar In each of the 5 studies, students reported greater satisfaction with using digital forms of cases during PBL Researchers reported the use of digital case scenarios requires decreased time for the students and educators
Zhang et al. (2018)	Researchers completed an analysis to compare the effectiveness of PBL and traditional teaching in Chinese radiology education	Design: Meta-analysis and systematic review Participants: Total of 1,487 medical students in a Chinese medical school Included 17 studies in meta-analysis	2 researchers reviewed articles Researchers searched the following databases: CNKI, Wanfang Data, VIP Information, CBM, English language databases (PubMed, Embase) Searched inception to November 2017 Inclusion criteria: • Medical students in a Chinese medical school	All studies published between 2009 and 2016 Sample sizes ranged from 15 to 90 students in experimental and control groups Most studies completed with 5-year medical students Majority of studies favored the use of PBL over traditional teaching for development of many skills

(continued)

Case-Based Learning Instructional Methods Evidence Table (continued)

Author/Year	Study Objectives	Design and Participants	Intervention and Outcome Measures	Results
			• Used intervention of PBL as experimental group • Compared to traditional teaching or lecture-based learning in control group • Used theoretical scores or skill scores related to radiology as outcome measures • Used controlled trial design	16 of the 17 studies reported knowledge scores with exams; demonstrated significant difference in knowledge scores in favor of PBL 13 of the 17 studies included outcomes of skills test for reading film; demonstrated significant difference in skill scores in favor of PBL Statistical analysis demonstrated no evidence of bias on the analysis of knowledge/skill scores

Due to large volume of studies related to PBL, we included systematic reviews from other health professional education literature. We included PBL studies with quantitative designs in occupational therapy education. We recognize there are several mixed-methods and qualitative designs in occupational therapy education related to PBL.

Adapted from American Occupational Therapy Association. (2002). AOTA's evidence-based literature review project: An overview (D. Lieberman & J. Scheer, Eds.). *American Journal of Occupational Therapy, 56,* 344-349. https://doi.org/10.5014/ajot.56.3.344

REFERENCES

American Occupational Therapy Association. (2002). AOTA's evidence-based literature review project: An overview (D. Lieberman & J. Scheer, Eds.). *The American Journal of Occupational Therapy, 56,* 344-349. https://doi.org/10.5014/ajot.56.3.344

Azer, S. A., & Azer, D. (2015). Group interaction in problem-based learning tutorials: A systematic review. *European Journal of Dental Education, 19*(4), 194-208.

Bassir, S. H., Sadr-Eshkevari, P., Amirikhorheh, S., & Karimbu, N. Y. (2014). Problem-based learning in dental education: A systematic review of literature. *Journal of Dental Education, 78*(1), 98-109.

Galvao, T. F., Silva, M. T., Neiva, C. S., Riberio, L. M., & Pereira, M. G. (2014). Problem-based learning in pharmaceutical education: A systematic review and meta-analysis. *The Scientific World Journal, 2014,* 1-7.

Jay, J. (2014). Problem-based learning—a review of students' perception in an occupational therapy undergraduate curriculum. *South African Journal of Occupational Therapy, 44*(1), 56-61.

Jin, J., & Bridges, S. M. (2014). Educational technologies in problem-based learning in health science education: A systematic review. *Journal of Medical Internet Research, 16*(12), 1-13. http://dx.doi.org/10.2196/jmir.3240

Kong, L. N., Qin, B., Zhou, Y. Q., Mou, S. Y., & Gao, H. M. (2014). The effectiveness of problem-based learning on development of nursing students' critical thinking: A systematic review and meta-analysis. *International Journal of Nursing Studies, 51,* 458-469. http://dx.doi.org/10.1016/j.ijnurstu.2013.06.009

Li, Y., Wang, X., Zhu, X. R., Zhu, Y. X., & Sun, J. (2019). Effectiveness of problem-based learning on the professional communication competencies of nursing students and nurses: A systematic review. *Nurse Education in Practice, 37,* 45-55.

Liu, L., Du, X., Zhang, Z., & Zhou, J. (2019). Effect of problem-based learning in pharmacology education: A meta-analysis. *Studies in Educational Evaluation, 60,* 43-58. https://doi.org/10.1016/j.stueduc.2018.11.004

Ma, Y., & Lu, X. (2019). The effectiveness of problem-based learning in pediatric medical education in China: A meta-analysis of randomized controlled trials. *Medicine, 98*(2), 1-8. http://dx.doi.org/10.1097/MD.0000000000014052

Merisier, S., Larue, C., & Boyer, L. (2018). How does questioning influence nursing students' clinical reasoning in problem-based learning? A scoping review. *Nurse Education Today, 65,* 108-115.

Niemiec, C. P., & Ryan, R. M. (2009). Autonomy, competence, and relatedness in the classroom: Applying self-determination theory to educational practice. *Theory and Research in Education, 7*(2), 133-144.

Nkosi, Z., & Thupayagale-Tshweneagae, G. (2013). Effectiveness of problem-based learning among student nurses: A system review (2005-2012). *African Journal for Physical, Health Education, Recreation and Dance, 19*(Suppl. 1), 11-21.

O'Donoghue, G., McMahon, S., Doody, C., Smith, K., & Cusack, T. (2011). Problem-based learning in professional entry-level therapy education: A review of controlled evaluation studies. *Interdisciplinary Journal of Problem-Based Learning, 5*(1), 5.

Qin, Y., Wang, Y., & Floden, R. E. (2016). The effect of problem-based learning on improvement of the medical educational environment: A systematic review and meta-analysis. *Medical Principles and Practice, 25,* 525-532. http://dx.doi.org/10.1159/000449036

Royeen, C. B. (1995). A problem-based learning curriculum for occupational therapy education. *American Journal of Occupational Therapy, 49*(4), 338-346.

Sayyah, M., Shirbandi, K., Saki-Malehi, A., & Rahim, F. (2017). Use of problem-based learning teaching model for undergraduate medical and nursing education: A systematic review and meta-analysis. *Advances in Medical Education and Practice, 8,* 691-700. http://dx.doi.org/10.2147/AMEP.S143694

Schmidt, H. G., & Moust, J. H. C. (2000). Factors affecting small-group tutorial learning: A review of research. In D. H. Evensen & C. E. Hmelo (Eds.), *Problem-based learning: A research perspective on learning interactions* (pp. 19-51). Lawrence Erlbaum Associates Publishers.

Shin, I. S., & Kim, J. H. (2013). The effect of problem-based learning in nursing education: A meta-analysis. *Advances in Health Science Education, 18,* 1103-1120. http://dx.doi.org/10.1007/s10459-012-9436-2

Tsigarides, J., Wingfield, L. R., & Kulendran, M. (2017). Does a PBL-based medical curriculum predispose training in specific career paths? A systematic review of the literature. *BMC Res Notes, 10*(24), 1-9. http://dx.doi.org/10.1186/s13104-016-2348-0

Zarea Gavgani, V., Hazrati, H., & Ghojazadeh, M. (2015). The efficacy of digital case scenario versus paper case scenario on clinical reasoning in problem-based learning: A systematic review and meta-analysis. *Research and Development in Medical Education, 4*(1), 17-22.

Zhang, S., Xu, J., Wang, H., Zhang, D., & Zhang, Q. (2018). Effects of problem-based learning in Chinese radiology education: A systematic review and meta-analysis. *Medicine, 97*(9), 1-6. http://dx.doi.org/10.1097/MD.0000000000010069

BIBLIOGRAPHY

Allen, D. D., & Toth-Cohen, S. (2019). Use of case studies to promote critical thinking in occupational therapy students. *Journal of Occupational Therapy Education, 3*(3), Article 9.

Azer, S. A. (2005). Challenges facing PBL tutors: 12 tips for successful group facilitation. *Medical Teacher, 27*(8), 676-681.

Barrett, T., & Moore, S. (2010). *New approaches to problem-based learning: Evitalising your practice in higher education.* Routledge.

Barrows, H. S. (1996). Problem-based learning in medicine and beyond: A brief overview. In L. Wilkerson & W. H. Gijselaers (Eds.), *Bringing problem-based learning to higher education: Theory and practice* (pp. 3-12). Jossey-Bass Inc.

Barrows, H. S., & Tamblyn, R. M. (1980). *Problem-based learning: An approach to medical education.* Springer.

Boud, D., & Feletti, G. (1997). *The challenge of problem based learning* (2nd ed.). Kogan Page.

Deci, E. L., Koestner, R., & Ryan, R. M. (1999). A meta-analytic review of experiments examining the effects of extrinsic rewards on intrinsic motivation. *Psychological Bulletin, 125*(6), 627.

Deci, E. L., & Ryan, R. M. (2000). The "what" and "why" of goal pursuits: Human needs and the self-determination of behavior. *Psychological Inquiry, 11,* 227-268.

Fain, E. (2017). Case based game: Integrating the practice framework with cases. *International Archives of Nursing and Health Care, 3,* 077. http://dx.doi.org/10.23937/2469-5823/1510077

Fleming, H. (1991). The therapist with the three-track mind. *American Journal of Occupational Therapy, 45,* 1007-1014.

Hung, W., Jonassen, D. H., & Liu, R. (2008). Problem-based learning. *Handbook of Research on Educational Communications and Technology, 3*(1), 485-506.

Kassirer, J. P. (2010). Teaching clinical reasoning: Case-based and coached. *Academic Medicine, 85*(7), 1118-1124.

McCaughan, K. (2015). Theoretical anchors for Barrows' PBL tutor guidelines. In A. Walker, H. Leary, C. Hmelo-Silver, & P. A. Ertmer (Eds.), *Essential readings in problem-based learning: Exploring and extending the legacy of Howard S. Burrows.* Purdue University Press.

Muller, S. (1984). Physicians for the twenty-first century: Report of the project panel on the general professional education of the physician and college preparation for medicine. *Journal of Medical Education, 59*(11, part 2), 1-208.

Onyon, C. (2012). Problem-based learning: A review of the educational and psychological theory. *The Clinical Teacher, 9*(1), 22-26.

Scaffa, M. E., & Wooster, D. M. (2004). Effects of problem-based learning on clinical reasoning in occupational therapy. *American Journal of Occupational Therapy, 58*(3), 333-336.

Srinivasan, M., Wilkes, M., Stevenson, F., Nguyen, T., & Slavin, S. (2007). Comparing problem-based learning with case-based learning: Effects of a major curricular shift at two institutions. *Academic Medicine, 82*(1), 74-82.

Thistlethwaite, J. E., Davies, D., Ekeocha, S., Kidd, J. M., MacDougall, C., Matthews, P., Purkis, J., & Clay, D. (2012). The effectiveness of case-based learning in health professional education. A BEME systematic review: BEME Guide No. 23. *Medical Teacher, 34*(6), e421-e444.

VanLeit, B. (1994). Problem-based learning: A strategy for teaching undergraduate occupational therapy students. *Education Special Interest Section Newsletter of the American Occupational Therapy Association, 4*(4), 2-3.

Whitcombe, S. W. (2013). Problem-based learning students' perceptions of knowledge and professional identity: Occupational therapists as "knowers." *British Journal of Occupational Therapy, 76*(1), 37-42.

Williams, B. (2005). Case based learning—a review of the literature: Is there scope for this educational paradigm in pre-hospital education? *Emergency Medicine Journal, 22*(8), 577-581.

GAME-BASED INSTRUCTIONAL METHODS

Whitney Henderson, OTD, MOT, OTR/L

BASIC TENETS

Educational literature uses the term *serious games* to describe any method that combines the features of a game with pedagogical approaches. In other words, educators do not simply use games for entertainment purposes but instead pair the game with the processes of learning—objectives, assessment, and feedback. Educators implement this instructional method for a variety of reasons:

> Additional Names in Literature: educational games, game-based learning, board games, simulated games, virtual games

- To tailor games so students acquire new skills and to gain deeper knowledge of concepts in an enjoyable learning environment
- To foster motivation, as games have a competitive component—even if the student is simply comparing their own performance against a prior performance
- To provide a safe environment for the student to engage in trial and error without serious consequences
- To deliver immediate feedback that informs the student and the educator

Educators cater to a variety of learning styles while advancing various skills and knowledge when they use games. They provide an experience that requires the students to actively conceptualize and experiment with concepts so they can solve problems and learn from their actions. Educators design games to engage students in low levels (recall) or high levels (application) of thinking. In addition, they may enhance the students' communication and collaborative skills needed to work in team environments. Educational literature suggests linking the entertainment feature with the effective aspects of teaching and learning to produce high-quality games. Educators achieve this outcome when they capture their students' attention and motivation to repeatedly interact with

Henderson, W. (Ed.). *Effective Teaching: Instructional Methods and Strategies for Occupational Therapy Education* (pp. 317-342).

TABLE 13-1	
Nine Essential Characteristics of Serious Games	

CHARACTERISTIC	DESCRIPTION
1. An action language	The game offers communication between the student and the serious game; the student interacts with the game to understand the rules and to play with intention.
2. Assessment	The game provides feedback to the student during participation.
3. Conflict or challenge	The game presents problems that adequately challenge the students and require them to adapt their actions.
4. Control	The student has a degree of interaction and freedom within the game.
5. Environment	The game represents the context.
6. Game fiction	The game has a world or story.
7. Human interaction	The game offers opportunities for communication between two individuals.
8. Immersion	The students have a perceptual and affective relationship to the game.
9. Rules and goals	The game possesses clear rules and goals.

course content, promote problem solving while exploring in-game tasks, and provide effective feedback and positive experiences. In their study, Bedwell and colleagues (2012) establish a taxonomy for serious game with nine essential characteristics (Table 13-1).

Educators create a powerful learning environment when they implement serious games in their courses. One of the most frequently cited characteristics of serious games that contributes to learning is student motivation. Because of the playfulness and entertainment features, students are motivated to remain engaged with the game for long periods of time (Figure 13-1). In addition, they typically experience higher motivation in a competitive (but relaxed and nonthreatening) atmosphere. Serious games are becoming an increasingly interactive and social environment, which promotes collaborative learning through a community of players. In this active experience, well-designed and implemented games facilitate and enhance student learning.

BACKGROUND

Interestingly, when writing this book, we originally intended to discuss game-based instructional methods in the chapters on simulation (Chapter 7) or technology (Chapter 14). However, once we began to dig deeply, we found numerous game-based instructional methods and a rapidly growing body of literature. We also recognized that not all games are grounded in technology or simulation. Therefore, we felt educators could benefit from a chapter devoted to game-based instructional methods.

The idea of games began in the 1800s when consumers earned trading stamps to spend at supermarkets and other shops. Educators' use of games to teach and learn in an educational context is by no means a new phenomenon. Elementary and secondary school teachers have used educational games to teach students a variety of concepts across many different grade levels for many

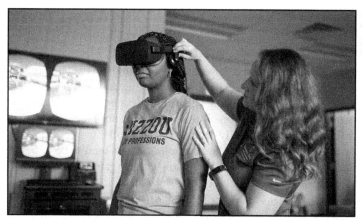

Figure 13-1. Student engaged in fun virtual reality game (Reproduced with permission from Keith Borgmeyer/ University of Missouri, 2019.)

years. In higher education, business and management education possesses a long history of game use during the teaching and learning process. In the 1960s, educators in medical education began to use games to teach students, and 2 decades later, nursing education introduced game show and board and card game formats into their teaching practices.

Despite these early beginnings, the coining of the term *gamification* occurred in 2003, but was not commonly used in educational literature until 7 years later. Therefore, many scholars still consider educator use of game-based instructional methods as an emerging practice, particularly in health professional education. However, we do note a large influx of games in medical education literature in recent years, and nursing education increasingly considers the use of games as a main-stream learning practice. Because of society's growing acceptance of digital games for entertainment purposes and technological advances in the computer, application, and game industries, educators should consider how to take advantage of these tools for educational purposes.

THEORY

Educational literature reports difficulty formulating a single theory for the development and implementation of serious games in educational settings. Many scholars believe educators can design games using several different models or theories of learning and often use many in com-bination (e.g., behaviorist, constructivist, cognitive). However, we commonly see educators and researchers reference Mihaly Csikszentmihalyi's theory of flow in serious game literature. The theory of flow explains the interactions between the players (students) and games and the level of engagement and immersion they experience while playing.

Students experience *flow* when they are entirely engrossed in the learning (e.g., they lose awareness of self and time). When in a flow state, they achieve a certain level of concentration and engagement as they complete a task that appropriately challenges their knowledge and skills. When they experience good flow, they enjoy playing and spend prolonged time participating in the game. Students need to experience this level of engagement (e.g., a flow state) to truly and effectively achieve learning. Csikszentmihalyi proposed nine dimensions of flow:

1. Balance between challenge and skill
2. Merge action and awareness
3. Establish clear goals
4. Provide unambiguous feedback (direct and immediate)
5. Use complete concentration
6. Experience a sense of control

7. Lose self-consciousness

8. Experience a transformation of time

9. Complete for an autotelic experience (desire to experience for own sake)

Educators consider these nine dimensions during game development to facilitate student achievement of flow. One of the biggest factors (and perhaps the best starting point) to achieve flow is the balance between challenge and skill. If the game challenges the student beyond their skills or knowledge, they experience frustration, anxiety, or stress. If the game does not provide adequate challenge, the students experience boredom and are easily distracted (e.g., similar to Lev Vygotsky's zone of proximal development discussed in Chapter 10). In addition, students tend to be in better flow when they play a game as a team rather than individually. As you design a game, return to these nine dimensions to ensure you are maximizing potential for flow.

In addition, Plass and colleagues (2015) report in order for games to reach maximum potential for learning, educators need to take many perspectives into consideration—cognitive, affective, motivational, and sociocultural factors. They believe serious games engage students in these areas in ways other instructional methods or learning contexts cannot achieve. From a cognitive perspective, educators design games with the goal to facilitate student construction of mental models. They consider how to include important content within the game and the processing demand of tasks (e.g., scaffold) so students achieve desired learning outcomes. From the affective perspective, educators consider how the game tasks, interactions, and environment impact students' emotions, attitudes, and beliefs. When educators view serious games from a motivational perspective, they provide experiences the students enjoy and desire to continue playing (e.g., intrinsic motivation, interests, reward, feedback). Lastly, from the sociocultural perspective, educators design games that afford opportunities for peer and social interactions and cultural experiences to successfully complete the game. When educators elicit multiple perspectives, they create powerful student learning experiences.

IMPLEMENTATION

In serious game literature, we do not find a conclusive or comprehensive structure for creating this instructional method. Therefore, similar to other instructional methods, we must rely on the components of evidence-based teaching when designing games for educational purposes. Despite the lack of a consistent framework, we note several common themes and important attributes for the development of a serious game, whether it be an element or the entirety of a game. We recognize the challenges to developing and implementing a framework, which covers a wide range from board games to larger budget digital games. Therefore, we combine several sources of information with Clarke and colleagues' (2016) EscapeED framework and Lameras and colleagues' (2017) essential features of serious games. This broad and adapted framework aligns games and educational strategies to balance play and deep learning. It is our hope this structure will support the production of clear, well-designed serious games, which achieves effective outcomes for both you and your students.

Step 1: Consider Students and Time

In the first step of development, you will want to carefully consider the students playing the game and the available time frame to engage in this experience. When considering your students, you should select an appropriate mode (or type) and level of difficulty based on the narrative you desire to convey, what content you have covered, what knowledge the students possess from prior courses, and the availability of resources to facilitate achievement or competency. If you are

TABLE 13-2

Four Purposes of Serious Games

PURPOSE	DESCRIPTION	EXAMPLE
1. Prepare for future learning	Students share experiences of engaging in a game so they can use for later learning.	Students play an online game to demonstrate competency of reading so they can better engage in class discussion.
2. Teach new knowledge and skills	Students acquire skills or knowledge as a result of playing the game.	Students learn about certain conditions through a "Family Feud" game.
3. Practice or reinforce prior knowledge of skills	Students practice various skills or strengthen understanding of concepts by participating in a game.	Students reinforce or practice communication skills required for successful completion of game.
4. Provide opportunities to develop 21st century skills	Students develop more complex socioemotional skills related to professional practice.	Students from different health care professions participate in "Breakout" game to foster collaboration and problem-solving skills.

implementing the game within a class period, we suggest you allow time to brief your students about the explicit rules, directions, and learning objectives for the game (10 to 15 minutes) and debrief with your students following completion (20 to 25 minutes). You can use the rest of class time to allow your students to participate in the game.

As you consider your students' abilities and time it will take, you can begin thinking about the purpose of the game before moving to the next step of developing your learning objectives. Serious games generally serve four purposes (Table 13-2).

Step 2: Write Desired Learning Outcomes

In the next step of development, you will write your learning objectives—what you want your students to achieve by engaging in a serious game. You can use the course and/or module outcomes to shape the learning objectives. Your learning outcomes drive the decisions you make when developing the game in the following steps. Educational literature suggests designing a game focused on a narrow and specific objective versus a random assortment of content to assist students to direct their focus to a particular skill or concept. In addition, educators need to strike a balance. If the game is too complex or competitive or it is too fun, the students will not learn. In order to achieve your learning objectives, you must maintain focus on learning while also having fun.

Educators often assume the learning objectives of a game are obvious to their students. It is critically important you clearly state the learning objectives prior to the start of the game. If you experience challenges in defining the objectives to your students, you should consider not playing the game until you have revisited your learning goals.

Step 3: Select the Theme

You are ready to select the game mode and theme that matches your desired learning objectives. We will provide several examples of different types of games later in this section. One of the easiest ways to select a game mode and/or theme is to brainstorm games you enjoy playing. Use the box below to list a few games. You can look for ways to match your learning objectives to these games.

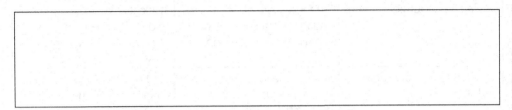

In this step, you will carefully consider the theme of the game. For example, do you want to write a single narrative that increases in complexity as the students advance through the game (e.g., scaffold), or do you want your students to collect tokens in a treasure quest when they correctly recall course concepts? In educational literature, you will see the terms emergence and progression to describe game themes. When educators employ an *emergence* structure, they create a game by combining a small set of rules with a large number of potential variations (e.g., board games). When they use a *progression* structure, educators design the experience in which the students have to perform a set number of actions for successful completion of the game.

Regardless of the theme you select, you will need to carefully consider the flow of the game. As we discussed before, flow immerses the individual in the game (e.g., loses awareness to time and self). Educators design a game to maintain students in as much flow as possible. They achieve this state by creating a game that is neither too easy nor too hard, so the students are in a consistent cycle of cognitive disequilibrium and resolution. Pitt and colleagues (2015) also suggest for educators to select a theme that affords students opportunities to create memories. Students demonstrate deeper learning when they are able to connect the content to a memory.

Step 4: Design the Game Mechanics

In Step 4, you will consider numerous aspects of game mechanics to facilitate a rich learning experience. *Game mechanics* are the collective tools, techniques, and applications essential to complete the learning experience. You will likely find this step the most challenging and time consuming. In Table 13-3, we list several elements of game design for you to consider. You do not have to use all of these elements in one game.

A *learning task* is an activity oriented to the outcomes that your students complete during the game. You will create several learning tasks, which can encompass cognitive, affective, physical, and game elements. In addition, some of the results of tasks serve as inputs for other learning tasks. Your learning tasks should provide your students an adequate challenge, but also possess different levels of difficulty.

In Table 13-4, we provide a list of questions for you to contemplate while designing the mechanics to ensure a natural flow within the game and a fit with your learning objectives. Please use the space next to the table to write your initial thoughts. After you have answered these questions, you can begin crafting the story, questions, rules, and answers. If you are electing to use a mode of high technology, we encourage you to connect with an instructional designer with experience in digital gaming during this step.

Table 13-3

Elements of Game Mechanics

ELEMENT	DESCRIPTION
Content and Skills	The educator designs the game to teach desired content and skills. This element influences other elements.
Incentive Structure	The educator designs incentives to motivate students to engage with the game and to provide feedback to modify or continue behavior. Game designers recommend the use of a variety of incentives to meet the preferences of many different students.
Musical Score	The educator designs background sounds to direct the students' attention to specific events or important moments. Sounds can warn students of danger or opportunities, induce emotions, or recognize the success of failure of a learning task. This element also includes any voices in the game.
Narrative Design	The educator designs the storyline with various features (e.g., scenes, actions, dialogues). This element provides the information for learning to occur by connecting rules, tasks, events, or characters. A good narrative design contributes to a game's *stickiness*—the students' desire to play or return to gameplay.
Visual Aesthetic Design	The educator designs many visual elements of the game, such as how the characters, cues, feedback, or incentives look and feel.

Step 5: Determine the Logistics

After you have completed the game mechanics, you are ready to arrange the logistics of the experience. Prior to the implementation of the game, you might need to secure equipment and space. If you are using a game grounded in technology, you will want to select a location with dependable internet. In addition, depending on the game mechanics, you might need to secure props, actors, or paper reports (medical reports, insurance records, pictures). For example, Largo and colleagues (2014) incorporated a patient's referral letter, medical history, and physical examination at the start of the game. Students made decisions about which labs, tests, or therapies they wanted to order based on these documents. Educators provided students the results of their decision (lab values, test results) and feedback via email, so they could further determine next actions. In addition, if using a digital game, you might need to consider developing and providing an orientation session for your students to complete prior to the game.

Step 6: Devise an Evaluation Plan

As with any other instructional method, you will need to devise a plan for evaluating the game and the students. Some educators ask their students to complete a survey or engage in the debrief process to offer feedback and suggestions for future game use. In a majority of situations, the game itself evaluates your students and provides them with important feedback. One reason why scholars believe games are effective is because games allow for graceful failure. Therefore, scholars suggest educators create an evaluative plan that allows for failure and to tell students it has the potential for learning. You can select evaluation methods that do not formally grade answers to reduce stress

TABLE 13-4

Game Mechanics Considerations

✓ What is the student doing within the game?	
✓ What are the learning tasks within the game?	
✓ What is the sequence of learning tasks?	
✓ Will the students solve a puzzle?	
✓ What questions will your students have to answer (e.g., multiple choice, short answer, select appropriate item on screen)?	
✓ Will they need to find clues to solve problems?	
✓ Will you provide in-game hints or descriptions to help them navigate the game?	
✓ What choices will the students make in the learning tasks?	
✓ What are the game rules?	
✓ How will the students answer the questions?	
✓ Will the students interact or collaborate during the game to complete the learning tasks?	
✓ How many learning tasks are feasible within your time frame?	
✓ Will there be milestones throughout the game?	
✓ How will the students receive feedback?	
✓ How will the students receive rewards?	

and anxiety. In fact, students explore areas, try new things, and take risks with lower consequences. Educators should also highlight powerful learning can occur from collaboratively discussing incorrect answers. We will discuss additional ways to monitor progress, provide feedback, and facilitate reflection later in the chapter.

ADDITIONAL IMPLEMENTATION NOTES

In this section, we provide a few additional strategies for successful implementation of game-based instructional methods. Educational literature strongly emphasizes the need for students to perceive the game as useful and easy to use. Therefore, we highly encourage you (and perhaps a colleague or student from another cohort) to participate in a mock game prior to use in the classroom. By taking the time to try the game, you will be able to modify game mechanics to improve flow and avoid any disruptions from design inconsistencies. In addition, you will also be more aware of potential areas of complexity and poorly defined attributes that can potentially cause your students to feel frustrated. By completing a mock game, you will also be better equipped to provide clear instructions for participation and prepared to communicate how the game aligns with the learning objectives. Lastly, each cohort of students could have different learning preferences, experiences, and academic preparation. Therefore, we recommend you revisit Step 1 each time you implement this method so you can evaluate your students and adapt the game if needed.

TIPS AND TRICKS

- Aim for the sweet spot—design a game where students can succeed, but also experience some struggle.
- Do not reinvent the wheel. Educators model many educational games after existing mainstream games.
- Consider the use of nontrivia games to stimulate higher-level thinking and participation (versus trivia-based games, which require a lot of recall).
- Raise the bar by incorporating a discussion or group teaching method after the game.
- Seize the opportunity to use incorrect responses as a catalyst for further learning and discussion.
- Consider the use of games that have more than one answer to reduce stress and anxiety (e.g., "Family Feud"—teams try to guess the most common answers).
- Play the role of the host by soliciting the collective knowledge of the group through the use of open-ended questions.
- Trivia games work best with smaller groups of students and problem-solving games work best with bigger groups of students.

> Ask your students to take turns answering questions to ensure participation in bigger teams.

TYPES OF GAMES

No Technology

Board Game

Students play a tabletop game by moving pieces according to certain ways along a marked board. In occupational therapy education, Mitchell and Booker (personal communication, September 13, 2019) modified a "Snakes and Ladders" game (board game known as "Chutes and Ladders") to facilitate their students' understanding of research concepts. In this serious game, the educators asked their students questions that required them to actively retrieve, apply, analyze, and evaluate research concepts (Figure 13-2A). The students rolled dice to move forward spaces on the board and could potentially land on the head of a snake or the foot of a ladder. If they answered the question correctly, they "stunned the snake" and remained in place or advanced up the ladder. If they answered incorrectly, they moved backward in the game by sliding down the snake or remained at the base of the ladder. The first student to reach the last space on the board game won the game. The educators also engaged the students in a debrief session following completion of the game (Figure 13-2B).

Card Game

Although literature on the use of this card game is found in nursing education, "BARNGA" is a perfect fit with occupational therapy education. Educators use this game in conjunction with a planned debrief to teach students cultural awareness. The educator arranges the students into small groups and provides them with a modified deck of cards and a list of rules for playing a new card game. The group has a few minutes to practice playing the game according to the written rules. After the students have had time to study the rules and practice the game, the educator collects the list of rules and establishes a strict new rule that the students can no longer have verbal communication. The students can gesture or draw pictures but cannot communicate verbally (Figure 13-3). Similar to a tournament when teams move to other sides of a bracket to play new opponents, the educator informs students to move to a different table while still following the same no verbal communication rule. The educator continues to move students around for approximately 10 minutes. What the students do not know is at the beginning of the game, every table received a slightly different version

Figure 13-2A. Students play "Snakes and Ladders" game to learn research concepts.

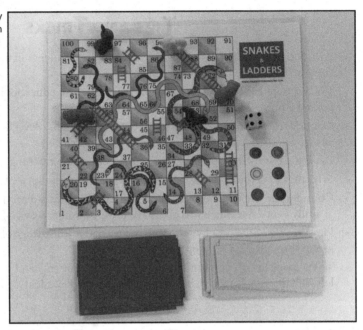

Figure 13-2B. Educators provide students feedback during board game.

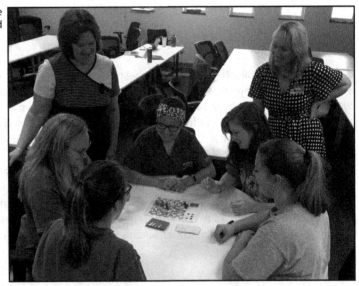

of the same game. These small differences spark great energy and discussion for the hidden aspects of culture! One great feature about this card game is that the format is readily available online and requires no to little modification. We have also used this game to teach occupational therapy students about bias during the evaluation process. In addition, inexperienced educators can easily implement this game because of the resources available to guide the implementation and debrief discussion time for reflecting-on-action.

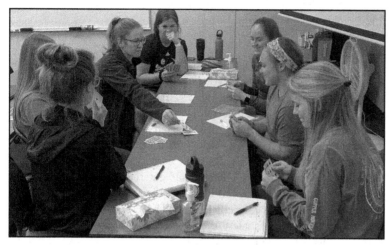

Figure 13-3. Students play "BARNGA" to understand assessment bias.

Breakout

In educational literature, we find a framework for fabricating a game based on the escape room businesses that have gained popularity over the last couple of years. In fact, educators can even purchase kits and share games via the BreakoutEDU website (https://www.breakoutedu.com). Humphrey (2017) created a BreakoutEDU game for students in sport psychology education to understand applied research skills. The author wrote a real-world scenario in which the students had to recommend 10 players to serve as coaches at a local football club. The students had 60 minutes to find clues and unlock new pieces of information, such as player information or nonplayer dialogues. Throughout the game, the educator provided in-game hints to help the students advance through the experience. Each group of students wrote an executive summary and list of recommendations and justification by the end of the game.

Low Technology

PowerPoint Games

Educators can transform many television game shows and board games (e.g., "Trivial Pursuit") to innovative social and cooperative learning tools. If you search the internet, you will find numerous free templates and instructions for creating a game using a PowerPoint presentation. In educational literature, we see examples of educators using a "Family Feud" template to teach infection control or "Jeopardy" template to teach medical terminology. You can find other game show templates, such as "Who Wants to Be a Millionaire," "The Price is Right," or "Deal or No Deal."

App

We understand there are several apps available for educational use; however, we will highlight the use of GooseChase (http://www.goosechase.com) for occupational therapy education. With this application, educators use a web browser to write missions and assign points in order to create the scavenger hunt. The students use their phones to complete a mission and win points by uploading a photograph or 10-second video or by providing a text entry. In turn, the educator can provide feedback or give bonus points for additional or well-thought out answers. Grant (2019) used this app to afford her students opportunities to develop skills in adaptive equipment use and prescription in a local teaching clinic.

High Technology

Home Simulation

Online Game Development Tools
- Scratch
- GameMaker
- Alice
- Adventure Maker
- Kodu

(Sera & Wheeler, 2017)

Many sites offer educators an online community where they can discuss and support game development.

Our students live in a high technology society. Therefore, we find an emergence of digital games in educational literature. In a 2018 systematic review, Gorbanev and colleagues (2018) reported a small majority (52.4%) of games occurred in a web-based environment. In medical education, Duque and colleagues (2008) created a video game to teach their students how to perform home visits with the geriatric population. They designed a highly interactive video game using a software application and bidimensional illustrations. The students entered the home of an older patient and explored different rooms using their own strategy and at their own pace. If the student correctly identified a factor that could potentially compromise the patient's safety, they clicked on it and received 10 points. If they incorrectly identified and clicked a concern, they lost 10 points. The students attempted to achieve a score of 500 points within 10 minutes of engaging with the game.

OPPORTUNITIES FOR FEEDBACK AND REFLECTION

Games provide an interactive environment and immediate feedback which attracts students' attention and challenges them to effectively demonstrate mastery of the learning objectives. Educators inherently give feedback to students because the game often offers immediate responses about correctness of answers or decisions. If the game contains more checkpoints, educators can better monitor student progress and use this information to understand where they need clarification, improvements, or resources. Educational literature offers many different mechanisms for the provision of feedback. For example, educators can ask students to upload evidence of achievement or short answers within the game. They provide students with individualized feedback before giving approval to advance to the next stage of the game. In another example, the educator can design a feedback system that rewards students a token when they correctly answer content questions.

An additional feedback and reflection strategy educators can implement is called "around the room in 80 seconds." During a game, the educator asks a question. When a student successfully answers the question, they state something they know about the topic. The educator goes around the room asking students to add another point they know about the topic until the group exhausts all relevant points. The educator listens as students continue to generate new ideas, examines any inaccuracies in thinking, redirects their attention, and fills in knowledge gaps (as needed). During this student-driven strategy, the educator has the learning objectives in mind and runs a mental checklist of the key points to ensure the goals are met.

Many scholars highlight a concern that serious games do not always foster the transfer of skills or knowledge to another learning or practical experience. Therefore, it is recommended educators employ debriefing to further scaffold content outside of the game. They may ask their students to write a narrative story to encourage awareness to their understanding of experiences, decisions, or events after completing the game. In this strategy, educators invite students to freely write an answer to a question for 5 minutes. Examples of questions include:

- Describe a time in the game or situation when you were confused.
- Explain a few inner resources you can use to deal with your limitations.
- What did you learn from the game that will impact the individuals you serve in your future practice?

You could also encourage your students to share their writings with a partner or the class, so they understand each other's different patterns of thinking or meaning.

APPLICATION TO OCCUPATIONAL THERAPY PRACTICE

In the current landscape, there is an increasing desire to involve patients and families in their own health care through the use of health games. In addition, patients and families have access to more and more tools to assist them to manage their health. Health care professionals use *health games* to investigate behavioral change and train various physical and mental behaviors and skills. The literature provides two examples of ways occupational therapy practitioners can potentially incorporate games into their practice.

Example 1: Use of Board Games for Social Skills or Health Education

For several of our clients and families, games might be a desired leisure or social participation occupation. Therefore, we can incorporate this meaningful occupation in our treatment sessions to address a variety of topics or concerns. Perhaps you are working with a group of young children in a preschool setting. You can use the broad framework outlined above to select a game to help teach the children in the class the important social skills of following rules, taking turns, staying seated in their chairs, and listening. We can also use board games to provide health education. Viggiano and colleagues (2014) offers an example of using a board game to help children and adolescents learn healthy eating habits, and Khazaal and colleagues (2013) show us how we can use a board game to teach the health promotion topic of smoking cessation.

Example 2: Use of Digital Games to Manage Health

Kumar and colleagues (2004) developed a handheld application called the Daily Automated Intensive Log for Youth to assist children and families with diabetes management. Researchers provided each individual with a device equipped with a health management logging system and a motivational game to help youth predict blood sugars. Occupational therapy practitioners could implement similar digital games to education and train clients in medication or financial management and in a self-management program.

Advantages

- Can potentially increase students' curiosity and interest level
- Increases energy level, engagement, and interaction
- Can adapt to address cognitive, affective, and psychomotor skills
- Enhances collaborative and communication skills and a sense of community when played in teams
- Provides a relaxed atmosphere and safe space for learning
- Typically promotes improved attitudes about learning when compared to traditional methods
- Can use for larger or smaller class sizes
- Provides opportunities for repetitive or scaffold learning
- Availability of wide variety of low- and high-technology options
- Allows for customizability and flexibility
- Students familiar with games
- Opportunities for low-cost options
- Opportunities to apply concepts to practice and engage in higher forms of learning (application, analysis)
- Increases in number of studies
- Provides the student with familiarity
- Allows students to recall knowledge from the game experience

Challenges

- Can be resource intensive (cost, time, space)
- Potentially causes the students to experience anxiety, embarrassment, or intimidation
- Can potentially be boring to some students
- Need for further conclusive evidence and well-designed studies (see Game-Based Instructional Methods Evidence Table)
- Challenges to develop an engaging game that also aligns with learning objectives
- Requires committed people with knowledge and skills beyond the course content

> If using these types of games, it is essential that you collect data to demonstrate the benefits of this method.

In the space below, list any additional advantages or challenges.

Brainstorm strategies for overcoming these challenges when implementing the use of game-based instructional methods.

THREE THINGS YOU CAN DO TOMORROW TO IMPLEMENT GAME-BASED INSTRUCTIONAL METHODS WITH YOUR STUDENTS

1. Explore websites that provide templates for games.
2. Connect with a game-based teaching and learning community on your campus (e.g., game designer, educators that use games).
3. Review a few educational applications and find one you can incorporate into your course.

Game-Based Instructional Methods Evidence Table

Author/Year	Study Objectives	Design and Participants	Intervention and Outcome Measures	Results
Agudelo-Londono et al. (2019)	Researchers tested the pedagogical effect and technological acceptance of CODIFICO (a serious game) in training medical students on International Classification of Diseases (ICD)-10 diagnosis coding	Design: Cohort study Participants: 61 undergraduate medical students from medicine at Pontifical Javeriana University	The researchers presented students with the game, the study methodology, and an overview of the ICD-10 coding Students completed a multiple-choice test using Blackboard Learn After the test, students downloaded and installed the CODIFICO mobile application on their phones After 7 days of using the phone application, the students completed a posttest Outcome measures: • Learning performance • Student perception of the serious game	Overall, students reported the serious game was useful There was no statistically significant difference found in learning performance for those who participated in the study
Bayram & Caliskan (2019)	Researchers aimed to determine the effects of a game-based virtual reality phone application on tracheostomy care education for nursing students	Design: Randomized controlled trial Participants: 118 first-year nursing students enrolled in the Fundamentals of Nursing II course at Gazi University; 59 nursing students were assigned to the control group, while another set of 59 nursing students were assigned to the experimental group	Intervention: Experimental group accessed virtual reality phone application following their first objective clinical exam Outcome measures: • Students' knowledge on tracheostomy care • The descriptive characteristics questionnaire • Tracheostomy care information test • Tracheostomy care skill checklists	The researchers found a greater increase in the knowledge score of students using the phone application as compared to that of the control group However, there was no statistical difference between the experimental and control groups in regard to the final knowledge scores

(continued)

Game-Based Instructional Methods Evidence Table (continued)

Author/Year	Study Objectives	Design and Participants	Intervention and Outcome Measures	Results
		Inclusion criteria: • Students enrolled in Fundamentals of Nursing II for the first time • Students with an Android mobile phone • Students with internet access • Students without previous experience in tracheostomy care		
Bigdeli & Kaufman (2017)	Researchers focused on digital games in medicine and aimed to explain benefits, flaws, and engagement factors influencing gamification instruments for health education	Design: Systematic review Participants: Health professions students	Databases searched: CINAHL Complete, Cochrane Library, EBSCOhost, Science Direct, Education Resources Information Center, PsycINFO, PsycArticles, PubMed, PubMed Central, MedLine Dates of publication: 2010 to 2015 Researchers collected various studies from the health professions disciplines to gather data on advantages and disadvantages of digital games as a form of education Inclusion criteria: • Full-text peer-reviewed papers in English • Health professions students were study participants	Advantages for digital games as an educational tool included: • Feasibility for adult learning • Engagement of learners, which further promotes knowledge acquisition, attitude, and practice • Learner individualization • Increased learning process and learner outcomes • Practicality for teachers, learners, and the health system

(continued)

Game-Based Instructional Methods Evidence Table (continued)

Author/Year	Study Objectives	Design and Participants	Intervention and Outcome Measures	Results
			Digital games in health professions education disciplines of medicine, nursing, pharmacy, and dentistry Outcome measures: Determining advantages and disadvantages of a game-based learning environment	Additionally, digital games encourage more collaboration between teachers and learners through the development of a safe virtual curricular and extracurricular educational space beyond ordinary teaching and learning contexts Disadvantages included: • Games could be intimidating for some students due to the competitive nature of games • There is dependency on interdisciplinary expertise, time consumption, and learning style dependency • Potential boredom • Lack of widely accepted guidelines • Students' lack of desire to cooperate leading to game failure • Potential negative reaction of learners to the game design • Physical harm risks
Diehl et al. (2017)		Design: Randomized controlled trial (RCT) Participants: 170 primary care physicians (PCPs) working within public health care units	Intervention: Researchers provided access to InsuOnline program on personal desktops to teach the PCPs on insulin use with patients in a public health care unit The control group participated in a traditional-format onsite learning session taught by a clinical endocrinologist	This study found no significant difference concerning game applicability between the 2 groups The game group reflected greater increases in competence scores immediately postintervention as compared to the control group

(continued)

Game-Based Instructional Methods Evidence Table (continued)

Author/Year	Study Objectives	Design and Participants	Intervention and Outcome Measures	Results
	Researchers assessed applicability, user acceptance, and educational effectiveness of InsuOnline (an electronic serious game for insulin education) compared with a traditional continuing medical education activity	Inclusion criteria: • Participants included medical doctors with an active register at a regional Council of Medicine in Brazil • Participants were currently working at a public health care unit as a PCP, and they were directly involved in the treatment of patients with diabetes in those facilities • Some degree of computer or gaming literacy	Additionally, the traditional-format session had same duration of the game Outcome measures: Score in the competence subscale in the postintervention self-assessment	Both the game group and the control group reported positive satisfaction with the educational mediums
Drummond et al. (2017)	Researchers identified the effects of an online course versus a serious game on management of sudden cardiac arrest in medical students	Design: RCT Participants: 82 second-year medical students from French medical facilities	Researchers randomized students into 2 different groups. The control group participated in the online course, while the intervention participated in a serious game	There were no statistically significant differences between the online course group and the serious game-based group regarding median training time needed to reach the minimum passing score of a cardiac arrest simulation

(continued)

Game-Based Instructional Methods Evidence Table (continued)

Author/Year	Study Objectives	Design and Participants	Intervention and Outcome Measures	Results
		Students were greater than 18 years old and participated in a 1-hour course on sudden cardiac arrest during their first year of the program	Researchers required both groups to participate in a hands-on simulation of cardiac arrest to compare education retention between the 2 groups on cardiac arrest management Outcome measures: Median training time needed by the different groups of students to reach the minimum passing score during a hands-on session of cardiac arrest	
Gorbanev et al. (2018)	Researchers highlighted the quality of evidence produced from various articles, and make developers aware of the importance of the pedagogical strategy during game design	Design: Systematic review Researchers included 21 articles for the effectiveness of serious games in medical education and the quality of the evidence supporting games in education Most games included in these articles were developed in the United States Participants: Medical students	Intervention: A multidisciplinary team of researchers used the Cochrane Collaboration Guidelines to conduct this systematic review Databases searched: Web of Science, Scopus, ProQuest, EBSCO Host, and OvidMedline Publication dates: 2011 to 2015 The Medical Education Research Study Quality Instrument (MERSQI) was used to determine the quality of evidence in the use of games Inclusion criteria: • Peer-reviewed journal articles that described or assessed the use of serious games or gamified apps in medical education • Studies included under- and postgraduate-level medical students and doctors Outcome measures: • Acquired skills and knowledge • Learner satisfaction and attitude • Quality of evidence	16 of the articles collected focused primarily on skill and knowledge, while the other 5 articles focused on learner satisfaction and attitude The MERSQI assessed the quality of the evidence from the gaming articles, and the researchers found that the quality of evidence was moderate, even though most articles reported some positive influence of games for student education The researchers classified the majority of the game developers' pedagogical strategies as behaviorists or cognitivists The majority of game designs were coherent with pedagogical strategies

(continued)

Game-Based Instructional Methods Evidence Table (continued)

Author/Year	Study Objectives	Design and Participants	Intervention and Outcome Measures	Results
Karbownik et al. (2016)	Researchers identified the effects of an educational board game on student knowledge of pharmacology as compared to a lecture-based seminar	Design: RCT Participants: 124 Polish third-year medical students from the Medical University of Lodz	Researchers randomly assigned to the intervention group (played an educational game) or the control group (participated in a lecture-based seminar) Both the control and intervention groups participated in a 90-minute session regarding pharmacology education in the format of either the lecture or the game Outcome measures: • Knowledge of pharmacology • Knowledge retention • Learning preference	While both the game-based group and the lecture-based group had improved short-term knowledge retention following the study, the game-based group had greater long-term retention as compared to the lecture-based group Both groups reported greater short-term retention following the study, but the game-based group reported that their educational game improved perceived education to a greater extent as compared to the lecture-based group
Lagro et al. (2014)	Researchers aimed to determine if GeriatriX (a serious game designed to address the complexity of decision making in geriatrics) would have positive effects on the ability to deal with complex geriatric decision making with medical students	Design: RCT Participants: 145 fifth-year medical students of the Radboud University Medical Center	Intervention: The control group participated in the standard geriatric education The intervention group played 3 cases of online GeriatriX in conjunction with the standard geriatric education Outcome measures: • Needs assessment scale • Questionnaire to test geriatric knowledge • Geriatric knowledge and cost effectiveness	Study found no significant difference between intervention and control groups in geriatric knowledge; rather, both groups improved their geriatric knowledge after participating in study. However, the intervention group reported greater self-perceived knowledge compared to control group Students who participated in GeriatriX more frequently chose the correct cost category for various medical procedures as compared to their control group counterparts
Luchi et al. (2017)	Researchers aimed to identify effect of an educational game on students' learning regarding action potentials	Design: RCT	This study was divided into 2 different experiments. Both experiments used the same population sample of first-year undergraduate students	The students that participated in the game activities had higher scores and fewer errors regarding resting membrane potential as compared with the control group

(continued)

Game-Based Instructional Methods Evidence Table (continued)

Author/Year	Study Objectives	Design and Participants	Intervention and Outcome Measures	Results
		Participants: 148 first-year students of the undergraduate course in dentistry at the School of Dentistry at Piracicaba of the University of Campinas	*Experiment 1 (n = 67):* Evaluated the effect of games on learning about resting potential by comparing the group that attended a lecture and studied the topic at home (control group) to the group that completed everything the control group did plus they completed an educational game *Experiment 2 (n = 81):* This experiment compared performances of the group that attended a lecture and studied the action potentials at home (control group) and the group that studied action potentials at home and completed the game activity	For the questions concerning action potentials, the students participating in the game group once again had higher scores and fewer mistakes as compared to the control group Students who participated in the game reported that the activity helped clarify content, increased understanding, and was a fun way to learn material
Nakao (2019)	Researchers aimed to clarify the possible roles of board game use in psychosomatic medicine	Design: Systematic review Researchers found 83 studies/articles to understand roles of board game use: 56 targeted education/training, 6 observed basic brain mechanisms, 5 examined preventative measures for dementia/healthy aging, and 3 assessed communication/public health policies	Databases searched: PubMed Publication dates: 2012 to 2018 Inclusion criteria: • Articles published after 2012 • Studies associated with board games and medicine Primary outcomes: • Health • Brain activity • Satisfaction	Several studies found that the basal ganglia are vital in one's ability to determine subsequent moves in game situations Board games were also found to have relatively positive impacts on health; symptoms of panic attacks, attention-deficit hyperactivity disorder, and Alzheimer's disease were shown to improve upon gaming intervention Board game use may decrease illness-prone behaviors in children and adults, as well as prevent cognitive impairments in older adults Studies found that board games can be an effective and fun medium for medical and safety education for students

(continued)

Game-Based Instructional Methods Evidence Table (continued)

Author/Year	Study Objectives	Design and Participants	Intervention and Outcome Measures	Results
Polivka et al. (2019)	Researchers determined the efficacy, usability, and desirability of a home health care interactive virtual simulation training system (VSTS) to train health care workers and students in responding to health and safety hazards in the home	Design: RCT Participants: 74 home health care workers and health professions students Inclusion criteria: • Students of health professional programs (speech therapy, occupational therapy, etc.) • Workers of home health care • Participants of 18 years of age or older	Intervention: Researchers assigned 39 participants to the experimental group, which participated in the home health care interactive VSTS The control group consisted of 36 participants that completed paper-based education Outcome measures: A questionnaire to assess usability, usefulness, and desirability	Students of the experimental group reported that the home health care interactive VSTS was both usable and useful The majority of students reported the simulation training system as desirable The researchers found the accuracy of detection of hazards within the home of the client to be high in both the intervention and control groups, indicating efficacy of training for both methods
Sipiyaruk et al. (2018)	Researchers sought to identify high-quality evidence regarding impacts of serious games on health care education (Part I); secondly, the study aimed to explore evidence regarding impacts of serious games in dental education (Part II)	Design: Systematic review Researchers included 9 systematic reviews to identify high-quality evidence associated with serious games and health care education (Part I)	Databases Searched: Embase, MedLine, PsycINFO, PubMed, CINAHL, Education Resources Information Center, British Education Index, British Nursing Index, Scopus, Cochrane Database of Systematic Reviews Publication dates: Part I: 2015 to 2016 Part II: 1975 to 2016	Participants partaking in serious games showed significant improvements in knowledge as compared to traditional approaches or no intervention; this was the most common outcome of the study A couple of systematic reviews reported increased knowledge retention for those who participated in the serious game interventions as compared to traditional methods

(continued)

Game-Based Instructional Methods Evidence Table (continued)

Author/Year	Study Objectives	Design and Participants	Intervention and Outcome Measures	Results
		Researchers included 2 RCTs to explore the evidence regarding serious games and their influence on dental education (Part II)	Part I inclusion criteria: • Systematic reviews or meta-analyses that analyzed outcomes of serious games in health care education • Studies were designed for learning and training of undergraduate or postgraduate students, or qualified professionals Part II inclusion criteria: • Any type of empirical study • Articles studying computer-based serious games in dental education • Articles presenting outcomes of serious games Primary outcomes: • Knowledge retention • Acquired skills • Satisfaction	2 of the systematic reviews found that serious games improved skills in medical students and that these games could be used for skill training in medical fields Several studies found that serious games tend to be associated with greater satisfaction as compared to traditional approaches, presenting a significant benefit for this medium of education The 2 RCT studies found that serious games could be an effective learning tool for dental education; however, there were no significant differences between the serious game groups and the traditional methods groups

Adapted from American Occupational Therapy Association. (2002). AOTA's evidence-based literature review project: An overview (D. Lieberman & J. Scheer, Eds.). American Journal of Occupational Therapy, 56, 344-349. https://doi.org/10.5014/ajot.56.3.344

REFERENCES

Agudelo-Londono, S., Gorbanev, I., Delgadillo, V., Munoz, O., Cortes, A., González, R. A., & Pomares-Quimbaya, A. (2019). Development and evaluation of a serious game for teaching ICD-10 diagnosis coding to medical students. *Games for Health Journal, 8*(5), 349-356. http://dx.doi.org/10.1089/g4h.2018.0101

American Occupational Therapy Association. (2002). AOTA's evidence-based literature review project: An overview (D. Lieberman & J. Scheer, Eds.). *The American Journal of Occupational Therapy, 56,* 344-349. https://doi.org/10.5014/ajot.56.3.344

Bayram, S. B., & Caliskan, N. (2019). Effect of a game-based virtual reality phone application on tracheostomy care education for nursing students: A randomized controlled trial. *Nurse Education Today, 79,* 25-31. https://doi.org/10.1016/j.nedt.2019.05.010

Bedwell, W. L., Pavlas, D., Heyne, K., Lazzara, E. H., & Salas, E. (2012). Toward a taxonomy linking game attributes to learning: An empirical study. *Simulation & Gaming, 43*(6), 729-760. http://dx.doi.org/10.1177/1046878112439444

Bigdeli, S., & Kaufman, D. (2017). Digital games in health professions education: Advantages, disadvantages, and game engagement factors. *Medical Journal of the Islamic Republic of Iran, 31*(117), 1-6. https://doi.org/10.14196/mjiri.31.117

Clarke, S., Arnab, S., Keegan, H., Morini, L., & Wood, O. (2016). EscapeED: Adapting live-action, interactive games to support higher education teaching and learning practices. In *International Conference on Games and Learning Alliance* (pp. 144-153). Springer. http://doi.org/10.1007/978-3-319-22960-7

Diehl, L. A., Souza, R. M., & Coelho, C. M. (2017). InsuOnline, an electronic game for medical education on insulin therapy: A randomized controlled trial with primary care physicians. *Journal of Medical Internet Research, 19*(3), e72. https://clinicaltrials.gov/ct2/show/NCT01759953

Drummond, D., Delval, P., Abdenouri, S., Truchot, J., Ceccaldi, P. F., Plaisance, P., Hadchouel, A., & Tesniere, A. (2017). Serious game versus online course for pretraining medical students before a simulation-based mastery learning course on cardiopulmonary resuscitation: A randomized controlled study. *European Journal of Anesthesiology, 34,* 836-844. http://dx.doi.org/10.1097/EJA.0000000000000675

Duque, G., Fung, S., Mallet, L., Posel, N., & Fleiszer, D. (2008). Learning while having fun: The use of video gaming to teach geriatric house calls to medical students. *Journal of the American Geriatrics Society, 56*(7), 1328-1332.

Gorbanev, I., Agudelo-Londono, S., Gonzalez, R. A., Cortes, A., Pomares, A., Delgadillo, V., Yepes, F. J., & Munoz, O. (2018). A systematic review of serious games in medical education: Quality of evidence and pedagogical strategy. *Medical Education Online, 23*(1), 1438718. https://doi.org/10.1080/10872981.2018.1438718

Grant, T. (2019). Using technology enhanced learning to promote the acquisition of practical skills in occupational therapy. *Journal of Occupational Therapy Education, 3*(2), Article 12. https://doi.org/10.26681/jote.2019.030212

Humphrey, K. (2017). The application of a serious, non-digital escape game learning experience in higher education. *Sport & Exercise Psychology Review, 13*(2), 48-54.

Karbownik, M. S., Wiktorowska-Owczarek, A., Kowalczyk, E., Kwarta, P., Mokros, L., & Pietras, T. (2016). Board game versus lecture-based seminar in the teaching of pharmacology of antimicrobial drugs—a randomized controlled trial. *FEMS Microbiology Letters, 363,* 1-9. http://dx.doi.org/10.1093/femsle/fnw045

Khazaal, Y., Chatton, A., Prezzemolo, R., Zebouni, F., Edel, Y., Jacquet, J., Ruggeri, O., Burnens, E., Monney, G., Protti, A. S., Etter, J. F., Khan, R., Cornuz, J., & Zullino, D. (2013). Impact of a board-game approach on current smokers: A randomized controlled trial. *Substance Abuse Treatment Prevention Policy, 8*(1), 3.

Kumar, V. S., Wentzell, K. J., Mikkelsen, T., Pentland, A., & Laffel, L. M. (2004). The DAILY (Daily Automated Intensive Log for Youth) trial: A wireless, portable system to improve adherence and glycemic control in youth with diabetes. *Diabetes Technology & Therapeutics, 6*(4), 445-453.

Lagro, J., van de Pol, M. H. J., Laan, A., Huijbregts-Verheyden, F. J., Fluit, L. C. R., & Olde Rikkert, M. G. M. (2014). A randomized controlled trial on teaching geriatric medical decision making and cost consciousness with the serious game GeriatricX. *Journal of the American Medical Directors Association, 15*(957), 957.e1-957.e6. http://dx.doi.org/10.1016/j.jamda.2014.04.011

Lameras, P., Arnab, S., Dunwell, I., Stewart, C., Clarke, S., & Petridis, P. (2017). Essential features of serious games design in higher education: Linking learning attributes to game mechanics. *British Journal of Educational Technology, 48*(4), 972-994.

Luchi, K. C. G., Montrezor, L. H., & Marcondes, F. K. (2017). Effect of an educational game on university students' learning about action potentials. *Advanced Physiology Education, 41,* 222-230. http://dx.doi.org/10.1152/advan.00146.2016

Nakao, M. (2019). Special series on "effects of board games on health education and promotion" board games as a promising tool for health promotion: A review of recent literature. *BioPsychoSocial Medicine, 15*(5), 1-7. https://doi.org/10.1186/s13030-019-0146-3

Pitt, M. B., Borman-Shoap, E. C., & Eppich, W. J. (2015). Twelve tips for maximizing the effectiveness of game-based learning. *Medical Teacher, 37,* 1013-1017.

Plass, J. L., Homer, B. D., & Kinzer, C. K. (2015). Foundations of game-based learning. *Educational Psychologist, 50*(4), 258-283. http://dx.doi.org/10.1080/00461520.2015.1122533

Polivka, B. J., Anderson, S., Lavender, S. A., Sommerich, C. M., Stredney, D. L., Wills, C. E., & Darragh, A. R. (2019). Efficacy and usability of a virtual simulation training system for health and safety hazards encountered by healthcare workers. *Games Health Journal, 8*(2), 121-128. http://dx.doi.org/10.1089/g4h.2018.0068

Sipiyaruk, K., Gallagher, J. E., Hatzipanagos, S., & Reynolds, P. A. (2018). A rapid review of serious games: From healthcare education to dental education. *European Journal of Dental Education, 22*(4), 243-257.

Viggiano, A., Viggiano, E., Di Costanzo, A., Viggiano, A., Andreozzi, E., Romano, V., Rianna, I., Vicidomini, C., Gargano, G., Incarnato, L., Fevola, C., Volta, P., Tolomeo, C., Scianni, G., Santangelo, C., Battista, R., Monda, M., Viggiano, A., De Luca, B., & Amaro, S. (2014). Kaledo, a board game for nutrition education of children and adolescents at school: Cluster randomized controlled trial of health lifestyle promotion. *European Journal of Pediatrics, 174*, 217-228. http://dx.doi.org/10.1007/s00431-014-2381-8

BIBLIOGRAPHY

Abdulmajed, H., Park, Y. S., & Tekian, A. (2015). Assessment of educational games for health professions: A systematic review of trends and outcomes. *Medical Teacher, 37*, S27-S32. http://dx.doi.org/10.3109/0142159X.2015.1006609

Adamson, M. A., Chen, H., Kackley, R., & Micheal, A. (2018). Game-versus lecture-based learning with generation Z patients. *Journal of Psychosocial Nursing, 56*(2), 29-36.

Akl, E., A., Pretorius, R. W., Sackett, K., Erdley, W. S., Bhoopathi, P. S., Alfarah, Z., & Schunemann, H. J. (2010). The effect of educational games on medical students' learning outcomes: A systematic review: BEME guide no 14. *Medical Teacher, 32*, 16-27. http://dx.doi.org/10.3109/01421590903473969

Alblas, E. E., Foldvord, F., Anschutz, D. J., van 't Riet, J., Granic, I., Ketelaar, P., & Buijzen, M. (2018). Investigating the impact of a health game on implicit attitudes towards food and food choice behavior of young adults. *Appetite, 128*, 294-302. https://doi.org/10.1016/j.appet.2018.05.141

Blakely, G., Skirton, H., Allum, P., & Nelmes, P. (2010). Use of educational games in the health professions: A mixed-methods study of educators' perspectives in the UK. *Nursing and Health Sciences, 12*, 27-32.

Blumberg, F. C., & Pagnotta, J. N. (2014). Gameplay and educational outcomes: Reminders for education game development. *Games for Health Journal, 3*(2), 115-116. http://dx.doi.org/10.1089/g4h.2014.0012

Boeker, M., Andel, P., Vach, W., & Frankenschmidt, A. (2013). Game-based e-learning is more effective than a conventional instructional method: A randomized controlled trial with third-year medical students. *PLoS ONE, 8*(12), e82328. http://dx.doi.org/10.1371/journal.pone.0082328

Bourgonjon, J., Valcke, M., Soetaert, R., & Schellens, T. (2010). Students' perceptions about the use of video games in the classroom. *Computers and Education, 54*, 1145-1156. http://dx.doi.org/10.1016/j.compedu.2009.10.022

Charlier, N., & De Fraine, B. (2013). Game-based learning as a vehicle to teach first aid content: A randomized experiment. *Journal of School Health, 83*(7), 493-499.

Davidson, S. J., & Candy, L. (2016). Teaching EBP using game-based learning: Improving the student experience. *Worldviews on Evidence-Based Nursing, 13*(4), 285-293.

Graham, I., & Richardson, E. (2008). Experiential gaming to facilitate cultural awareness: Its implications for developing emotional caring in nursing. *Learning in Health and Social Care, 7*(1), 37-45.

Kreutzer, C. P., & Bowers, C. A. (2016). Making games for health engaging: The influence of cognitive skills. *Games for Health Journal, 5*(1), 21-26. http://dx.doi.org/10.1089/g4h.2015.0048

Lowenstein, A. J., & Bradsaw, M. J. (2001). *Fuszard's innovatie teaching strategies in nursing* (3rd ed.). ASPEN.

Rondon, S., Sassi, F. C., & Furquim de Andrade, C. (2013). Computer game-based and traditional learning method: A comparison regarding students' knowledge retention. *BMC Medical Education, 13*(30), 1-8. http://www.biomedcentral.com/1472-6920/13/30

Sera, L., & Wheeler, E. (2017). Game on: The gamification of the pharmacy classroom. *Currents in Pharmacy Teaching and Learning, 9*, 155-159. http://dx.doi.org/10.1016/j.cptl.2016.08.046

Wang, C. H., Wu, K. C., & Tsau, S. Y. (2019). Flow learning experience: Applying marketing theory to serious game design. *Journal of Educational Computing, 57*(2), 417-447. http://dx.doi.org/10.1177/0735633117752454

14

TECHNOLOGY-BASED
INSTRUCTIONAL METHODS

Megan Edwards Collins, PhD, OTR/L, CAPS, CFPS

BASIC TENETS

In the 21st century, educators have endless access to technology. Their pedagogical approach impacts how they use technology in their courses, inside and outside the classroom. Educators who tend to believe that knowledge should be transmitted to students typically utilize technology as a way to pass on information (e.g., PowerPoints, podcasts). In contrast, educators who view students as active constructors of their own knowledge may use technology options to support and facilitate their learning process (e.g., as a way to obtain information and work on group activities). It is helpful for educators to reflect on their pedagogical approach and how technology may enhance their approach when exploring the possibility of teaching with these instructional methods.

When educators utilize technology appropriately, they can provide enriching and engaging learning experiences for their students. However, the challenge and charge are to ensure they are appropriately and effectively utilizing it as a learning tool and not simply a means to entertain. They must recognize technology cannot be a substitute for effective teaching and should take many considerations when determining whether to utilize it in their courses. One of these considerations includes selecting the appropriate technology to enhance the learning environment. Technology-based instructional teaching methods include using digital platforms, such as computers, tablets, and smartphones; software applications; camcorders; digital cameras; the internet; and audio and video conferencing. In this chapter, we will discuss concepts and ideas educators should take into account when exploring technology options and provide an overview of some common technology tools for teaching and learning.

Henderson, W. (Ed.). *Effective Teaching: Instructional Methods and Strategies for Occupational Therapy Education* (pp. 343-357).

BACKGROUND

Technology is becoming increasingly prevalent in today's society. For example, in 2019, approximately 58.8% of the world's population used the internet—a 1,157% increase from the year 2000 (International World Stats, 2019). In North America, 89.4% of the population used the internet in 2019—a 203% increase from 2000 (International World Stats, 2019). Today's society also commonly participates in smartphone use with 93% of millennials, 90% of Gen Xers, 68% of baby boomers, and 40% of the Silent Generation owning a smartphone (Vogels, 2019). Furthermore, 72% of Gen Z has access to mobile services (Jenkins, n.d.). Individuals' use of tablets or smartphones has increased from 0.3 hours a day in 2008 to 3.3 hours a day in 2017 (Marvin, 2018). Because technology is commonplace in today's society, occupational therapy educators and practitioners will undoubtedly serve students, clients, and families who have frequent access and utilization of technology.

Throughout history, technology has impacted educational practices by providing more opportunities and options for educators and students. This includes modern-day students and educators now being able to communicate virtually (either asynchronously or synchronously) across the globe. As society has made advances, technology has transformed the classroom to keep up with the needs and preferences of students. From the invention of the printing press in 1436 to the development of cloud-based resources in the late 1990s to early 2000s, educators and students have access to a wide range of resources. These options are essential to help prepare students for the technological expectations they may encounter upon entering the workforce. Examples of technology used throughout the years include printed books, sandboxes (introduced in 1806), chalkboards (introduced in 1841), lead pencils (introduced at the beginning of the 20th century), film (first used in education around 1902), radio (first used in education in the early 1920s), overhead projectors (first used in education around the 1930s and 1940s), typewriters (first used in education in the 1920s), televisions (introduced in education in 1939), computers (largely used in classrooms beginning in the 1980s), learning management systems (used starting in the early 2000s), and the internet (used in classrooms starting in the mid to late 1990s).

The use of technology in occupational therapy education is no different. Breines (2002) noted that, "Technology is linked to occupational therapy practice through occupation. This link helps to guide a modern curriculum" (p. 467). The use of technology in occupational therapy curriculum is essential to stay current with social and cultural norms so future practitioners can best meet the needs of the clients they will serve. Current Accreditation Council for Occupational Therapy Education standards also mandate that occupational therapy programs prepare students for the use of technology in practice, including the ability to utilize electronic documentation systems, virtual environments, and telehealth technology (Technology in Practice, Standard B.4.15; American Occupational Therapy Association, 2018). In addition, Accreditation Council for Occupational Therapy Education Standard A.2.14 specifically mentions that educational programs must have adequate instructional aids and technology to support program learning objectives and teaching strategies. Unfortunately, literature suggests a lack of information and description of specific technology in occupational therapy. Common technology found in occupational therapy literature include learning management systems, online library resources, clinical virtual simulations, online quizzes, and posting class resources and online lectures.

Educators of other health care disciplines also have a history of utilizing technology. For example, starting in the early 1990s, nursing literature discusses the use of personal digital assistants. Personal digital assistants have now morphed into more current technology, such as computer tablets and smartphones. The use of such devices in academic programs has been noted in an effort to enhance communication and to prepare future nurses to utilize them in clinical settings. Physical therapy education reports employing technology such as websites, chatrooms and discussion boards, web-based tutorials, blogs, video podcasts, and high-fidelity computer-enhanced mannequins.

THEORY

Educators that desire to explore technology in their classrooms and courses can use the technology acceptance model (TAM) as a guide. Developed by Fred Davis in 1985, the TAM examines all stages of technology use, including initially considering technology, training on the technology, and implementing and using technology. This model provides a framework for examining how beliefs regarding technology (e.g., how effective it can be and how easy it is to learn) can impact attitudes toward technology (e.g., technology is worth pursuing or too much effort to pursue). These attitudes and beliefs impact an individual's intentions and motivations to use technology.

The TAM considers three core principles: (1) perceived usefulness, (2) perceived ease of use, and (3) attitudes toward technology. Research has demonstrated the reliability and validity of the variables:

- *Perceived usefulness (PU)* describes the degree to which an individual views technology as an effective and efficient method to complete a task
- *Perceived ease of use (PEU)* explores the degree to which individuals believe they can easily and readily learn and use the technology
- *Attitudes toward technology* is "a person's evaluation of technology or specific behavior associated with the use of technology" (Scherer et al., 2019, p. 15)

PU and PEU are the primary influencers on two outcome variables—behavioral intention and technology use. *Behavioral intention* describes the potential individual's intentions or plans to use technology. Meanwhile, *technology use* is an individual's actual use of technology. For example, an individual who has no intention of using technology will most likely not use technology.

The TAM also identifies the external variables that can impact views and beliefs regarding technology, such as subjective norms, computer self-efficacy, and facilitating conditions. With *subjective norms*, the individual believes those in their personal or professional circle believe they should or should not use technology (e.g., the individual's perception of societal expectations regarding technology use). *Computer self-efficacy* includes the individual's belief regarding the ability to use a computer. Finally, *facilitating conditions* relate to the individual's perception of whether there are external resources to support technology use (e.g., resources for training or troubleshooting). The TAM model recognizes several other external variables and factors that impact an individual's decision to use technology. However, individuals who had a successful experience using technology are more likely to explore and try other options compared to individuals who had challenging times or poor outcomes.

Occupational therapy educators can apply the TAM to their use of technology in their classroom and courses. For the core variable of PU, educators are more likely to use various forms of technology if they believe it has the potential to be an effective and beneficial way to enhance the environment and learning. Educators who do not feel they can successfully implement technology for learning are less likely to use it in their classes. Looking through the lens of the PEU variable, educators who feel technology can be relatively easy to use are more likely to implement it during a learning experience. Each of these variables impact behavioral intention. For example, if educators feel technology can be an effective part of a course without a great deal of effort, they are likely to have strong intentions. Educators with intentions to use technology are more likely to actually implement it in their courses than those who have no intention of utilizing technology. Finally, external variables also play a role in their final decision to use technology. Educators who feel their students and/or colleagues expect them to use technology (subjective norms) and have the skillset (self-efficacy) and available resources (facilitating conditions) are more likely to implement and utilize technology than educators who experience opposite views and feelings.

Take a moment to reflect on your beliefs about technology in the box below. What forms of technology do you feel you should use given your professional and personal contexts? What forms of technology are easy to use or more challenging to use? What current beliefs do you have about the use of technology in classrooms? How does your access to resources and support impact the way you use technology?

IMPLEMENTATION

When they implement technology-based instructional methods, educators encourage a learning environment that views students as active participants in their educational process. The educator must always remember that technology is **not** a replacement or supplement for an effective teacher or effective pedagogy. When selecting technology, they must carefully reflect on their learning objectives and what students might discover to guide their decision. In addition, educators must remember that students possess different learning styles and should present content with a variety of different methods. While at times traditional methods may best suit the needs of students given course content or learning objectives, educators can utilize technology in innovate ways to cover most areas. For example, when discussing and working on soft skills, such as body language or rapport building, educators can record students engaging with clients or role playing in simulated scenarios. Students can view and reflect on their performance to identify areas of strength and address areas for improvement. We provide an overview of the process educators can use to select and implement technology.

Step 1: Selecting Technology

Educators consider many areas when determining whether and how to utilize technology, such as:

- How options can alter and/or enhance the learning environment
- The evidence available to support the use of technology
- How the culture and policies at all levels (e.g., departmental to institutional) support or do not support the use of technology
- How to implement a particular method

In addition, they should also contemplate the students' ability to use technology, the targeted learning outcomes, and the potential benefits, drawbacks, and overall abilities of the technology. Educators must also address the need for students to evaluate the reliability and appropriateness of sources found using technology. Similar to pragmatic reasoning, they explore technology options in terms of financial cost, access, and comfort of all involved individuals (Table 14-1). In the end, educators remain student-centered (Chapter 1) when they ensure they are thinking about the advantages to the students and not just themselves.

TABLE 14-1

Factors to Consider When Selecting Technology

FACTOR	DESCRIPTION
Cost	Educators and students have access to many technology resources; some are free while others are limited unless the educator or student purchases the upgrades or technology. Educators experience challenges because many appealing options have a significant cost or require a subscription. However, they can explore if the company offers group or student rates to reduce the cost.
Access	Educators consider the ability and overall accessibility of technology options to meet the needs of a wide range of students. They need access to the equipment and the required infrastructure to implement a selected piece of technology. In addition, educators must contemplate what students can reasonably be expected to possess and use. For example, if educators or students lack access to a web camera, microphone/speakers (e.g., for recording videos or virtual meetings), reliable internet, or an adequate quantity of devices, they may have a limited number of possible technology options. An institution may not allow the use of certain technologies for a number of reasons, such as privacy or security concerns or the inability to integrate with the institution's current technology. The financial cost may also make it unlikely that the educator's organization will be able to provide such equipment and infrastructure.
Reliability	It is important for educators to recognize technology may not always work as they planned. When designing technology-based instructional methods, they should always have a plan of action in case the internet is not adequately working, the students are unable to access the server, or a website is down for maintenance.
Privacy and confidentiality	There is a need for educators to inform students that they (or anyone else) will not access or utilize their information outside the course unless informed otherwise. Educators should review the security levels of the technology they are considering, utilize strong passwords, and follow other guidelines that the technology developer may provide (e.g., frequently changing passwords or ensuring to log out of a site when done). Educators should instruct students to follow these same tips.
Comfort	Educators and students experience greater success with technology when they have support or training to increase comfort. Educators' knowledge of options and use is a major factor in whether or how they implement technology-based instructional methods. Their decisions often depend on their personal and professional experiences as student and educator and their beliefs on whether technology can or should be used given the content. They need to demonstrate comfort and familiarity with the technology they use and view the method as something useful for the learning process.

(continued)

TABLE 14-1 (CONTINUED)

Factors to Consider When Selecting Technology

FACTOR	DESCRIPTION
	Educators also need to be aware that many students are familiar and comfortable with using technology but may sometimes still experience challenges utilizing a selected piece of technology. In addition, they should be cognizant that not all students may be comfortable using a certain piece of technology or find that technology best meets their learning needs. Literature suggests certain technology trends, such as female students are less comfortable than male students when utilizing technology. Students from a younger generation and more affluent backgrounds have more experience and access than others. The educator must also remember the priority is for students to master the course material and achieve the learning objectives—not learn how to use the technology (unless learning the technology is a learning objective!) They must understand their students' experiences and consider how they can provide support, so the students are not so time-consumed with learning how to navigate the technology that they miss important content.

Step 2: Implementing Technology

After selecting an appropriate method, educators determine what is the most effective way to introduce the students to the material and how students will practice using and applying technology. We want to warn you that some students may perceive that the use technology is an educator's mechanism to remove self from teaching. Therefore, they should explicitly explain to the students the intent and purpose for using technology in the course. They should also make their expectations for appropriate technology use, the benefits of using the technology, and how to functionally use the technology clear to their students. In addition, educators should ensure technology is not a distraction (e.g., this encourages the students to utilize the technology during class time in ways unrelated to the learning process).

When planning to implement technology, educators must allow enough time to set up the needed technology to ensure everything is ready for use and working properly. They should also have a backup plan in case something goes wrong with the technology. One strategy educators can use for successful implementation is to work with individuals in the institution's information technology department (or equivalent department). Finally, educators should be prepared to assist students with troubleshooting technology challenges, as well as account for time it might take for students to get their technology devices or programs started. By alerting students of how you will use the technology beforehand and asking them to have everything ready when class begins will help you decrease the amount of time needed to initiate technology use.

The educator can implement technology in the classroom to explore and present classroom content, to demonstrate and offer the opportunity for students to practice with options that are available for clients, and to open up a discussion on using technology as part of the occupational therapy process. This can include how practitioners use technology to provide education to clients and to promote and select for occupational engagement. Finally, educators can have students use various types of technology for assignments, such as creating a video or other resource.

TECHNOLOGY-BASED INSTRUCTIONAL METHODS

Educators can use many types of technology in the courses they teach. In this section, we provide a basic overview of and resources for various types of technology. Regardless of the technology used, educators must also consider how it can provide users with feedback and the opportunity for reflection.

Classroom Response Systems and Other Student Polling Resources

One way for educators to actively engage students and to identify where they are in the learning process is to utilize classroom response systems and similar technologies. With classroom response systems, the educator poses multiple-choice questions and the students select an answer. The educator quickly views the students' answers to the question, which provides opportunities to review content, reinforce key points, and rectify any misconceptions as needed. When determining which option is best to use, the educator considers the cost (for both the educator and students) and the functionality of the program. They can ask questions, such as:

- Can we access the program on a smartphone or computer tablet?
- Can I incorporate pictures and videos?
- Can I ask open-ended questions or only closed-ended questions?

Polling Options
- iClicker (https://www.iclicker.com/)
- Poll Everywhere (https://www.polleverywhere.com/)
- Kahoot (https://kahoot.com/)

When educators use open-ended response systems, such as Poll Everywhere, they gain information about the opinions of many students. In addition, educators can use response systems to help their students focus their attention on areas to study. Many students find this technology nonthreatening (e.g., their responses are anonymous and ungraded) and report a fun and engaging experience due to the sometimes competitive nature of the programs.

Online Resources

As previously mentioned, educators have access to a variety of online resources to enhance student learning and engagement (Table 14-2). Some of these resources are as simple as locating an online video, which students view and discuss inside or outside the classroom. They may range from a TED talk (https://www.ted.com/talks) to videos found searching the internet. Educators can also create engaging videos for students to view. The use of electronic medical record software, such as Fusion Web (https://www.fusionwebclinic.com/), is another online tool that can help students effectively document their evaluations, interventions, and goals in preparation for professional practice.

Apps

Educators are increasingly using mobile apps as an effective way to engage students with content and to achieve learning outcomes. Apps continue to grow and rapidly improve in the breadth of content. Educators can review and explore options in the various stores depending on the platform they use (e.g., Android versus iOS). The American Occupational Therapy Association also provides a list of apps according to practice areas for educators to review and access (https://www.aota.org/Practice/Manage/Apps.aspx).

Examples of Apps
- MOBI and GONI are two examples of apps (found at http://www.rehablearning.com/) that are beneficial when students are learning and determining mobility devices and mastering goniometry.
- 3D 4Medical has a variety of helpful apps related to anatomy and other aspects of health (found at https://3d4medical.com/apps).

TABLE 14-2

Online Resources

RESOURCE	DESCRIPTION
International Clinical Educators, Inc. Learning Center https://www.icelearningcenter.com/ice-video-library	Provides educators with videos of practitioners and clients of varying diagnoses and in various settings to engage students inside or outside the classroom; educators receive access to lesson plans and other resources with strategies on how to utilize the videos in the classroom. Access requires a subscription.
Panopto https://www.panopto.com/	Provides educators access to an online video platform; also possesses other features (e.g., quizzes). Access requires a subscription.
Screencast-O-Matic https://screencast-o-matic.com/	Provides educators with a video recording and editing platform. Has a basic free recording option and subscription plans.
PlayPosit https://go.playposit.com/	Enables educators to embed questions at various points in a video; can use a video found online or a created one; allows educators to see responses. Students answer questions before advancing the video, creating a more interactive learning experience. Integrates with many learning management systems; has a basic free option and subscription plans.
VoiceThread https://voicethread.com/	Allows educators and students to create and post documents, photos, videos, and other resources; they can comment on postings in various ways, fostering interaction. Access requires a subscription.
Flipgrid https://info.flipgrid.com/	Allows educators to create a "grid" for students. The educator posts prompts that the students are then expected to reply to via a video. Students can also respond to peers' responses. Does not require a subscription.
Piazza https://piazza.com/	Offers a platform where educators and students can post questions and other discussion prompts to encourage online interaction and collaboration. Does not require a subscription.

(continued)

TABLE 14-2 (CONTINUED)

Online Resources

RESOURCE	DESCRIPTION
Adobe https://www.adobe.com/creativecloud.html	Offers a wide range of programs, such as Adobe Spark, which allows educators and students to create websites to present content in an engaging manner; other Adobe programs enable educators or students to create and edit videos (Adobe Premiere Pro) and pictures (Adobe Photoshop), depending on the needs. It is important for educators to be aware that they cannot always access everything they created on Adobe after they or the students leave an institution. Some programs are free, and some require a paid subscription.
Google Drive https://www.google.com/drive/	Includes Google Docs, Sheets, and Slides, which enable students and educators to share and collaborate on documents and presentations. Offers 15 GB of free storage with the option to purchase more storage space.

Tutorials

Educators have the option to use tutorials to create and post videos and additional information online. They can embed questions or other learning activities throughout the tutorial that students must complete before moving forward or only post following completion. Educators often use tutorials to supplement traditional class time and students can review material at their own pace (refer to Chapter 5). Educational literature suggests tutorials to increase student satisfaction.

Social Media and Other Collaboration Options

As the use of social media increases, so does the potential for educators to use these forms of technology (e.g., Twitter, Facebook) in the classroom. The majority of students use social media platforms for personal use and may also find this option beneficial for learning content. Educators can post class content and due dates on social media platforms or create assignments that require students to use or discuss social media.

In addition, there are many options for educators to integrate technology within a learning management system or online resources to facilitate collaboration with others (e.g., Blackboard Collaborate, Skype, Zoom, Google Hangout Meets, Kubi). Using these forms of technology, they can virtually meet students for class and invite guest speakers from all over the world! They may use collaborative options to enable students to hear firsthand from practitioners and others who might not be able to physically come present to their class for a variety of reasons, such as time constraints and geographical distance.

TIPS AND TRICKS

- Educators should provide guidelines, instructions, training, and strategies to students on how they plan to use the technology.
- Educators should practice using technology options before integrating them into the classroom, so they can make informed decisions and have a solid understanding.
- Educators can attend conferences that discuss and review technology options (e.g., Appalachian State University offers a free e-learning conference [in-person or online]).
- Educators and students should utilize librarians and other resources that can provide guidance and assistance on identifying and implementing technology (e.g., universities and colleges often have a department on campus to focus on faculty development).
- Educators and students need to be aware of resources and technology support the developers may provide and utilize as needed.
- Educators can also use technology options to help monitor academic integrity, such as:
  - Limiting or controlling what students have access to while in the classroom (e.g., locking areas on the internet so the students only access what they need to complete learning activities).
  - Checking for signs of plagiarism through technology (e.g., Turnitin; https://www.turnitin.com).
- Educators should frequently dialogue with students to determine what technology they are personally and professionally using to ensure relevance of potential options and to understand access and resources.
- Educators can ask colleagues about technology they are successfully integrating into their courses to minimize the learning curve and expense for students.

OPPORTUNITIES FOR FEEDBACK AND REFLECTION

Educators frequently utilize technology to provide feedback and opportunities for reflection. Remember from Chapter 1, students desire more feedback. Technology affords educators numerous opportunities to provide students with this critical information. Depending on the type of technology, they may have the option to enter comments that students can view upon submission to provide a rationale for correct or incorrect responses. Educators can also use learning management systems and other technologies to ask students to submit assignments. Following submission, the educator offers feedback electronically by providing comments on a rubric or within the actual assignment. Both educators and students easily provide and view feedback. Educators may also wish to have students provide access to assignments or other learning activities so the entire class can view to provide feedback and reflection to one another. Examples include asking students to review and critique documentation completed in an electronic health record. Finally, educators have the option of using technology to have students engage in reflective activities that further explore course concepts (e.g., blogs) or to demonstrate activity growth throughout the curriculum (e.g., e-portfolio).

In addition to using technology for assignments, educators also incorporate technology to provide feedback and reflection opportunities for students while they are actually completing classroom activities. For example, they use technology to input questions within a video that students answer before progressing to the next phase. In doing so, they provide students with feedback about content mastery or areas for further review. Similarly, educators may also add reflective questions or learning activities that require students to reflect on a course concept. They may have the ability to see student reflection and performance, which they can continually use to adjust or review course content.

Seeking feedback from students immediately after using technology can help educators gauge the effectiveness and perceptions they have. This can help educators make any needed changes or adjustments to their technology use to best meet the needs of students and to best ensure that learning objectives are being met. When students provide positive feedback, educators better understand what technology is perceived effective and should be used more frequently. As previously stated throughout this chapter, it is critical for educators to frequently communicate with students to ensure they have a positive experience with a selected piece of technology. They should ask students if technology is facilitating their learning, what challenges they are experiencing, and if they are effectively using the technology. Educators can use the feedback to make necessary changes and address concerns. They must also reflect on their use of technology and whether a particular method is facilitating achievement of desired learning outcomes. This reflection includes frequently reviewing technology options to make sure they are using the most effective and relevant forms.

APPLICATION TO OCCUPATIONAL THERAPY PRACTICE

Educational literature provides numerous benefits and reasons for educators' use of technology-based instructional methods to prepare students to successfully meet the needs of society. Regardless of physical and/or cognitive abilities, many individuals use technology as a part of their daily routines and occupations. Therefore, it is essential for occupational therapy educators to enhance their students' understanding of common technologies and their ability to use and provide services in new and innovative ways. For example, occupational therapy practitioners are increasingly using technology to track and monitor client progress, health, and safety, such as asking a client to wear a mobile device (such as a smartwatch or Fitbit) to track vital signs or activity level or to detect falls. Many educators and practitioners are also utilizing 3D printers to make adaptive equipment and other devices for clients.

Example 1: Use of Telehealth to Provide Occupational Therapy Services

Occupational therapy practitioners can use telehealth to provide services to clients in remote areas where it is challenging to provide services in person or in situations when a client may not be able to leave home or lacks transportation to get to a therapy session. They can provide services related to education on adaptive equipment for activities of daily living, recommendations for home modifications, explanations of proper body mechanics, or reviews of a home exercise program. Occupational therapists are also able to provide supervision of occupational therapy assistants via telehealth. Telehealth affords health care professionals opportunities for effective communication and collaboration for the provision of efficient and safe client-centered care.

Example 2: Use of Apps to Increase Independence in Occupations

An occupational therapy practitioner can incorporate the use of many apps to increase a client's independence and participation in valued occupations. As previously stated, many individuals have and are familiar with the use of smart technology and apps. Therefore, the addition of an app on a client's phone offers a simple intervention strategy. For example, for individuals experiencing challenges in cognition, apps related to money management, transportation systems (e.g., bus schedule), or medication management could be beneficial. In addition, occupational therapy practitioners can encourage clients to use their phones to set timers for weight shifting, stretching, or breaks and can take pictures or videos of transfers, exercises, body mechanics, or work stations.

Advantages

- Students overwhelmingly support the use of technology
- Provides students and educators with user-friendly options
- Offers great resources for information
- Provides options for personalization and interaction
- Reports of appreciation for an environmentally friendly option
- Allows students to share knowledge and resources with each other
- Increases ease of communication and collaboration from any location at any time
- Offers sources of support
- Provides an enhanced sense of connectedness
- Provides easy access to course resources
- Affords students opportunities to review and master content at their own pace
- Allows for active and collaborative learning
- Provides educators with enhanced ways to integrate and assess learning
- Increases students' intrinsic motivation and critical thinking
- Encourages persistence during difficult tasks
- Provides educators a potentially easier way to monitor and provide feedback to students to clarify/adjust learning assignments and instructions
- Enables educators to reach students and speakers from a wider geographical range

Challenges

- Requires students and educators to remain current on options and changes
- Requires students and educators to stay alert; as new options emerge, other technology options may become obsolete
- Potentially requires updates and new infrastructure
- Necessitates a time commitment for educators to research options, learn new technology, restructure the classroom design and/or assignments, and ensure appropriate equipment and infrastructure is in place to work properly
- Lacks current evidence supporting the use and effectiveness of technology options (particularly social media)
- Experiences practical and logistical challenges, such as slow systems and the size of technology devices
- Challenges students because of uncertainty about the reliability of information, the need for electricity and internet access, and concerns about availability and accessibility of supports
- Concerns for the need to be in constant contact and communication may make it challenging for the student and/or educator to take needed time away from the classroom content
- Concerns for being overwhelmed with the amount of information, increasing the cognitive load, surface-level professing of information, and difficulty appraising the quality and accuracy of resources

In the space below, list any additional advantages or challenges.

Brainstorm strategies for overcoming these challenges when implementing technology-based instructional methods.

THREE THINGS YOU CAN DO TOMORROW TO IMPLEMENT TECHNOLOGY-BASED INSTRUCTIONAL METHODS WITH YOUR STUDENTS

1. Meet with the instructional design team at your institution to learn about what technology options are available on your campus.
2. Review three learning apps from the previous resources.
3. Make one of your lectures into a polling game (e.g., iClicker, Kahoot, Poll Everywhere).

REFERENCES

American Occupational Therapy Association. (2018). 2018 Accreditation Council for Occupational Therapy Education (ACOTE) standards and interpretive guide. *American Journal of Occupational Therapy, 72*(Suppl. 2), 7212410005p1-7212410005p83.

Breines, E. (2002). Occupational therapy education in a technological world. *American Journal of Occupational Therapy, 56*(4), 467-469.

International World Stats. (2019). Internet world stats: Usage and population statistics. https://www.internetworldstats.com/stats.htm

Jenkins, R. (n.d.). How Generation Z uses technology and social media. *Ryan Jenkins: Next Generation Speaker.* Retrieved from https://blog.ryan-jenkins.com/how-generation-z-uses-technology-and-social-media

Marvin, R. (2018). Tech addiction by the numbers: How much time we spend online. *PCMag.* Retrieved from https://www.pcmag.com/article/361587/tech-addiction-by-the-numbers-how-much-time-we-spend-online

Scherer, R., Siddiq, F., & Tondeur, J. (2018). The technology acceptance model (TAM): A metal-analytic structural equation modeling approach to explaining teachers' adoption of digital technology in education. *Computers & Education, 128*, 13-35. http://dx.doi.org/10.1016/j.compedu.2018.09.009

Vogels, E. (2019). Millennials stand out for their technology use, but older generations also embrace digital life. *Pew Research Center.* Retrieved from https://www.pewresearch.org/fact-tank/2019/09/09/us-generations-technology-use/

BIBLIOGRAPHY

Apple. (2019). Apple watch. Helping your patients identify early warning signs. Retrieved from https://www.apple.com/healthcare/apple-watch/

Carlos, C., Alejandro, Q., & Francisco, P. (2017). The information and communications technology in higher education: A YouTube channel as a resource. *Gymnasium: Scientific Journal of Education, Sports, and Health, 18*(1), 194-199.

Cason, J. (2012). Telehealth opportunities in occupational therapy through the affordable care act. *American Journal of Occupational Therapy, 66*(2), 131-136. http://dx.doi.org/10.5014/ajot.2012.662001

Cervera, M., & Johnson, L. (2015). Education and technology: New learning environments from a transformative perspective. *RUSC Universities and Knowledge Society Journal, 12*(2), 1-13. http://dx.doi.org/10.7238/rusc.v12i2.2570

Durodolu, O. (2016). Technology acceptance model as a predictor of using information system' to acquire information literacy skills. *Library Philosophy and Practice* (e-journal), 1450. https://digitalcommons.unl.edu/libphilprac/1450

Englund, C., Olofsson, A., & Price, L. (2017). Teaching with technology in higher education: Understanding conceptual change and development in practice. *Higher Education Research & Development, 36*(1), 73-87. http://dx.doi.org/10.1080/07294360.2016.1171300

Fitbit. (2019). https://www.fitbit.com/home

Gee, B., Salazar, L., Porter, J., Clark, C., & Peterson, T. (2017). Overview of instructional technology used in the education of occupational therapy students: A survey study. *The Open Journal of Occupational Therapy, 5*(4), Article 13. http://dx.doi.org/10.15453/2168-6408.1352

Haran, M. (2015). A history of education technology. *Institute of Progressive Education & Learning.* http://institute-of-progressive-education-and-learning.org/a-history-of-education-technology/

Haughton, N., Yeh, K., Nworie, J., & Romero, L. (2013). Digital disturbances, disorders, and pathologies: A discussion of some unintended consequences of technology in higher education. *Educational Technology, 53*(4), 3-16.

Huffman, A., Whetten, J., & Huffman, W. (2013). Using technology in higher education: The influence of gender roles on technology self-efficacy. *Computers in Human Behavior, 29,* 1779-1786. http://dx.doi.org/10.1016/j.chb.2013.02.012

Hung, H., & Yuen, S. (2010). Educational use of social networking technology in higher education. *Teaching in Higher Education, 15*(6), 703-714. http://dx.doi.org/10.1080/13562517.2010.507307

Jaaskelä, P., Häkkinen, P., & Rasku-Puttonen, H. (2017). Teacher beliefs regarding learning, pedagogy, and the use of technology in higher education. *Journal of Research on Technology in Education, 49*(3-4), 198-211. http://dx.doi.org/10.1080/15391523.2017.1343691

Jain, D., Sharma, S., & Shelly, G. (2012). Problem & aspects of technology in higher education (with special reference to professional courses). *International Journal of Management Research and Review, 2*(9), 1584-1589.

Jones, A., Dean, E., & Hui-Chan, C. (2010). Comparison of teaching and learning outcomes between video-linked, web-based, and classroom tutorials: An innovative international study of profession education in physical therapy. *Computers & Education, 54,* 1193-1201.

Jones, M. (2018). HealthCare: How technology impacts the healthcare industry. *Healthcare in America.* Retrieved from https://healthcareinamerica.us/healthcare-how-technology-impacts-the-healthcare-industry-b2ba6271c4b4

Kirkwood, A. (2014). Teaching and learning with technology in higher education: Blended and distance education needs "joined-up" thinking rather than technological determinism. *Open Learning, 29*(3), 206-221. http://dx.doi.org/10.1080/02680513.2015.1009884

Kirkwood, A., & Price, L. (2013). Missing: Evidence of a scholarly approach to teaching and learning with technology in higher education. *Teaching in Higher Education, 18*(3), 327-337.

Kurt, S. (2015). Educational technology: An overview. *Educational Technology.* Retrieved from https://educationaltechnology.net/educational-technology-an-overview/

Lee, H., Min, H., Oh, S., & Shim, K. (2018). Mobile technology in undergraduate nursing education: A systematic review. *Healthcare Informatics Research, 24*(2), 97-108. http://dx.doi.org/10.4258/hir.2018.24.2.97

Macznik, A., Ribeiro, D., & Baxter, G. (2015). Online technology use in physiotherapy teaching and learning: A systematic review of effectiveness and users' perceptions. *BMC Medical Education, 15,* Article 160.

Mica Zen Technology. (2019). What is the cloud and when did it start? Retrieved from https://www.micazen.com/what-is-the-cloud-and-when-did-it-start/

Mueller, J., Wood, E., De Pasquale, D., & Cruikshank, R. (2012). Examining mobile technology in higher education: Handheld devices in and out of the classroom. *International Journal of Higher Education, 1*(2), 43-54.

Proffitt, R., Schwartz, J., Foreman, M., & Smith, R. (2019). Role of occupational therapy practitioners in mass market technology research and development. *American Journal of Occupational Therapy, 73*(1), 7301347010p1-7301347010p6. http://dx.doi.org/10.5014/ajot.2019.028167

Purdue University. (2019). The evolution of technology in the classroom. Retrieved from https://online.purdue.edu/blog/evolution-technology-classroom

Siwicki, B. (2017). Advanced tech is evolving nursing education to meet hospital demand. *Healthcare IT News*. Retrieved from https://www.healthcareitnews.com/news/advanced-tech-evolving-nursing-education-meet-hospital-demand

Smith, N., Prybylo, S., & Conner-Kerr, T. (2012). Using simulation and patient role play to teach electrocardiographic rhythms to physical therapy students. *Cardiopulmonary Physical Therapy Journal, 23*(1), 36-42.

Smith, R. (2017). Technology and occupation: Past, present, and the next 100 years of theory and practice. *American Journal of Occupational Therapy, 71*(6), 7106150010p1-7106150010p15. http://dx.doi.org/10.5014/ajot.2017.716003

Srivastava, T., Waghmare, L., Jagzape, A., Rawekar, A., Quazi, N., & Mishra, V. (2014). Role of information communication technology in higher education: Learners perspectives in rural medical schools. *Journal of Clinical and Diagnosis Research, 8*(6), 1-6. http://dx.doi.org/10.7860/JCDR/2014/8371.4448

Tri Anni, C., Sunawan, S., & Haryono, H. (2018). School counselors' intention to use technology: The technology acceptance model. *The Turkish Online Journal of Educational Technology, 17*(20), 120-124.

University of Texas Arlington Online. (2017). Technology's role in nursing education. Retrieved from https://academicpartnerships.uta.edu/articles/healthcare/technologys-role-in-nursing-education.aspx

U.S. Department of Education. (n.d.). Use of technology in teaching and learning. Retrieved from https://www.ed.gov/oii-news/use-technology-teaching-and-learning

FINANCIAL DISCLOSURES

Bailey Baucum has no financial or proprietary interest in the materials presented herein.

Kelli Bayne has no financial or proprietary interest in the materials presented herein.

Bailey Bremser has no financial or proprietary interest in the materials presented herein.

Dr. Cynthia Clough has no financial or proprietary interest in the materials presented herein.

Dr. Megan Edwards Collins has no financial or proprietary interest in the materials presented herein.

Dr. Meredith Gronski has no financial or proprietary interest in the materials presented herein.

Paige Headlee has no financial or proprietary interest in the materials presented herein.

Dr. Whitney Henderson has no financial or proprietary interest in the materials presented herein.

Haley Homan has no financial or proprietary interest in the materials presented herein.

Dr. Leigh Neier has no financial or proprietary interest in the materials presented herein.

Dr. Stacy Neier has no financial or proprietary interest in the materials presented herein.

Lyndi Plattner has no financial or proprietary interest in the materials presented herein.

INDEX

Printed in the United States
by Baker & Taylor Publisher Services